Well-Being

Also by John Haworth

WORK AND LEISURE: An Interdisciplinary Study in Theory, Education and Planning (*co-editor*)

COMMUNITY INVOLVEMENT AND LEISURE (*editor*)

WORK, LEISURE AND WELLBEING

PSYCHOLOGICAL RESEARCH: Innovative Methods and Strategies (*editor*)

Also by Graham Hart

THE SOCIAL ASPECTS OF AIDS SERIES (*co-editor*)

THE HEALTH, RISK AND SOCIETY SERIES (*general editor*)

Well-Being

Individual, Community and Social Perspectives

Edited by

John Haworth
Manchester Metropolitan University, UK

and

Graham Hart
University College London, UK

palgrave
macmillan

First published in hardback 2007
This paperback edition published 2012 by
PALGRAVE MACMILLAN

Palgrave Macmillan in the UK is an imprint of Macmillan Publishers Limited,
registered in England, company number 785998, of Houndmills, Basingstoke,
Hampshire RG21 6XS.

Palgrave Macmillan in the US is a division of St Martin's Press LLC,
175 Fifth Avenue, New York, NY 10010.

Palgrave Macmillan is the global academic imprint of the above companies
and has companies and representatives throughout the world.

Palgrave® and Macmillan® are registered trademarks in the United States,
the United Kingdom, Europe and other countries.

ISBN 978-0-230-00168-8 hardback
ISBN 978-0-230-35568-2 paperback

This book is printed on paper suitable for recycling and made from fully
managed and sustained forest sources. Logging, pulping and manufacturing
processes are expected to conform to the environmental regulations of the
country of origin.

A catalogue record for this book is available from the British Library.

Library of Congress Cataloging-in-Publication Data
Well-being : individual, community and social perspectives / edited by
    John Haworth and Graham Hart.
        p.   cm.
    Includes bibliographical references and index.
    ISBN-13: 978-0-230-00168-8 (cloth)
    ISBN-13: 978-0-230-35568-2 (pbk)
    1. Quality of life.   2. Well-being.   I. Haworth, John, 1937–
    II. Hart, Graham, 1957–
    HN25.W45 2007
    306.01—dc22   2006052975

Printed and bound in Great Britain by
Antony Rowe CPI, Chippenham and Eastbourne

Contents

v

List of Figures

List of Tables

Notes on Contributors

Dr Rosemary Abbott was a postdoctoral research associate in the Department of Psychiatry, University of Cambridge, UK. She currently works on the Leverhulme Trust grant, Human Flourishing: A Life Course Approach. Previously, she has collaborated with psychiatric researchers on longitudinal studies of depression, cognitive therapy and ageing.

Dr Dimitris Ballas is a Senior Lecturer in the Department of Geography, University of Sheffield, UK. His research interests include economic geography; social and spatial inequalities; social justice; exploring geographies of happiness; and socio-economic applications of Geographical Information Systems (GIS). He is currently working on a two-year ESRC mid-career research fellowship project, which started in February 2006 and aims at investigating different definitions of happiness and well-being and exploring the degree to which happiness varies over time and space.

Dr Margaret Boneham is Director of the School of Social and Life Sciences at the University of Bolton, UK. Her research interests include ageing and ethnicity, community health and social capital.

Dr Tim Croudace is a population-based quantitative psychologist and Senior Lecturer in Psychometric Epidemiology. He is a UK Department of Health Career Scientist in Public Health and specializes in the application of psychometric measurement and latent variable modelling approaches to epidemiological longitudinal studies. He is also trained in health services research/health technology assessment and analyses intervention/prevention trials in school and healthcare settings.

Antonella Delle Fave, M.D., is Professor of Psychology at the Medical School of the University of Milano, Italy. Her main research interests are the cross-cultural investigation of the quality of daily experience and its long-term developmental impact. She has been involved as supervisor in intervention projects on migration, disability and social maladjustment.

Danny Dorling is Professor of Human Geography in the Department of Geography, University of Sheffield, UK. He is currently studying the transformation of social inequality in the United Kingdom: 1945–2005, in the context of a British Academy Research Leave Fellowship. His current research interests include the visualization of spatial social structure through drawing atlases; the changing social, medical and political geographies of Britain as revealed by the 2001 Census; and from using a wide range of resources, trying to fathom the implications of rising housing market and wealth inequalities, the polarization of health and life chances and the prospects for new social policies based on evidence and advocacy from research.

David Haley, ecological artist, is a Research Fellow in MIRIAD at Manchester Metropolitan University, UK, where he co-founded the Social and Environmental Arts Research Centre, the Water & Well-Being Research Group; and leads the MA Art as Environment programme. He has artworks in the Tate Library Collection and Shrewsbury Museum & Art Gallery and has exhibited in London, New York, Kyoto and http://greenmuseum.org/c/enterchange, while writing for publications like *Water Encyclopaedia: Oceanography; Meteorology; Physics and Chemistry; Water Law;* and *Water History, Art, and Culture*, international journals and presenting keynote papers at international conferences.

Professor Graham Hart is Director of the Centre for Sexual Health & HIV Research, Royal Free and University College, London, UK. His main research interests are in risk behaviours for and interventions to prevent unwanted sexual health outcomes, including HIV infection. He has published widely in these areas. He is committed to positive sexual health and translational research for successful prevention programmes.

Dr Stephani Hatch is an adjunct Assistant Professor of Epidemiology, Mailman School of Public Health at Columbia University, USA and UK Medical Research Council Visiting Research Fellow with the National Survey of Health and Development (1946 Birth Cohort). Dr Hatch is a sociologist with background in medical sociology and postdoctoral training in psychiatric epidemiology. Dr Hatch's research interests have focused on the impact of social statuses and cumulative adversity and advantage on health, as well as theoretical links between social status and inequality in ageing.

Dr John Haworth is a Visiting Research Fellow in the Research Institute for Health and Social Change at Manchester Metropolitan University, and a Visiting Professor at Bolton University. He was a Research Fellow (part time) in the Department of Psychology, and an Honorary Research Fellow, Department of Fine Arts, Manchester Metropolitan University, UK. He has published extensively on work, leisure and well-being. Formerly at Manchester University, he co-founded the Leisure Studies

Association, and the international journal *Leisure Studies*. Recent funded projects on well-being, and creativity and embodied mind, can be seen at www.haworthjt.com

Dr Jane Henry is Head of the Open University Business School Human Resources and Change Management Centre and founder of the BPS Consciousness and Experiential Psychology Section. She co-organized the 1st European Positive Psychology Conference, is on the European Network for Positive Psychology steering committee, and was a consultant to the BBC TV series *Making Slough Happy*. Her research includes work on development strategies that take acount of individual and cultural differences. Her books include *Creative Management, Creativity and Perception in Management, Research into Exceptional Experience* and *European Positive Psychology*. She is a regular broadcaster and consults on well-being and creativity for various organizations here and abroad.

Professor Felicia A. Huppert is Professor of Psychology in the Department of Psychiatry, University of Cambridge and Director of the Well-Being Institute and the Cambridge Interdisciplinary Research Centre on Ageing (CIRCA), UK. Her principal research interest is positive aspects of psychological well-being and its determinants and consequences throughout the life course.

Carolyn Kagan is Professor of Community Social Psychology and Director of the Research Institute for Health and Social Change at Manchester Metropolitan University, UK. Her work includes participatory evaluation research with those marginalized by the social system and she has worked for many years supporting service developments involving people with learning difficulties and those living in poverty.

Amanda Kilroy RGN, BSc (Hons), MRes, Cert Ed, was a research associate in the Arts for Health Unit, Manchester Metropolitan University, UK. She was the research lead for a collaborative project exploring stakeholder perspectives of the impact of culture, creativity and the arts on health and well-being. Her background was in nursing and complementary medicine. She was also an experienced lecturer, group facilitator and participatory researcher whose work focuses on using action research and collaborative inquiry approaches to engage diverse participants in meaningful and relevant research and organizational and personal development.

Professor Diana Kuh is the Director of the MRC National Survey of Health and Development, UK, also known as the British 1946 Birth Cohort and

Professor of Life Course Epidemiology at University College London. She studies the independent, cumulative and interactive effects of biological, social and psychosocial risk factors across the life course that influence ageing, in terms of physical and cognitive capability and functioning of body systems, development of chronic disease, probability of survival, and quality of life.

Suzan Lewis is a Professor at Middlesex University Business School (formerly at Manchester Metropolitan University), UK. Her research and consultancy focuses on 'work-life balance' and workplace practice, culture and change, in diverse national contexts. She has led many national and international research projects on these topics. She is a founding editor of the international journal *Community, Work and Family*. Her numerous publications include: *The Flexible and Profitable Workplace: a Guide to Implementing Flexible Working Practices in Professional Services, Work-Life Integration: Case Studies of Organisational Change* and *The Myth of Work-Life Balance*. She has advised governments and worked with employers and policy-makers on work-life issues in the USA, Europe and Japan.

Ray Pahl was a Research Professor of Sociology at the Institute for Social and Economic Research at the University of Essex and Emeritus Professor of Sociology at the University of Kent, UK. He was the author of many books including *Whose City? Divisions of Labour, After Success* and, most recently, *Rethinking Friendship: Hidden Solidarities Today* (with Liz Spencer). His researches at Essex was on social comparisons and relative contentment in the middle mass.

Perri 6 is Professor of Social Policy at Nottingham Trent University, UK. His recent books include *Public Emotions* (with Squire, Radstone and Treacher), *Beyond Delivery: Policy Implementation as Sensemaking and Settlement* (with Peck), *Managing Networks of Twenty-first Century Organisations* (with Goodwin, Peck and Freeman), *E-governance: Styles of Political Judgment in the Information Age Polity* (2004) and *Towards Holistic Governance: the New Reform Agenda* (with Leat, Seltzer and Stoker). His research interests encompass governance, institutional viability, well-being and choice, the effectiveness and acceptability of public policies to change citizens' behaviour, organizational behaviour, privacy and data protection.

Dr John Pickering lectures in the Department of Psychology of Warwick University, UK. His interests began in cognition in general and in the cultural production of consciousness in particular. These topics have evolved over the years into more specific engagement with the cultural roles of technology, ecopsychology and Deep Ecology, and with the comparison and posible integration of Western psychology and Buddhism. His overall and ongoing goal is to apply what he discovers to the problem of finding more sustainable ways to live.

Dr George B. Ploubidis was a postdoctoral research associate in the Department of Psychiatry, University of Cambridge, UK. He worked on the Leverhulme Trust grant, Human Flourishing: A Life Course Approach. He was specialized in psychometric and applied statistics with applications in diabetes, mental health and individual psychological differences.

Isaac Prilleltensky is Dean of the School of Education at the University of Miami in Florida, USA. His interests include the interactions between social justice and well-being, and the concurrent promotion of personal, interpersonal, organizational and community well-being.

Ora Prilleltensky is a faculty member in the Department of Educational and Psychological Studies in the School of Education at the University of Miami, USA. Ora teaches counselling and her scholarly interests are in the fields of well-being and disabilities studies.

Christina Purcell has a first degree in Cultural Studies and an MA in International Politics from Manchester University. She was a Research Assistant at Manchester Metropolitan University.

Dr Marcus Richards is currently a Medical Research Council Programme Leader, a Reader in Cognitive Epidemiology at University College London, UK, and a senior member of the team responsible for the MRC National Survey of Health and Development, also known as the British 1946 Birth Cohort. A psychologist by background, he has had a long-standing interest and involvement in the epidemiology of cognitive development and ageing.

Peter Senior MBE was a Director of 'Arts for Health' at Manchester Metropolitan University, UK. He was a recognized as the pioneer of an international arts and health movement, which introduces the services of artists and designers to the world of healthcare. In 2001 he was co-chairman of the first European forum 'The Arts and Culture in Health and Hospitals' and has been instrumental in developing the second one with the Arts Council of Ireland, 24–26 June in Dublin in 2004. He has served on a wide range of national committees for the Arts Council of England, the Department of Health and several national charities.

Dr Mary Shaw is a Reader in Medical Sociology at the University of Bristol, UK. Her current research interests include: social and geographical inequalities in mortality and morbidity; the social and spatial accumulation of health inequalities; poverty and the health of disadvantaged groups (particularly homeless people); health and social policies; teenage pregnancy and parenthood; and photography in social science.

Professor Judith Sixsmith is Professor of Adult Social Care, Division of Psychology and Social Change at Manchester Metropolitan University in the UK. Her current research projects include work on men, masculinities and health, ageing and health, children's well-being and the relationship between social capital, gender and health in disadvantaged communities.

Professor Michael E. J. Wadsworth was the Director of the MRC National Survey of Health and Development, UK, also known as the British 1946 Birth Cohort from 1986 until 2006 and Professor of Social and Health Life Course Research at University College London. His interests include change in health and in health-related behaviour in relation to age, cohort and period differences in health and health-related behaviour; the effect of secular changes in educational attainment on health; health-related behaviour; and social participation.

Michael White is Emeritus Fellow at the Policy Studies Institute (PSI), University of Westminster, UK. He was formerly Head of Employment Studies and Principal Research Fellow at PSI. He co-directed two studies within the ESRC's Future of Work Research Programme, and in 2004 was co-author of a resulting book, *Managing to Change? British Workplaces and the Future of Work*, published by Palgrave Macmillan.

Introduction

John Haworth and Graham Hart

We are all interested in well-being, consciously or subconsciously, as together we create well-being. In recent years, researchers, educators, policy makers and politicians have been directly concerned with well-being, which has been viewed variously as happiness, satisfaction, enjoyment, contentment, engagement, fulfilment and flourishing, or a combination of these, and other, hedonic and eudaimonic factors. Well-being is also viewed as a process, something we do together, and as sense-making, rather than just a state of being. It is acknowledged that in life as a whole there will be periods of ill-being, and that these may add richness to life. It has also been recognized that well-being and the environment are intimately interconnected. Certainly, well-being is seen to be complex and multifaceted, and may take different forms.

The book has its origins in a series of transdisciplinary seminars on well-being funded by grants from the Economic and Social Research Council in the UK.[1] The objective of the seminars was not to replace, but provide an alternative to, and to complement, the overwhelming harm-based focus of much social scientific research into health. Well-being offers a paradigm that allows those in the academic, policy and user fields to focus on positive outcomes, and how best to realize them. The series, and related publications, show the importance of societal, environmental, and individual factors for well-being.[2] Contributors to the seminars, and others eminent in their field, were commissioned to write in-depth chapters for the present book. Each chapter is important for well-being in its own right. Together they present a new dynamic view of well-being, one which will be crucial for the way in which we will cope with the twenty-first century.

Well-being research

In recent years in the USA there has been a focus on 'Positive Psychology' (www.positivepsychology.org) concerned with factors leading to well-being and positive individuals (e.g. Kahneman, Diener and Schwartze, 1999; Special Edition of the *American Psychologist*, January 2000: Snyder and Lopez 2000; Keyes and Haidt 2002; Seligman 2003; Sheldon 2004; Csikszentmihalyi and Csikszentmihalyi 2006; Peterson 2006; Diener, Lucas, Schimmack, and Helliwell 2009; Seligman 2011) – Positive Psychology is seen as concerned with how normal people might flourish under benign conditions – the thriving individual and the thriving community. Positive Psychology changes the focus of psychology from preoccupation with repairing the worst things in life to building the best things in life. In the USA, the field of Positive Psychology at the subjective level is about positive experience: well-being, optimism, hope, happiness, and flow. At the individual level it is about the character strengths – the capacity for love and vocation, courage, interpersonal skill, aesthetic sensibility, perseverance, forgiveness, originality, future-mindedness, and genius. At the group level it is about the civic virtues and the institutions that move individuals toward better citizenship: leadership, responsibility, parenting, altruism, civility, moderation, tolerance, and work ethic.

In discussing 'Positive Psychology', Seligman and Csikszentmihalyi (2000) distinguish between pleasure and enjoyment. They note that 'Pleasure is the good feeling that comes from satisfying homeostatic needs such as hunger, sex, and bodily comfort. Enjoyment on the other hand, refers to the good feelings people experience when they break through the limits of homeostasis – when they do something that stretches them beyond what they were – in an athletic event, an artistic performance, a good deed, a stimulating conversation. Enjoyment, rather than pleasure, is what leads to personal growth and long term happiness.'

Csikszentmihalyi and Csikszentmihalyi (2006), in an edited book on what makes life worth living, highlight the importance of personally meaningful goals, individual strengths and virtues, and intrinsic motivation and autonomy, in what makes people happy and life meaningful. Positive emotions and the development of personal resilience are also important in optimal functioning (Fredrickson 2006). Further research is needed on the related topics of flow, meaning, bliss, mindfulness, and consciousness (www.flowpsychology.com/flow-of-life/Joseph-Campbell/www.consciousness.arizona.edu).

Seligman (2011) argues that while happiness is a part of well-being, happiness alone doesn't give life meaning. Central to well-being is what allows one to flourish. He proposes that Positive Emotion (of which happiness and life satisfaction are aspects) is one of the five pillars of Positive Psychology, along with Engagement, Relationships, Meaning, and Accomplishment – or PERMA, the permanent building blocks for a life of profound fulfilment. Some aspects of these five elements are measured subjectively by self reports, while other aspects are measured objectively. Seligman cites research by Huppert and So (2009) who made provisional operational definitions of flourishing and applied this to existing European Social Survey data 2006/7. This showed a wide variation in the prevalence of flourishing across countries, with the highest rates of flourishing being in northern Europe and the lowest rates in Eastern Europe. Huppert and So advocate a series of steps to be taken, including seeking an international consensus on an operational definition of flourishing. Seligman notes that as our ability to measure the elements improve, which he recognizes will be accompanied by vigorous debate, we can ask with rigour how many people in a nation, in a city, or in a corporation are flourishing. He sees the goal of positive psychology in well-being theory as measuring and building human flourishing. Diener et al. (2009), on the basis of their extensive international research with a range of measures of subjective well-being, advoctate their use, along with objective measures, as an aid to public policy formation.

An International Positive Psychology Association (IPPA) has been formed (www.ippanetwork.org); and a European positive psychology network has also been established (www.enpp.eu/) which promotes regular conferences and publications (e.g. Linley and Joseph 2004; Delle Fave 2006; Freire 2010). In Europe, a World Data Base of Happiness Research is freely available on the internet at http://www.eur.nl./fsw/research/happiness. In the UK the Centre for Applied Positive Psychology (CAPP) (www.cappeu.com) has developed Release 2, a world-leading strengths assessment and development tool, designed to unlock the performance potential of individuals, teams, and organizations through releasing their strengths.

The positive psychology programme is very praiseworthy, and is stimulating much needed research in many countries. However, it focuses primarily on individual influences on well-being. Yet recent advances in research in social neuroscience show the essential social nature of the human mind and brain (www.socialmirrors.org and the Social Brain project of the Royal Society for the Arts). The positive psychology programme could be enhanced by the study of the influence of social institutions on behaviour and well-being (e.g. Jahoda 1982). Haworth (in press) presents evidence of the need for a positive social psychology of organizations, one which includes a study of the reciprocal interaction between the person and the organization, including the public and the State. Prilleltensky (2001, 2008) argues from extensive studies that wellness is achieved by the simultaneous and balanced satisfaction of personal, interpersonal, and collective needs.

In the UK, the study of well-being is now a key element in the Economic and Social Research Council's Lifecourse, Lifestyle, and Health Thematic Priority 2000. UK perspectives on well-being and happiness include psychological (Argyle 2002), psycho-biological (Huppert et al. 2005; Huppert 2009a) and population based (Huppert 2009b), social (Halpern 2005), and economic approaches (Oswald 2003, 2010 pdf, 2011 pdf www.andrewoswald.com; Layard 2003, 2005 www.actionforhappiness. org; New Economics Foundation: www.neweconomics.org). Layard reviewed evidence showing that above a certain level, economic growth (GDP) does not increase overall societal well-being, as people evaluate their income in relation to changing standards. Research by Wilkinson (1996, 2000) and Wilkinson and Picket (2009) shows that increase in socio-economic inequalities in developed countries is associated with health inequality; which is likely to be detrimental to the well-being of individuals and communities. The Marmot Report (2010) gives extensive evidence in the UK for the importance of tackling health inequalities, and that the fair distribution of health, well-being, and sustainability are important social goals (www.ucl.ac.uk/gheg/marmotreview). Dorling (2010) shows dramatic differences in health and inequality across the UK. The Equality Trust has been established in the UK to promote a healthier, happier, more sustainable society. It campaigns to gain the widest public and political understanding of the harm caused by inequality (www.equalitytrust.org.uk). Doran and Whitehead (2004) also show from research in the UK that social policies and political context matter for health. The UK Cabinet Office has produced a report on Life Satisfaction (Donovan, Halpern, and Sargeant 2002). This found strong links between work satisfaction and overall life satisfaction, and also between leisure activities and overall satisfaction, concluding that there is a case for government intervention to boost life satisfaction, by encouraging a more leisured work–life balance. Another approach emphasizes a set of practices, rather than a state of happiness. For example, Perri (2002) argued that well-being is about what people recognize, within particular institutions, as a shared life – a life well lived and worth living together.

The study of both work and leisure has contributed significantly to the broader approach to well-being (e.g. Jahoda 1982; Warr 1987, 1999; Csikszentmihalyi and Le Fevre 1989; Roberts 1999; Taylor 2001,

2002; Haworth 1997; Haworth and Veal 2004; Haworth and Lewis 2005; Iso-Ahola and Mannell 2004; Stebbins 2004; Kay 2001, 2006; Haworth and Roberts 2010, Haworth 2011). Warr (1987) in his concept of mental health from a Western perspective, advocates the measurement of affective well-being, competence, autonomy, aspiration, and integrated functioning. However, it is the measure of affective well-being which has received the greatest empirical attention (Warr 1990). Delle Fave and Massimini (2003) note that creative activities in leisure, work, and social interaction can give rise to 'flow' or 'optimal' experiences. These experiences foster individual development and an increase in skills in the lifelong cultivation of specific interests and activities. Taylor (2002) in a report on the ESRC funded Future of Work programme advocates that a determined effort is required to assess the purpose of paid work in all our lives, and the need to negotiate a genuine trade-off between the needs of job efficiency and leisure. The report considers that class and occupational differences remain of fundamental importance to any understanding of the world of work. Arguably, class is also important in understanding the world of leisure. Critcher and Bramham (2004) state that 'Where access to leisure increasingly rests on the capacity to purchase goods and services in the market, the distribution of income becomes an important determinant of leisure life chances.' A recent European Union funded qualitative research project, Transitions (www.workliferesearch.org/transitions), examined the transition to parenthood among employees in changing European workplaces. It found a drive for more efficiency and an intensification of work across all the countries studied; a widespread implementation gap between policies to support the reconciliation of work and family, and actual practice; and persisting gender differences in work–life responsibilities and experiences. The study also highlighted the important role in well-being played by managers and work colleagues. The research showed that the study of well-being benefits from being located in a life domain.

Well-being: measurement and process in the UK

At the behest of the UK Government, the Office of National Statistics (ONS) (www.ons.gov.uk) is developing new measures of national well-being. The aim is that these new measures will cover the quality of life of people in the UK, environmental and sustainability issues, as well as the economic performance of the country. A national well-being consultation has been held, with people, organizations and business across the UK, for them to say what matters most to them and their sense of well-being, and what is important for measuring the nation's well-being.

The New Economics Foundation (Nef) (www.neweconomics.org) in a detailed downloadable report 'Measuring our progress' looks at what is needed, making comprehensive recommendations. Their approach to measuring well-being is based on the dynamic model they developed for the Government Office for Science's 2008 Foresight project, and uses the idea of flourishing. They consider that flourishing can be measured in the short term by including a small number of questions within an existing large scale population survey, and recommend five questions to assess the evaluative, hedonic, and functioning elements of well-being. In the longer term, flourishing should be measured using a tailor made survey to capture the richness of well-being in the UK. They consider that measuring well-being directly will enable policy makers to improve decisions, and identify inequalities in well-being.

The British Psychological Society response to the ONS consultation (*The Psychologist*, May 2011, p. 367) welcomes the approach combining both subjective and objective measures. However, it details the complexities involved, and considers that 'It will be essential for care to be taken to reflect the multidimensional (multimodal) character of any well-being index.' It emphasizes the importance of studying well-being in life domains, such as work. It also stresses that it is important to consider social inequalities and societal and structural influences on well-being.

The Leisure Studies Association response to the ONS consultation (*LSA Newsletter 89* 2011, www.leisure-studies-association.info) emphasizes that leisure is crucial to the state of health of the nation and to the well-being of individuals. It considers that leisure as a concept can and should be operationalized to understand the rich component parts that enable individuals to forge a life worth living. The response makes several proposals concerning measures of well-being, including adding the following question on enjoyment to surveys 'How much of the time in the last seven days did you enjoy what you were doing (in your leisure time)?' (answered on a 10 point scale from none of the time to all of the time).

The ONS will add four questions to its next annual Integrated Household Survey. These are: Overall, how satisfied are you with your life nowadays?; Overall, how happy did you feel yesterday?; Overall, how anxious did you feel yesterday?; Overall, to what extent do you feel the things you do in your life are worthwhile? The questions will be answered on a scale from 0–10. Smaller surveys addressing other aspects of well-being, will be conducted each month. Initially, results will be regarded as experimental to see if the questions work, and that they meet public policy and other needs, including international developments.

New technologies are emerging in social research, which may be of value in either the large or small scale in-depth measurement of well-being. For example, Nef in its National Accounts of Well-being has developed an online questionnaire for well-being, with immediate processing and visualization of results in comparison to others. Haworth (2010, www.well-being-esrc.com) and Kelock et al. (2011), have utilized the mobile phone/camera to develop a photo-ethnographic approach to daily life and well-being.

There are several important groups in the UK also concerned with the process of achieving well-being in individuals, groups, and society. For example, 'Action for happines' is a movement for positive social change (www.actionforhappiness.org). It considers that by choosing to live in a way that prioritizes things that really matter we can create a vital shift in societal values. The Equality Trust has been established to promote a healthier, happier, more sustainable society (www.equalitytrust.org.uk), and www.compassonline.org.uk campaigns for a more equal, sustainable, and democratic world. The document 'The Great Transition' downloadable from Nef, proposes a range of measures to attempt to achieve a just society where good lives do not have to cost the Earth. Demos (www.demos.co.uk) is a think-tank focusing on power and politics, giving a voice to people and communities, involving them closely in its research. Political parties in the UK are also debating the way forward for society, with different emphasis being placed on the role of the individual and the State.

Many of the chapters in this book arise from this milieu of research on well-being. They both develop and challenge existing concepts and approaches. Other chapters bring fresh perspectives to research on well-being from different disciplines. In Part 1 of the book the chapters have a primary focus on individual and community approaches to well-being. They show how these are inevitably intertwined, and that both homogeneity and diversity (or what may be termed 'constrained diversity') exist in society. In Part 2 individual and community perspectives are combined with a societal dimension, set in a global environmental context. Each chapter in the book is important for its own domain of enquiry, while reflecting the interconnectedness of domains. Summaries of the chapters are provided for each part, and presented together. These indicate not just the desirability, but the necessity of addressing well-being from individual, community, and societal perspectives, in an integrated manner; not least in tackling increasing social inequalities in societies (Navarro 2004; Marmot 2010).

Considered together, the chapters show the emergent influence on research into well-being of the experiential model of consciousness being proposed by Merleau-Ponty (1962), this model emphasizes the intertwining of experience and being, and the importance of both pre-reflexive and reflexive thought (see Haworth 1997, ch. 7). The chapters also reveal the importance of recognizing 'constrained diversity' in the human condition, and the necessity to consider the implications of this for research and policy in complex, uncertain situations, with associated unintended consequences of action. Such an approach to well-being could be used to implement several types of interventions or enhancements for well-being (Pawelsky 2006), including empowerment, which is a relatively neglected approach in positive psychology. The approach would also sit comfortably with the analysis and call for a social policy for the twenty-first century (Jordan 2006).

The introduction concludes by summarizing several key concepts relating to well-being identified in the book.

Part 1: Individual and community perspectives on well-being

Jane Henry in Chapter 1 on 'Positive Psychology and the Development of Well-Being' notes that positive psychology focuses on the *positive side of life*, and that despite an espoused concern with institutions in the sense of a concern with civic values, for example, the majority of positive psychology studies to date have focused at the level of the individual. In her chapter she gives an illustration of some of the positive psychology research on well-being, positive style and positive experiences. Both simple and multidimensional measures of well-being have been used effectively. Positive style includes important research into an individual's natural talents or *strengths*, though difficulties are associated with searching for a universal list of strengths. A positive explanatory style, such as optimism, is generally beneficial, though this may not always be the case for different personality types. From her research, Henry advocates that both working to accentuate the positive and to cope better with the negative have their place. She also notes that there is some evidence that positive and negative affect are two separate variables, not a unipolar one; thus reducing negative affect and increasing positive affect may be separate enterprises.

Research into the experience of 'flow' is recognized as important, though Henry notes that there are probably many states of optimal experience other than flow, notably varieties of contentment and other low arousal states of satisfaction. These types of experiences have been more thoroughly examined in spiritual practice than in psychology. She considers they deserve further research.

Henry discusses her research into what people thought had accounted for any long-term improvement in their own well-being. These studies suggest that intuitive, physically active and social approaches have been valued by more people than reflective routes. Henry considers that they challenge not only the dominance of talking therapy as the favoured route to self-improvement but the rather individualistic and goal-oriented route to well-being emphasized by many positive psychologists and other caring professionals.

Antonella Delle Fave in Chapter 2 on 'Individual Development and Community Empowerment: Suggestions from Studies on Optimal Experience' emphasizes the role of individuals as active agents in shaping their cultural environment and in promoting its complexity. In cultural evolution, psychological selection is important, with optimal experience playing an important role, fostering personal growth and cultural empowerment. Cross-cultural research on optimal experience by the author using a questionnaire showed that the activity categories associated with the most pervasive optimal experience were productive activities (work or study) and structured leisure (sports, arts and crafts, hobbies). Social and family interactions and the use of mass media followed with lower percentages. The findings also showed that optimal experience comprises a stable cognitive core (focus of attention, control of the situation) across activity categories, though wider variations across categories were detected in the values of affective (e.g. excitement) and motivational (e.g. wishing to do the activity) variables. While work can be important for optimal experience, the study showed that none of the blue-collar and white-collar participants in the present study (around 200 people) associated assembly line work or routine office tasks with the most pervasive optimal experiences.

Delle Fave considers that the extent to which a society provides its members with long-term, meaningful, intrinsically rewarding and engaging activities can be indicative of a successful cultural transmission, in that it facilitates the preferential replication of such activities through psychological selection. She advocates that information on people's perception of opportunities for optimal experiences in the daily domains is essential to design intervention programmes grounded in individual potential for empowerment. This can facilitate an effective match between individual needs and values, on the one side, and society development and integration, on the other. Also, from a broader perspective, in order to promote empowerment, the introduction of any cultural information – be it represented by an artefact, a law, a value, a philosophical outlook, an educational or organizational strategy – has to take into account its consequences for the well-being of individuals, of the ecosystem, and of other societies at the same time.

Isaac and Ora Prilleltensky in Chapter 3 discuss 'Webs of Well-Being: the Interdependence of Personal, Relational, Organizational and Communal Well-Being'. The main premise of the chapter is that what happens in any domain of well-being – collective, organizational, relational or personal – affects the others. They argue that to minimize the importance of contextual factors for well-being has adverse consequences for understanding psychological processes and efforts at social change.

The authors present a model of well-being consisting of sites, signs, sources, strategies and synergy, which captures the interdependence of personal, relational, organizational and communal well-being. The sites are where well-being takes place, for example, the personal, indicated by signs such as personal control. A clean environment, freedom from discrimination, safe neighbourhoods, good schools and employment opportunities are signs of community well-being. These are communal goods that benefit everyone. Well-being at the different sites is dependent on a variety of sources. For example, nurturance and early positve experiences of attachment influence relational well-being. The fourth S is for *strategies*. To promote well-being in each one of the sites of interest – persons, relationships, organizations and communities – a plan of action is needed. *Synergy*, the fifth S, comes about when an understanding of sources and strategies is combined. In accord with the concept of webs, the best results for any one site of wellness come about when work is done on all fronts at the same time.

The authors argue that the key to successful strategies is that they must be specific enough to address each one of the sites, signs and respective sources of well-being at the same time. Interventions that concentrate strictly on personal sites neglect the many resources that organizations and communities contribute to personal well-being. Paradoxically, strategies that concentrate exclusively on personal well-being undermine well-being because they do not support the infrastructure that enhances well-being itself. The authors believe that this has been a major gap in previous efforts to sustain individual well-being through strictly psychological means such as cognitive reframing, positive thinking, information sharing and skill building. Individuals cannot significantly alter their level of well-being in the absence of concordant environmental changes. Conversely, any strategy that promotes well-being by environmental changes alone is bound to be limited. The authors consider that there is ample evidence to suggest that the most promising approaches combine strategies for personal, organizational and collective change. It is not one or the other, but the combination of them all that is the best avenue to seek higher levels of well-being in these three sites.

Judith Sixsmith and Margaret Boneham in Chapter 4 on 'Health, Well-Being and Social Capital' examine the concept of social capital focusing on the key components of participation, trust and reciprocity, and social networks of bonding, bridging and linking ties. They review qualitative work which has begun to map out the different processes and mechanisms through which social capital is fundamental to an understanding of community relations and has implications for health and well-being.

Social capital may operate in different ways, reflecting heterogeneous community groups. Thus any analysis of social capital needs to pay attention to marginalized groups and how everyday lives are lived in diverse community contexts. Sixsmith et al.'s (2001) study of the relationship between social capital, health and gender in a disadvantaged community, found that intimate social bonds offered important opportunities for social support, paralleling Kagan et al.'s (2000) conclusions that, 'The poor neighbourhood may have weak and inward looking networks, which nevertheless offer strong support in adversity.' However, the relationship between bridging capital and individual well-being was more complex, with advantages for the community as a whole in the establishment of bridging ties to professional help but less benefit for individual community leaders whose expectations were poorly aligned to professional methods of communication. The lack of accessible bridging and linking capital to professional advice meant that more inventive ways of perceiving health and illness were not aired (Sixsmith and Boneham 2003). Sixsmith and Boneham's research also indicates that an understanding of the relationships between social capital, health and well-being must involve an appreciation of issues of gender and place.

The authors note that whilst poverty, discrimination and deprivation may exert their negative influence through undermining stocks of social capital, simply bolstering communities' stocks of social capital is no panacea. Indeed, it could be argued that emphasis on the role of social capital in enhancing health might divert attention away from the more urgent need to improve health through reducing income inequalities. They advocate that if the government is serious about reducing health inequalities and improving people's quality of life, there needs to be a genuine three-way partnership between people, local communities and government (DoH 1999). Social structures that cater for individual and social well-being, and which empower people and local communities in the face of an increasingly centralizing government agenda, need to be strengthened. It is only when people, communities and the government work equally together that social policy can make a real positive change to people's health and well-being.

Carolyn Kagan and Amanda Kilroy in Chapter 5 on 'Psychology in the Community' outline the key principles of community psychology, look at how community well-being is understood, and explore the role of boundary critique as a means of developing critical awareness about community interventions designed to enhance well-being. Community psychology is seen as a value-based practice that focuses its attention on those most marginalized by the social system The underlying principles of a radical community psychological praxis are seen as: articulation of an explicit value base (a just society and its underpinning values); use of ecological metaphor; adoption of a whole systems perspective; interdisciplinary working; understanding and working with the dialectic relationship between people and systems; and practices enhancing people's critical consciousness. The concept of well-being in the community, and of the community, is multifaceted. It recognizes that for people to lead truly flourishing lives they need to feel they are personally satisfied and developing; that eudaimonic well-being (personal development and fulfilment) is as important as hedonic well-being (satisfaction and happiness). At the same time a community psychological perspective, however, would suggest that both the hedonic and eudaimonic well-being of people who are socially excluded, are inseparable from not only their economic position, the environmental conditions in which they live and the political and ideological messages that confine them to poverty whilst enjoining them to break free and better themselves, but also from the human services that exist to both assist and to regulate them. Yet few attempts have been made to explore the interconnections.

The authors and their colleagues have been exploring the impact of participation in the arts on health and well-being from a community psychological perspective. They have drawn on critical systems thinking (CST) in their work on evaluation. In this chapter they discuss one aspect of this, namely, boundary critique. A particular brief was to examine how participation in arts projects leads to changes in well-being and mental health and to make recommendations for project improvement. The evaluations were to involve close collaboration between the artists and researchers. Early on, a number of boundary disputes became clear. For example, artists and researchers had different ways of understanding well-being, which led to an inability to agree how best to conceptualize well-being and describe it within the evaluation. Artists and researchers also disagreed about the relative importance of the aesthetic product and the processes of creation and creativity used within the projects, which meant that agreement could not be reached about a relevant evaluation framework. Discussing these boundary disputes just served to strengthen the impasse. An appreciative inquiry (AI) approach, described in the chapter, was chosen to encourage a deeper and more meaningful means of communication. The chapter discusses the concept of boundary and boundary critique, a topic of considerable importance to issues of communication and negotiation in community well-being.

David Haley in his contribution to Chapter 6 on 'Art, Health and Well-Being' argues that an expanded dynamic notion of art could provide the creative dialogue needed to value disparate readings of well-being. He notes that art, freedom and democracy mean different things to different people and are 'essentially contested'; and that these and other concepts, such as well-being and health, cannot, therefore, be defined in terms of formal, analytical philosophy. He cites George Lakoff and Mark Johnson, in *Philosophy in the Flesh* (1999), who argue 'for an experientially responsible philosophy, one that incorporates results concerning the embodiment of mind, the cognitive unconscious, and metaphysical thought'. His text explores some aspects of art, health and well-being to try to understand how they may resonate with each other to generate understandings of what a 'better quality of life' might be. Art in its broadest sense is seen as virtuous ways of making and understanding the world. It recognizes that art can be integral to everyday life, that there is an embodied need for all organisms to engage with their evolutionary development and participate in creative processes, and that the environment is part of our being and identity. Denial of this embodied ecology and these therapeutic creative activities can be experienced as chronic forms of personal, community and societal neuroses – an intrinsic lack of well-being.

Haley highlights an alternative to rationally based problem based learning, termed 'question based learning'. Here the premise is that we don't know, and that we have to listen and learn from a situation before acting. This approach informs a constantly evolving notion of well-being, achieved as a dynamic creative process. He cites scientists and artists advocating a form of free exchange of ideas and information fundamental for transforming culture and freeing it of destructive misinformation, so that creativity can be liberated.

Peter Senior in his contribution to Chapter 6 summarizes the important part played by the arts for health and well-being in the UK and elsewhere. He notes that the arts today can bring many benefits to the healing environment. They assist recovery by encouraging feelings of well-being and alleviating stress. They can improve the quality of healthcare environments by linking art, architecture and interior design. Through their involvement in the arts the lives of patients, visitors and staff can be enriched. Closer links between the health services and the community can be developed through arts and cultural activities. A wide range of arts activities in Britain's health service is now provided by partnerships between the health service and arts organizations from the state and voluntary sectors, and between artists, healthcare staff and local communities. Activities include performances of music, theatre, puppetry, poetry, environmental and decorative arts schemes, and participatory arts projects for patients, staff and public.

In 1988 Peter Senior established Arts for Health as a national centre, located in the Faculty of Art and Design at the Manchester Metropolitan University (www.mmu.ac.uk/artsforhealth/). Its aim was to unite artists, designers and health authorities in establishing arts for health projects as an integral part of the nation's healthcare culture. He advocates that just as the purpose of medicine is to restore the human being to a state of well-being, so the aim of art within healthcare should be to reflect beauty, harmony and delight in ways that echo that purpose. Research studies are referenced which indicate the important work done by artists of all kinds working in health settings to raise awareness of the effect of the physical and social environment on staff, public and patients.

Perri 6 in Chapter 7 on 'Sense and Solidarities: Politics and Human Well-Being' notes that well-being encompasses a wide range of subjective and objective measures, and that, typically, it is treated as a variable to be optimized. The chapter argues that this understanding of well-being is misguided. It proposes an alternative account which includes the following three propositions:

1. Well-being is about what people will recognize, under particular institutions, as shared life well lived and worth living together over the life course.
2. Well-being is achieved as much by the ways in which people, under different institutions, make sense of their lives and their social world as it is by material resources.

3. Well-being is a set of practices, not a state. Some ill-being may be necessary to well-being, understood as a richer process than mere contentment.

The author considers that well-being is something that we do together, not something that we each possess. An adequate account of well-being is thus seen to require a theory of the range of basic institutions of social organization, within which people can make viable sense of their lives. This chapter uses a neo-Durkheimian institutional approach. It argues, contrary to postmodern conceptions, that the forms of social organization – and hence of well-being – are not indefinitely various. Rather, there is a limited plurality of basic institutional forms, which support several hybrids or coalitions. In each form, quite distinct styles of sense-making and therefore of well-being are to be found. These basic forms of social organization are in perpetual conflict with each other. Each springs up in response to the others. None can be eliminated from any viable society: attempts to do so will result in the return of the suppressed form, often in corrupt, illicit or violent forms. The central challenge for policy and politics of well-being, then, is to find ways in which the basic commitments of each of the forms can be articulated in an overarching settlement.

Well-being is thus seen as plural, complex, even unstable. The author argues that social science can provide understanding of the institutional framework within which policy-makers must work. But it cannot promise, and policy-makers should not demand, any universally valid, apolitical prescriptions. Social science can provide invaluable tools with which to support – but never substitute for – political judgement, and it can identify some pitfalls. It can tell the policy-makers what to think about and how to think about those things, rather than telling them what to think.

One general maxim is given for policy-makers – where all good things do not go together, where complex trade-offs must be struck between the four institutional orders that yield different value systems and capabilities for well-being, each with its own weaknesses and risks, one can reasonably suggest that policy-makers ought to focus on the control of harms – accepting that there are always trade-offs between different harms – as a general priority before pursuing benefits.

An example is given of the practical use of the approach to public policy implied in the theoretical apparatus. The author suggests that the 'social capital' argument has misread and misconstrued the empirical literature; and that there is not a sound base of evidence upon which to make robust assessments of the efficacy of interventions, and the balance of intended and unintended consequences, for different forms of social organization. He advocates that policy-makers need to engage in iterative design, evaluation and redesign, in reaching for accommodations.

Part 2: Societal perspectives on well-being

The chapters in this section show the importance of the links between the individual, society and the environment for well-being, which itself is complex and multifaceted. Culture, social institutions and technological developments can influence well-being in both deleterious and beneficial ways. It is vitally important that research and analysis is undertaken at this level. Equally the chapters show that diversity permeates the relationship between the individual and society, requiring continued investigation in relation to well-being.

John Pickering in Chapter 8, 'Is Well-Being Local or Global?', brings a perspective from ecopsychology on well-being. Ecopsychology considers there to be an emotional bond between human beings and the environment. Well-being means the feeling of having a place in the world, of being at home in the world, and of living in balance with the trials of life. Pickering argues that our relationship with the environment is increasingly violent and destructive. We are beginning to realize that the effects of our technologized lifestyles are leading to damage on a global scale that we may not be able to repair. The unease that this creates is fundamentally detrimental to well-being. The effects may not be close to the surface of our conscious lives, but they are important nonetheless. In one sense, 'today's job' is what it has always been: to seek well-being and to feel whole, secure in a stable identity. But this is made more difficult when identity itself is open to indefinite redefinition. Selfhood is constructed using what the culture around it provides. What we take ourselves to be is in turn taken from what our cultural context defines a self to be. In the wealthy world selfhood is closely bound to the variety of lifestyles a rich and abundant culture can offer.

Pickering considers that a satisfying and sustainable relationship with the natural world has been, over the history of human kind, the basis of well-being. This is not a static condition but depends on a healthy balance between met and unmet needs. Yet advertising creates artificial needs which are designed to be permanently unmet. They act as an irritant, undermining our sense of balance between what we have, what we need and what we want. Much of what threatens well-being arises from the massive over-consumption required to meet pathological needs inflamed by media technology.

What some ecopsychologists have called the 'all-consuming self' is a narcissistic condition in which selfhood becomes too strongly defined by possession, having been detached from its more natural supports by a barrage of consumerist images in the media. If this need to possess is pathologically inflated, the self/world boundary becomes a moving frontier of greed. Cultures in which it has taken hold will violently wrest what they want from the environment and from other cultures. This violence can be concealed within hyper-reality to some extent, but preconsciously the news leaks out. Combined with preconscious needs for self-actualization that cannot be met, it makes for a powerful degradation of well-being. Pickering argues that well-being depends on a life in balance. He advocates that if our way of life is being driven deeply out of balance by artificial and unsustainable needs, this has to be addressed if we are to carry out research that is appropriate and useful.

Ballas et al. in Chapter 9 on 'Societal Inequality, Health and Well-Being' consider well-being at the ecological level and investigate the relationship between happiness and inequality across Britain. The chapter briefly reviews the theoretical background of happiness research and also considers its relevance to public policy. It can be argued that societies that are extremely polarized and divided are less desirable, and less 'well', than those which have elements of equity and communitarianism as their core values and principles. The chapter presents evidence for the recent widening of the gap between the rich and the poor leading to unprecedented post-World War Two socio-economic polarization and income inequalities in Britain. The geographies of income and wealth in Britain also show spatial dimensions of socio-economic polarization. Using data from the British Household Panel Survey the geographical distribution of happiness in England and Wales shows similarities to the spatial dimensions of income distribution. The authors consider that, on the basis of the evidence presented in this chapter, it becomes clearer that public policy that is aimed at income and wealth redistribution and societal equality would probably lead to higher overall levels of happiness and well-being.

Hatch et al. in Chapter 10 discuss 'A Life Course Approach to Well-Being'. They see well-being as characterized by the capacity to actively participate in work and recreation, create meaningful relationships with others, develop a sense of autonomy and purpose in life, and to experience positive emotions. Well-being varies with age, and with personality and age-related attributes such as educational attainment and health status that are known to be shaped by early life experience. They cite evidence from the 1946 British birth cohort study and other longitudinal studies, that developmental factors, the early social environment, early behaviour and temperament have long-term effects on adult physiological, cognitive and psychosocial well-being. An active pursuit of well-being over the life course implies a considerable amount of individual agency, which operates within the context of social structure that regulates access to fundamental resources (Link and Phelan 1995). They argue that a life course framework offers a dynamic model of the interplay over time between the individual and the environment that can be used to understand the factors that develop and maintain well-being and successful adaptation over the life course. They identify several theoretical constructs and processes concerning well-being that could be operationalized in longitudinal studies; with one objective being to develop social policy interventions.

Michael White in Chapter 11 on 'Organizational Commitment: a Managerial Illusion?' examines one of the main ways in which working life can become more fulfilling: through a sense of involvement with and commitment to an organization. This type of commitment, and the committed experience it can offer, is in principle available to most working-age people, and there is a widespread belief that it can be effectively fostered by certain kinds of management practice that are becoming increasingly prevalent. Organizational commitment (OC) vies with job satisfaction as the leading current indicator of well-being at work. By being committed, we demand more of ourselves and express more of our potential. Through our commitments taken as a whole, we also express the values that we wish to shape our lives. Our commitments define our selves, and so commitment is closely linked to two other foci of contemporary desire: personal choice and identity.

The chapter examines OC by means of two sample surveys of employed people, the Employment in Britain survey (EIB) of 1992, and the Working in Britain survey (WIB) of 2000/1. The surveys were nationally representative of people in paid work aged 20–60; the information was collected by means of personal interviews in the employed people's homes. The surveys show that while an increased number of employees experienced High Commitment Management (HCM) practices over the period aimed at increasing OC, the average level of OC expressed by employees decreased. Some practices in some companies increased OC, but the responses to HCM practices were variable. A detailed examination of the findings suggest that the managerial model of OC, whereby the employer can 'produce' or 'generate' OC by taking certain actions, is misconceived. A model that better fits the findings is one where employees actively look for what they can engage with and commit to because it matches their preferences. What attracts them towards a commitment at one time may attract them less at a later time, or vice versa. For some people, for example, the issue of work-life balance can influence OC. The author argues that in important respects people construct their own well-being, and one of the ways in which they do so is by choosing commitments which make them more fully or more actively the people they want to be. The chapter recognizes that HCM practices have some positive effect on OC, and suggests they may be linked with a 'diversity policy' that recognizes the diversity of personal circumstances and values among employees, which may possibly provide a more nurturing environment for employees' spontaneous commitments.

Suzan Lewis and Christina Purcell in Chapter 12 focus on 'Well-Being, Paid Work and Personal Life'. Positive well-being is increasingly conceptualized in terms of the satisfactory integration or harmonization of work and family – often referred to as 'work-life balance'. The authors draw on data from an EU Framework Five study (*Transitions*) which examined how young European women and men negotiate motherhood and fatherhood and work-family boundaries, and how this impacts on their well-being. This chapter draws on one case study of a finance sector organization in the UK, although the discussion of this case is contextualized within the wider study. The study shows the crucial role played by managers. Workplace policies and practices are shaped by national and local regulations, but are also increasingly a matter of daily and informal negotiation with managers in local organizations. Well-being for parents varied across departments, highlighting the discretionary application of informal, trust-based policies. However, even when managers and their working practices did enhance parents' flexibility and autonomy over work and family boundaries, this tended to be undermined by other factors, particularly long hours and the intensification of work. The study also showed that social comparison and sense of entitlement are important in determining expectations and subsequent well-being; and that the transition to parenthood reinforces traditional gender identity and roles within couples – women being under more pressure to be carers and men to be main wage-earners.

The study showed the important role of context on well-being. Access to high affordable quality childcare is crucial to attitudes to, and experience of, employed parenthood, although this concerned mothers rather than fathers. Finance was also a real issue for the lower paid employees in the context of high house prices and childcare costs. There was much evidence across all the case studies of an intensification of the expectations of parenting, which includes aspiration to provide not only more time and attention but also more material goods. To some extent the parents' sense of well-being reflected their expectations of work and of their ability to attain their aspirations for themselves and their children – based on consumerism rather than citizenship (Sointu 2005). However, the finance sector participants were very different in their expectations and ambitions than the social services participants in the UK public sector case study.

The study argues that well-being is complex, multifaceted, fluctuating over time and influenced by the many layers of context in which individuals' lives are embedded, which indicates the need for a multilayered approach to policy. Changes in legislation alone are of limited value for enhancing well-being of new parents without shifts in organizational, family and community values and practices. The authors advocate a life course approach to research into well-being

John Haworth in Chapter 13 on 'Work, Leisure and Well-Being in Changing Social Conditions' notes that the meanings and concepts of work and leisure are being reappraised, and the relationships between work, leisure, social structure and well-being have emerged as challenging concerns for researchers, educators and policy-makers. A recent government report in the UK on 'Life Satisfaction: the State of Knowledge and Implications for Government' cited strong links between work satisfaction and overall life satisfaction, and also between active leisure activities and overall satisfaction. Yet many people feel stressed because of financial difficulties and the dominance of work, and in such situations leisure is used primarily for recuperation from work.

Research into work and leisure has significantly informed the study of well-being. Jahoda (1982) has made a crucial case for the importance of the social institution of employment for well-being. She identified five categories of experience which employment automatically provides. These are: time structure, social contact, collective effort or purpose, social identity or status, and regular activity. Jahoda emphasizes that in modern society it is the social institution of employment which is the main provider of the five categories of experience. She considers that since the Industrial Revolution employment has shaped the form of our daily lives, our experience of work and leisure, and our attitudes, values and beliefs. Jahoda regards dependency on social institutions not as good or bad but as the *sine qua non* of human existence.

The categories of experience identified by Jahoda have been incorporated in the nine environmental factors proposed by Warr (1987) as important for well-being. These features of the environment, such as opportunity for control, are considered to interact with characteristics of the person to facilitate or constrain psychological well-being or mental health. Research by the author and colleagues shows strong associations between each of the nine factors and measures of mental health. An important development of the model is the inclusion of the role of enjoyment.

Extensive research shows that enjoyment in both work and leisure is important for well-being. Using the experience sampling method, the author and colleagues found that experiences which are challenging, met with equal skill and enjoyable (enjoyable 'flow' experiences), were associated with higher levels of well-being, measured by standard questionnaires. Enjoyable flow experiences come from both work and leisure. It has been argued that it is not possible to say what is a healthy work-life balance, and that a range of affective experiences should be examined in daily life.

Taylor (2002) considers that class and occupational differences remain of fundamental importance to any understanding of the world of work. Class is also important in understanding the world of leisure (Critcher and Bramham 2004). Haworth concludes with the following points: It is important to monitor the distribution of resources available for work and leisure in different groups in society. The social and economic institutions of work and leisure also need to be more in balance. Equally, in societies characterized by diversity, research is needed into the experiences and motivations of individuals with varying work and leisure lifestyles, as there is no one correct policy for work and leisure.

Ray Pahl in Chapter 14 on 'Friendship, Trust and Mutuality' notes that the importance of friends for well-being has long been understood. He also identifies the central paradox in the sociological theory of friendship. On the one hand there are those, such as Simmel and Bauman, who argue that the institutions and values of market society and consumerism destroy the conditions in which the true ideal of friendship can flourish. Yet, on the other hand, Silver argues that it is only under the conditions of modern society that the distinctive ideal can possibly emerge.

Pahl considers that if we limit ourselves to ideals and dispositions we are getting little understanding of the actual empirical reality of the friendly relationships most people have in their everyday lives. He draws on research undertaken by Liz Spencer and himself over the past decade concerned with 'Rethinking Friendship'. The research design was rigorously qualitative and at its heart was the exploration and analysis of the people whom respondents considered 'were important to them now'. The research showed the diverse nature of friendship in Britain today. For example, some of the friendly relationships were so close that they could be described as being quasi-family. Other friendships, by contrast, were casual, shallow and short-lived. Certain kinds of friends – associates, neighbours, 'fun friends' – may fade when people move, or follow different life course trajectories. Yet such fun friends can be immensely affectionate and last a lifetime. The research also showed the suffusion of family and non-family forms of relationship, and distinctive personal communities. Family-based communities were found to have less poor well-being than 'partner-based' and 'professional-based' personal communities. The author concludes that not only is friendship essential for our individual and collective well-being, its disciplined study and exploration can help us as a society to be more conscious of the processes of which we form a part. The author suggests that friendship should be studied in schools.

Conclusion

Several key concepts relating to well-being have been identified in the book. These include the following:

- Well-being is complex and multifaceted. It is considered as a state and a process. It is a contested concept.
- Well-being includes personal, interpersonal and collective needs, which influence each other.
- Well-being may take different forms, which may conflict across groups in society, requiring an overarching settlement. Well-being may also take different forms over the life course of an individual.
- Well-being is intimately intertwined with the physical, cultural and technological environment, and requires a global perspective.
- Interventions to enhance well-being may take different forms. They should be conducted at individual, community and societal levels, ideally in concert. Interventions need to recognize diversity and socio-economic inequalities in society, and be concerned with the unintended as well as the intended consequences of action.

Notes

1. The co-ordinators for the seminar series were: Dr John Haworth and Professor Graham Hart; and Professor Sarah Curtis from the Department of Geography, Queen Mary, University of London.
2. Papers from the seminars, and links to other research on well-being, can be found at the project website http://www.wellbeing-esrc.com.

References

American Psychologist (2000) Special Edition on positive psychology, 55, 1.

Argyle, M. (2002) *The Psychology of Happiness*. London: Methuen.

Critcher, C. and Bramham, P. (2004) 'The Devil Still Makes Work', in J. T. Haworth and A. J. Veal (eds), *Work and Leisure*. London: Routledge.

Csikszentmihalyi, M. and Csikszentmihalyi, I. S. (eds) (2006) *A Life Worth Living: Contributions to Positive Psychology*. Oxford: Oxford University Press.

Csikszentmihalyi, M. and LeFevre, J. (1989) 'Optimal Experience in Work and Leisure', *Journal of Personality and Social Psychology*, 56, 5: 815–22.

Delle Fave, A. (ed.) (2006) *Dimensions of Well-Being: Research and Intervention*. Milan: FrancoAngeli.

Delle Fave, A. and Massimini, F. (2003) 'Optimal Experience in Work and Leisure among Teachers and Physicians: Individual and Bio-cultural Implications', *Leisure Studies*, 22, 4: 323–42.

Diener, E., Lucas, R. E., Schimmack, U. and Helliwell, J. F. (2009) *Well-being for Public Policy*. Oxford: Oxford University Press.

DoH (1999) *Saving Lives: Our Healthier Nation* (CM4386). London: Stationery Office.

Donovan, N., Halpern, D. and Sargeant, R. (2002) *Life Satisfaction: the State of Knowledge and Implications for Government*. London: Strategy Unit, Cabinet Office, Downing Street.

Doran, T. and Whitehead, M. (2004) 'Do Social Policies and Political Context Matter for Health in the United Kingdom?' in V. Navarro (ed.), *The Political and Social Contexts of Health*. New York: Baywood.

Dorling. D. (2010) *Injustice: Why Social Inequality Persists*. Cambridge: Polity Press.

Fredrickson, B. L. (2006) 'The Broaden-and-Build Theory of Positive Emotions', in M. Csikszentmihalyi and I. S. Csikszentmihalyi (eds), *A Life Worth Living: Contributions to Positive Psychology*. Oxford: Oxford University Press.

Freire, T. (ed.) (2010) *Understanding Positive Life: Research and Practice on Positive Psychology*. Lisboa: Escolar Editora.

Halpern, D. (2005) *Social Capital*. Cambridge: Polity Press.

Haworth, J. T. (1997) *Work, Leisure and Well-Being*. London: Routledge.

Haworth, J. T. (2011) 'Life, Work, Leisure, and Enjoyment: The role of Social Institutions', *Leisure Studies Association News Letter*, 88: 72–80.

Haworth, J. T. (In press) Life, Work, and Enjoyment: The role of Social Institutions. In (eds) S. David, I, Boniwell, and A, Conley. The Oxford Handbook of Happiness. Oxford: Oxford University Press.

Haworth, J. T. and Lewis, S. (2005) 'Work, Leisure and Well-Being', *British Journal of Guidance and Counselling*, 33, 1: 67–79.

Haworth, J. T. and Roberts, K. (2010) 'Leisure: The Next 25 Years', Science review for the DTI Foresight project on Mental Capital and Mental Wellbeing. Report submitted July 2007. Published in C. Cooper et al. (eds) *Mental Capital and Mental Wellbeing*. John Wiley & Sons/Blackwell, pp. 697–703.

Haworth, J. T. and Veal, A. J. (eds) (2004) *Work and Leisure*. London: Routledge.

Huppert, F. A., Baylis, N. and Keverne, B. (eds) (2005) *The Science of Well-Being*. Oxford: Oxford University Press.

Huppert, F. A. (2009a) 'Psychological Well-being: Evidence Regarding its Causes and Consequences', *Applied Psychology: Health and Well-being*, 1, 2: 137–64.

Huppert, F. A. (2009b) 'A New Approach to Reducing Disorder and Improving Well-Being', *Perspectives on Psychological Science*, 4, 1: 108–11.

Huppert, F. A. and So T. T. C. (2009) *What Percentage of People in Europe are Flourishing and What Characterises Them*. The Well-being Institute: University of Cambridge.

Iso-Ahola, S. and Mannell, R. C. (2004) 'Leisure and Health', in J. T. Haworth and A. J. Veal (eds), *Work and Leisure*. London: Routledge.

Jahoda, M. (1982) *Employment and Unemployment: a Social Psychological Analysis*. Cambridge: Cambridge University Press.

Jordan, B. (2006) *Social Policy for the Twenty First Century*. Cambridge: Polity Press.

Kagan, C., Lawthom, R., Knowles, K. and Burton, M. (2000) 'Community Activism, Participation and Social Capital on a Peripheral Housing Estate', paper presented to European Community Psychology Conference: Bergen, Norway.

Kahneman, D., Diener, E. and Schwarz, N. (1999) *Well-Being: the Foundations of Hedonic Psychology*. New York: Russell Sage Foundation.

Kay, T. (2001) 'Leisure, Gender and Family: Challenges for Work-Life Integration'. ESRC seminar series 'Well-being: Situational and Individual Determinants', 2001–2002, www.wellbeing-esrc.com, Work, Employment, Leisure and Well-Being.

Kay, T. (2006) 'Where's Dad?' Fatherhood in Leisure Studies, *Leisure Studies*, 25, 2: 133–52.

Kellock, A., Lawthom, R., Sixsmith, J., Duggan, K., Mountian, I., Haworth, J., Kagan, C., Brown, D. P., Griffiths, J. E., Hawkins, J., Worley, C., Purcell, C., Siddiquee, A. (2011) 'Using Technology and the Experience Sampling Method to Understand Real Life', in S. Hesse-Biber (ed.) *Emergent Technologies in Social Research*. Oxford: Oxford University Press, pp. 542–62.

Keyes. C. L. and Haidt. J. (eds) (2002) *Flourishing: Positive Psychology and the Life Well-Lived*. Washington DC: American Psychological Association.

Lakoff, G. and Johnson, M. (1999) *Philosophy in the Flesh: the Embodied Mind and its Challenge to Western Thought*. New York: Basic Books.

Layard, R. (2003) 'Happiness: Has Social Science a Clue?' A series of three lectures which can be accessed at the website cep.lse.ac.uk.

Layard, R. (2005) *Happiness: Lessons from a New Science*. London: Allen Lane.

Link B. G. and Phelan, J. C. (1995) 'Social Conditions as Fundamental Causes of Disease', *Journal of Health and Social Behavior (Extra Issue)*: 80–94.

Linley, P. A. and Joseph, S. (eds) (2004) *Positive Psychology in Practice*. Hoboken, NJ: Wiley.

Marmot Report (2010) (www.ucl.ac.uk/gheg/marmotreview).

Merleau-Ponty, M. (1962) *Phenomenology of Perception*. London: Routledge & Kegan Paul.

Navarro, V. (ed.) (2004) *The Political and Social Contexts of Health*. New York: Baywood.

New Economics Foundation (www.neweconomics.org).

Oswald, A. (2003) 'How Much Do External Factors Affect Well-Being? A Way to Use "Happiness Economics" to Decide', *The Psychologist*, 16: 140–1.

Pawelsky, J. (2006) 'A Philosophical Look at Positive Interventions', paper presented at the Third European Conference on Positive Psychology, Braga, Portugal.

Perri 6 (2002) 'Sense and Solidarities: a Neo-Durkheimian Institutional Theory of Well-Being and its Implications for Public Policy'. ESRC seminar series 'Wellbeing: Situational and Individual Determinants', 2001–2002, www.wellbeing-esrc.com, Research and Policy for Well-Being.

Peterson, C. (2006) *A Primer in Positive Psychology*. Oxford: Oxford University Press.

Prillentensky, I. (2001) Personal, Relational, and Collective Well-being: an integrative approach. ESRC seminar series 'Wellbeing: situational and individual determinants' 2001–2002 www.wellbeing-esrc.com Wellbeing: interaction between person and environment.

Prilleltensky, I. (2008) 'The Role of Power in Wellness, Oppression and Liberation: the Promise of Psychopolitical Validity', *Journal of Community Psychology*, 36, 2: 113–268.

Roberts, K. (1999) *Leisure in Contemporary Society*. Wallingford, UK: CABI Publishing.

Seligman, M. E. P. (2003) *Authentic Happiness*. London: Nicholas Brealey.

Seligman, M. E. P. (2011) *Flourish: A Visionary New Understanding of Happiness and Well-Being*. London: Free Press.

Seligman, M. E. P. and Csikszentmihalyi, M. (2000) 'Positive Psychology: an Introduction', *American Psychologist*, 55, 1: 5–14.

Sheldon, K. M. (2004) *Optimal Human Being: an Integrated Multi-level Perspective*. Mahwah, NJ: Lawrence Erlbaum.

Sixsmith, J. and Boneham, M. (2003) 'Social Capital and the Voluntary Sector: the Case of Volunteering', *Voluntary Action*, 5, 3: 47–60.

Sixsmith, J., Boneham, M. and Goldring J. (2001) 'Accessing the Community: Gaining Insider Perspectives from the Outside', *Qualitative Health Research*, 1 (3: 4): 578–89.

Snyder, C. R. and Lopez, S. J. (eds) (2000) *Handbook of Positive Psychology*. Oxford. Oxford University Press.

Sointu, E. (2005) 'The Rise of an Ideal: Tracing Changing Discourses on Well-Being', *Sociological Review*: 255–74.

Stebbins, R. A. (2004) 'Serious Leisure, Volunteerism and Quality of Life', in J. T. Haworth and A. J. Veal (eds), *Work and Leisure*. London: Routledge.

Taylor, R. (2001) 'The Future of Work-Life Balance'. ESRC Future of Work Programme Seminar Series. Economic and Social Research Council, Polaris House, Swindon, UK.

Taylor, R. (2002) 'Britain's World of Work-Myths and Realities'. ESRC Future of Work Programme Seminar Series. Economic and Social Research Council, Polaris House, Swindon, UK.

Totikidis, V. and Prilleltensky, I. (2006) 'Engaging Community in a Cycle of Praxis: Multicultural Perspectives on Personal, Relational and Collective Wellness', *Community, Work and Family*, 9, 1: 47–67.

Transitions. Final Report. Research Report No. 11. Manchester Metropolitan University: Research Institute for Health and Social Change. www.workliferesearch.org/transitions.

Warr, P. (1987) *Work, Unemployment and Mental Health*. Oxford: Clarendon Press.

Warr, P. (1990) 'The Measurement of Well-Being and Other Aspects of Mental Health', *Journal of Occupational Psychology*, 63: 193–210.

Warr, P. (1999) 'Well-Being and the Workplace', in D. Kahneman, E. Deiner and N. Schwartz (eds), *Well-Being: the Foundations of Hedonic Psychology*. New York: Springer-Verlag.

Wilkinson, R. G. (1996) *Unhealthy Societies: the Afflictions of Inequality*. London: Routledge.

Wilkinson, R. G. (2000) *Mind the Gap: Hierarchies, Health and Human Evolution*. London: Weidenfeld & Nicolson.

Wilkinson, R. and Pickett, K. (2009) *The Spirit Level: Why More Equal Societies Always do Better*. London: Allen Lane.

Part 1

1
Positive Psychology and the Development of Well-Being

Jane Henry

Positive psychology

Positive psychology burst onto the stage in 1999. It focuses on the *positive side of life* studying well-being, positive experiences such as flow, positive emotions such as satisfaction and happiness, positive strengths such as courage and wisdom, positive explanatory styles such as optimism and hope, positive coping such as resilience and post-traumatic growth and positive development such as creativity and positive ageing.

The charge is that since World War Two psychology and indeed most of the rest of social science, education, health and business have *focused on the negative* side of life and neglected research into ways in which normal people can learn to function particularly well in the world. In organizational studies there are lots of papers on stress, burnout and the glass ceiling and few on organizational well-being; health psychology is almost entirely devoted to the study of illness; adult development draws on strategies borrowed from psychotherapeutic techniques designed to help neurotics; and education is currently dominated by a model centred around inputting competencies that individuals are deficient in rather than building on people's natural talents.

New movements rarely take place in isolation. A shift in interest in the positive side of life is seen in other areas: in counselling, for example, solution-focused therapy is popular, and cognitive-behavioural therapists are becoming interested in mindfulness; in education we find a renewed interest in creativity; and business is beginning to see increasing interest in appreciative inquiry (AI) and allied approaches. With US estimates that about a quarter of the population are languishing compared to only a fifth who could be judged as flourishing

(Keyes 2002), rates of depression on the increase, satisfaction at work declining, and the threat of global warming making it urgent that the affluent citizens of the world learn to appreciate life in a less energy-intensive fashion, it is time to accelerate the development of the science of well-being.

Positive psychology asserts that we are not giving enough attention to studying what works well and has vigorously set about making good this deficiency. Of course this movement builds on earlier work on well-being such as Bradburn's (1969) work on affect, Jahoda's (1982) and Warr's (1999) work on well-being at work, Argyle's (2001) studies of the social correlates of happiness, Kahneman et al.'s (1999) work on well-being, Veenhoven's World Database of Happiness studies (2003), Seligman's (1998) work on learned optimism, Csikszentmihalyi's (1990) work on flow and creativity and Vallaint's (1993) long-term study of positive ageing. Positive psychology has drawn together much of this work and one of the founders, Seligman, has given the field a considerable injection by securing substantive funds for work in the area. Humanist psychologists may charge that positive psychology is merely continuing their programme on self-actualization and peak experiences but many key researchers in positive psychology come from a background that owes more to Bandura (1997) than to Maslow (1970).

The positive psychology movement was initiated in the US and is dominated by US researchers, but it has attracted a European following from early on. Many of the Americans are researchers interested in or influenced by work on social cognition. Despite an espoused concern with institutions in the sense of a concern with civic values for example, the majority of positive psychology studies to date that have caught the public imagination have focused at the level of the individual. In contrast, the European positive psychology movement has attracted individuals who value a *multidisciplinary* and *applied* perspective that takes greater cognizance of cultural context. Practitioners in education, counselling, coaching, business, economics and public policy have seen the potential of the field for spin-offs.

Well-being research

Below I give an illustration of some positive psychology research on well-being, positive style and positive experiences.

Considerable work has gone into attempts to measure well-being. For example, work on life satisfaction and the quality of life, global measures of happiness and well-being such as those to be found in successive Gallup polls, facet measures of well-being and studies in specific domains such as work or health, e.g. Warr's work on satisfaction at work or the WHOQOL inventory. Global measures of well-being do not necessarily show much correlation with facet measures. Currently, subjective well-being is often estimated by a measure incorporating life satisfaction and an assessment of positive and negative mood (Deiner 1984). An objection to the simple measures often used in surveys of well-being is that well-being is a multidimensional construct better assessed via a combination of various sub-dimensions. Ryff and Keyes (1995), for example, suggest six: positive relations with others, self-acceptance, personal growth, purpose in life, autonomy, environmental mastery (managing one's life and immediate environment).

Despite their simplicity, global measures of well-being have produced some very interesting results. For example, the fact that although GDP has more than doubled in the past 50 years, in the US and UK a roughly constant proportion of about a third of the population rate themselves as very happy. Over the same period depression rates have risen, with young people apparently experiencing more depression than older adults when they were younger. Within countries, above a certain minimum, currently about £15,000, *life-satisfaction* ratings show very little correlation with income. Relationships, on the other hand, appear much more critical for well-being than income. About two-fifths of married people rate themselves as happy compared to just over a fifth of the never married (Myers 2000). In individualistic countries more cohabiting couples rate themselves as very happy than single people. The distinguishing feature of the happiest 10 per cent of college students in Deiner and Seligman's (2002) US study was also characterized by a rich and fulfilling social life (see Chapter 14 for elaboration).

Interestingly the *weak correlation between income and well-being* has helped catalyse certain economists and policy-makers into advocating that governments pay less attention to materialist advance and more attention to social factors. Layard (2005), a prominent economist, advocates greater investment in cognitive-behavioural techniques to decrease the incidence of depression and increase the happiness of the population. The New Economics Foundation, a UK think-tank, advocates, amongst other things, that UK employees take productivity gains as time off, to move towards a shorter working week, so allowing employees to spend more time with their family (Marks 2004); an activity that

NEF judges is more likely to enhance the individual's and their family's well-being. Bhutan, perhaps because of its Buddhist heritage, already takes account of social well-being in setting policy, banning plastic bags and Coca-Cola on the grounds that there are perfectly fine indigenous alternatives for example.

The comparative studies of well-being also point up longstanding differences in life satisfaction and happiness ratings between different countries. Scandinavia comes out consistently high despite its cold climate and high taxes. One interpretation notes that inequality between people is among the lowest in Scandinavia. The ex-communist countries such as Russia and Romania still come out poorly. The lack of stability in these countries and the fact that people may have less control over their lives are assumed to be contributing factors to their relatively low scores. Veenhoven's (2003) World Database of Happiness provides an excellent source of material on cross-cultural measures of happiness and well-being in this area.

It must be noted that there is also great individual variation in well-being. There are clear correlations with personality, independent of social conditions. Extroverts, for instance, tend to rate themselves as considerably happier than introverts. Indeed extroversion has about a 0.7 correlation with positive affect. There is also considerable consistency in measures over the life course. Even lottery winners and those who experience a bad accident tend to revert back close to their baseline level of happiness, normally within a year (Brickman 1978).

Positive psychologists acknowledge that genetic factors appear to account for about half the variability in life-satisfaction ratings. Nevertheless whatever one's set point for happiness one can still try to move it up somewhat. Some positive psychologists have estimated that life circumstances such as our income, marital status and environment only account for about 10 per cent of the variance in happiness within an individual and go on to claim that there is scope for intentional improvement in the remaining 40 per cent. Intentional activities could range from adopting a positive attitude, taking exercise and being kind to others to pursuing personally meaningful goals (Sheldon and Lyubomirsky 2004).

Positive style

Positive psychologists are interested in characteristics associated with a positive disposition and a positive explanatory style.

Strengths

One line of work looks at positive traits, specifically individual talents or strengths like courage, curiosity, wisdom, kindness and patience. Peterson and Seligman (2004) have produced the VIA (virtues in action) inventory with a view to assessing individual strengths. The six overarching categories they use are wisdom, love, temperance, courage, justice and transcendence. Under wisdom they include curiosity, love of learning, perspective, judgement and creativity; and under love, intimacy, kindness and social intelligence, for example. This focus on natural talents rather than the abnormal symptoms typically categorized in psychiatric and treatment manuals seems a much-needed counter to the dominance of manuals of symptoms and characteristics like the *DSM* (*Diagnostic and Statistical Manual of Mental Health*). Given so much of our behaviour appears to be genetically determined it seems an excellent idea to place more emphasis on developing strengths than trying to develop in areas we will always find difficult.

However, searching for a universal list of strengths is not easy. The Europeans and Indians I have worked with find Peterson's list very American in its individual and active qualities. Some British people have commented on the lack of qualities like patience and forbearance. Several Indians felt it needed more interpersonal virtues like harmonious or supportive. A South African team are currently developing a list of interpersonal virtues (Van Eeden et al. 2006).

There are many other collections of personality traits and values. The dominant personality model at present is the Five-Factor model (Costa and McCrae 1992). Its main dimensions are extroversion, openness to experience, agreeableness, conscientiousness and stability/neuroticism. A positive score on its dimensions can also be seen as strengths, so for example a positive score on openness could include the strengths of warmth, forgiveness and modesty and a positive score on stability/neuroticism could include strengths of kindness, calmness and resilience. However, it is arguable whether it is so easy to label certain strengths as positive characteristics in all circumstances. For example, humour is a great quality but being funny all the time can be irritating. The descriptions of the MBTI (Myers Briggs Type Indicator) types, whose dimensions correlate with Five-Factor measures such as NEO (Neuroticism, Extroversion, Openness), offer a different form of analysis. They present all personality preferences as having both strengths and weaknesses, for example people who are good at completing tasks are often not so flexible and people who are adaptable may incline to be off-task on other occasions.

Although Seligman and Peterson expected working from your strengths to be a or the key factor in improving well-being, those people logging onto Seligman's (2004) website (authentichappiness.org) have rated the more interpersonally oriented *gratitude* exercise as more helpful initially in web-based studies. This exercise entails visiting someone to tell them how grateful you are to them and why. Follow-up work showed that a gratitude exercise involving delivering a letter to someone explaining why you grateful to them had a very large effect in the first month but after six months the two exercises with a larger effect involved making a point of appreciating three things each day and thinking why you valued them and using one of your strengths in a new way each day for a week or more (Seligman et al. 2005).

There is an abundance of evidence linking a happy disposition and positive outlook on life with health. Two long-term studies make the point rather well. A study by Danner et al. (2001) related subjective well-being as identified in an application letter to be a nun at 18 and longevity. At 85, 90 per cent of the nuns whose subjective well-being was rated in the top 25 per cent were alive compared to a third of those who were least happy. At 94 just over a half of those in the top quarter were still alive compared to about a tenth of those in the bottom quarter. All the nuns were unmarried teachers who ate a similar diet, and none smoked or drank. Harker and Keltner's (2001) study involved rating yearbook pictures of females at single sex colleges in the mid-1960s for smiling behaviour. A genuine Duchenne smile in which the corners of the eyes crease, along with a wide smile, was strongly predictive of happiness decades later.

Optimism

It has long been known that a positive explanatory style such as optimism and the capacity to view difficulties or even trauma as an opportunity for growth, generally offers a helpful attitude for life. Optimists and pessimists are known to have different reasoning styles. On the whole optimists view bad things that happen to them as specific and transitory events caused by the circumstances rather than their own failings whereas pessimists are more likely to attribute a negative event as occurring at least in part because of their long-standing failings, i.e an internal, stable and generalizable deficiency in themselves.

Seligman (1998) encourages pessimists to apply the cognitive-behavioural techniques of challenging and disputing negative interpretations of events in an attempt to challenge negative attributions and learn to be more optimistic. Given that so much of personality and cognitive style is genetic, this comes very much more easily to some than others. Carol Craig is currently implementing a programme of education in Scotland designed to encourage Scottish children to adopt a more positive explanatory style both to increase their self-confidence and self-esteem but also as a counter to what she sees as a rather pessimistic culture in Scotland (centreforconfidence.co.uk).

An optimistic explanatory style is assumed to be desirable. And in many circumstances it is: optimism is known to correlate with happiness ratings, for example. However, an optimistic attitude is often maintained through a series of positive illusions about the self and its prospects, documented by Taylor (Taylor and Brown 1994). One of the downsides of these illusions is that optimists are more likely to underestimate risk than pessimists. In addition, some psychologists argue that a pessimistic attitude can be beneficial for certain types of people, in particular the naturally anxious. Rubenstein (1999), for example, outlines the merits of defensive pessimism, explaining how an anxious person can feel better prepared and comforted by rehearsing things that can go wrong. In a study of 14 different happiness inducing techniques Fordyce (1983) also found large differences in what worked for different people. What worked seemed to be at least partially determined by people's weaknesses. So the way to achieve well-being may be quite different for different personality types.

There is also the question of how far one can aid growth purely by developing the positive. Most qualities run on a continuum and what can be stubbornness in one context might be persistence in another. Lazarus (2003) charges that positive psychology is making a mistake if it concentrates solely on the positive, arguing that both positive and negative approaches have their place. Acting as a facilitator attempting to improve the well-being of 50 people for a recent BBC series I found that many people were aware of positive approaches to living, such as counting your blessings. For some less assertive members of the group, however, the rudiments of assertiveness training such as the broken record technique were more useful to them than work on strengths, appreciation and gratitude exercises. (In essence the broken record technique involves repeating your main point, e.g. 'I do not have time to do this extra work', rather than being drawn in to answering other side issues.) It seems that both working to accentuate the positive and to cope better with the negative have their place.

Positive experiences

Another arm of positive psychology research is the study of positive experiences. Below I outline some work on positive emotion, the state of flow and creativity.

Positive emotion

There is evidence that positive and negative affect are two separate variables not a unipolar one. Reducing negative affect and increasing positive affect may be separate enterprises.

One promising line of work has been taken up by Fredrikson (2002). She terms her theory on the positive effect of *positive emotion* the broaden and build theory. Negative emotion is known to narrow the range of attention and associations making it harder to come up with a variety of ideas. The broaden and build theory asserts that positive emotion increases the range of associations in the brain making it easier to come up with more ideas and solve problems, and further that this broadening effect builds positive resources which have a positive effect in the future, for example enhancing resilience. The experience of positive emotion may indeed form the base for an upward development spiral but recent work by Kaufmann (2003) suggests that the relationship between mood and task is more complex as he finds that positive mood is not always beneficial for creative problem solving. David (2006) also reported studies on doctors' diagnostic abilities where a positive mood was helpful for some tasks but not all. The benefits of particular moods seem to vary according to the situation.

Flow

The work on *flow*, a state of engaged absorption, provides a fascinating series of studies (Csikszentmihalyi 1990; Haworth 2004; Delle Fave and Massimini 2004). A helpful feature of this work is that it moves beyond intercorrelations of attitude statements and links to real experiences. The flow state of contented absorption is characterized by seven features including loss of sense of self. It occurs when people are undertaking activities that offer some challenge and where they get feedback on their progress. It can be experienced in diverse activities ranging from looking after children to gardening and dancing (Csikszentmihalyi 1990). It is argued that the state of flow occurs more frequently when people are active and engaged, i.e. running rather than passively watching TV or undertaking housework which lacks challenge. This research suggests that if we want to be happily absorbed in life we would be well advised to get actively involved in things we enjoy. However, watching TV 50 hours a week is common in the US and UK, though falling among the young who spend increasing time on the internet. Admittedly Argyle (2001) found that people did report flow watching soaps, presumably as the characters are experienced as surrogate friends. In recent longitudinal work Csikszentmihalyi has shown that the time spent in flow as a young teenager links positively to the level of self-esteem four years later (Csikszentmihalyi and Rathunde 1997).

There are probably many other states of optimal experience other than flow, notably varieties of contentment and other low arousal states of satisfaction. These types of experiences have been more thoroughly examined in spiritual practice than psychology. They deserve further research.

Positive psychology is a young science and to date the bulk of the work has been addressed at the level of the individual, looking at the subjective experience of well-being, the characteristics and experiences of those living happy and fulfilled lives and ways of developing desirable positive qualities, though the founders are also interested in the development of positive institutions. Clearly more work needs to be done at levels other than that of the individual, notably that of the group, organization and community. Well-being is an area that is of interest to many disciplines and it is impacted by a variety of factors. At the 3rd European Positive Psychology Conference in Portugal earlier in 2006 Csikszentmihalyi made a plea for positive psychology to retain a wide perspective on influences on well-being that take account of situational as well as individual factors. He went on to articulate a case for taking account of the built environment as one such factor.

Creativity

Creativity is an example of a quality that used to be perceived as something deriving from the individual and that is now seen as a more socially rooted activity that emerges naturally from activity within groups over time. Systems theories of creativity now take account of individual and situational factors but this has not always been the case. In the 1950s research centred on the individual qualities that led to certain individuals possessing creativity. This resulted in research oriented to identifying what these qualities were and organization policies entailing testing people for their capacity for creative thinking, often measured by that extremely poor approximation to it – divergent thinking. This approach came naturally in a Western culture that privileged the innovative approach to creativity of starting afresh and doing things differently. In contrast, cultures like Japan have long recognized the merits of an adaptive form of creativity that focuses more on building on what has gone before. These different styles of creativity can be related to different cognitive styles, essentially a preference for openness, looking at the big picture and searching in a wide area versus a preference for completion, searching in a narrower area and doing things better.

One characteristic of creative people is that they spend more time at the front end looking for the important problem that is worth devoting their time to. The theoretical explanation for this is that creativity is a form of *expert recognition*. The policy implication is that creative people are only likely to be creative in areas they know about. Creativity also takes persistence and often involves going against the status quo. People are generally more prepared to do this in areas they care about, hence it is no surprise that people are more likely to be creative in areas that interest them. In organizations creative projects generally involve a group of people with different expertise. An open culture where contributions are recognized and people are encouraged to experiment seems to make it much more likely that participants will be willing to share their ideas with others. Open cultures also aid creativity by allowing people more flexibility to do things their own way (Henry 2001).

Many creative flourishings seem to have happened around a hub of creative people engaged in related enterprise – art in Florence in medieval times, pop music in Liverpool in the 1960s, personal computing in Silicon valley in the late twentieth century and now biotech around Cambridge for example. Hubs like this give people a chance to *network* with each other, keep up to date, be challenged and build on others' ideas. The science of complexity studies the emergence of new patterns and processes in complex adaptive systems, i.e. any system where the agents within it are capable of learning and changing their behaviour, be this system a brain, the stock market or an organization. These studies show that new creative behaviours emerge naturally in all adaptive systems including human ones. This has led some organizations to redirect policies for encouraging creative endeavour to nurturing and supporting ideas that emerge naturally rather than trying to predetermine what these might be or who might be creative. Nowadays people studying creativity look at the community of practice from which it emerges, adopting more of a systems lens that looks at the interaction between the creative individual, the domain they are working in and the norms of the field this occurs within over time (Csikszentmihalyi 1999).

Positive development

In contrast a lot of the positive psychology approaches advocated so far aim at improving the well-being of individuals, for instance, identifying your natural strengths and trying to find work which allows you to exercise them or reframing work to give you a chance to exercise one of your main strengths, e.g. seeing most encounters as an opportunity to be kind to others. Another approach encourages people to be more appreciative and to count their blessings, for example to be thankful for several good things that happen each day before going to bed. One exercise encourages people to be explicitly grateful, for example to make a point of telling someone how grateful you are to them and why.

Many positive psychology strategies stress the importance of finding and acting on *meaning* to obtain a fulfilled and useful life. Fava's well-being therapy, Seligman's work on learned optimism and Snyder's work on developing hope use variants of cognitive-behavioural techniques to encourage people to work towards desired *goals*. This is of course a very Western notion of the route to happiness and well-being. Eastern spiritual practitioners would be much more likely to advocate detachment from emotion and desires and the development of compassion towards others.

One interesting theoretical approach is Ryan and Deci's (2000) self-determination theory. This argues that autonomy, a feeling of competence or mastery and relatedness with others are central human needs and that well-being is more likely when these needs are met and less likely when they are not.

If we look at correlates of well-being it seems clear that interpersonal factors appear to be critically important. More of the socially embedded and supported repeatedly rate themselves as happier than single people. As mentioned earlier people who are married and cohabitating report themselves as more satisfied than those who are single. Those who belong to social groups are also more likely to rate themselves happier than those who do not belong to social groups. The socially supported also fare better on various health measures. People are also more likely to rate themselves happier in the present when they are with friends than alone (Argyle 1999). Indeed it seems that satisfying relationships could be the key factor in maintaining well-being for most people.

Approaches aiding the development of lasting well-being

Curious to find out what people thought had accounted for any long-term improvement in their own well-being, I have conducted a series of studies over the last ten years asking people how they've changed if they feel they have and what they feel helped them improve their well-being over a ten-year period (Henry 2006).

The participants are several hundred mainly European managers, educators and psychologists, with an average age of thirty-something, and with a gender ratio of three males to two females. In this non-random sample the approach considered most helpful so far is *quietening the mind*. Narrowly defined this has been cited by about a fifth of the group. By quietening the mind I mean some attempt to alter the state of consciousness through formal practices such as mindfulness, meditation or contemplation, or more informal intuitive practice; for example going to bed confident that the way forward will come to them in the morning. In a couple of cases people cited fishing. Angling is the most popular sport yet people rarely catch fish. They do, however, regularly sit still for hours, often in quiet locations, so it offers a great opportunity for peace. Though not yet very prominent in the positive psychologist's armoury, mindfulness is beginning to make itself felt as an effective and alternative route to increased well-being in therapeutic circles (Kabat-Zhin 1996). Another favoured approach was self-acceptance. Some people found their sense of well-being increased once they had accepted the way they were and started working with their foibles rather than striving after goals or doing so more effortlessly. About a tenth of my sample cited self-acceptance and/or becoming more oriented to others as the most important route for improving their well-being.

We also know that exercise, diet and time spent outside in the light can impact on well-being. Csikszentmihalyi's work on flow suggests that being actively engaged in activities that absorb our attention helps. Yet these active and embodied routes to well-being, along with more social strategies, seem to get very little attention from caring professionals, most of whom offer talking therapy of one kind or another. In my studies physical and active approaches, including walking, dancing or being out in nature, were seen as effective routes to improving well-being. We know that running raises endorphins that can directly improve mood. There are claims that being out in nature is uplifting in itself, though this may be culturally relative. My Brooklyn friend's young children who were used to a concrete play area, cried when first introduced to grassy open spaces and some visiting Chinese students seemed happier in densely crowded Tottenham Court Road in London than the green fields that surround my university! Weather does not seem to be as critical as one might expect judging by the fact that Californians rate themselves no happier than Midwesterners living in much colder climates.

About a fifth of my sample cited physical activity, getting actively absorbed in the world or garnering social support of one kind or another as the most helpful approach to maintaining their well-being. These are all characteristics known to be associated with those exhibiting well-being anyway.

Another fifth cited strategies more reminiscent of strategies emphasized in therapy, counselling and coaching, for example reflecting, reframing, developing more mastery and a better balance in life. About a tenth cited strategies associated with positive psychology, coaching and self-help such as developing a more positive attitude, and being future- and goal-oriented. Some cited other approaches including the use of humour and drugs.

The striking thing about these results is the frequency with which non-analytical approaches to improving well-being were cited. These studies suggest that intuitive, physically active and social approaches were valued by more people than reflective routes. They challenge not only the dominance of talking therapy as the caring professional's favoured route to self-improvement but the rather individualistic and goal-oriented route to well-being emphasized by many positive psychologists and other self-development professionals.

Conclusion

To date positive psychologists have focused primarily at the level of the individual. They have made a fantastic start in drawing together work on social cognition and allied fields, and in garnering an unprecedented level of funding to support these endeavours. Yet epidemiological studies of well-being suggest it is the socially embedded rich in significant relationships and social support that fare particularly well on measures of well-being.

The European Network for Positive Psychology (enpp.org) comprises a multidisciplinary, culturally and historically aware group with an applied orientation. Hopefully this stance will help positive psychology develop in a manner that takes full account of interpersonal, cultural and environmental influences on the development of well-being alongside individual factors.

References

American Psychologist (2000) Special Edition on positive psychology, 55, 1.

Argyle, M. (1999) 'Causes and Correlates of Happiness', in E. Deiner and N. Schwarz (eds), *Wellbeing: the Foundations of Hedonic Psychology*. New York: Russell Sage.

Argyle, M. (2001) *The Psychology of Happiness*. 2nd edn. London: Routledge.

Bandura, A. (1997) *Self-efficacy*. New York: Freeman.

Bradburn, N. M. (1969) *The Structure of Psychological Well-being*. Chicago: Aldine.

Brickman, P. (1978) 'Lottery Winners and Accident Victims: Is Happiness Relative?' *Journal of Personality and Social Psychology*, 36: 917–27.

Carr, A. (2004) *Positive Psychology: the Science of Happiness and Human Strengths*. Hove: Brunner-Routledge.

Costa, P. T and McCrae, R. (1992) 'Normal Personality Assessment in Clinical Practice: the NEO Personality Inventory', *Psychological Assessment*, 4, 1: 5–13.

Csikszentmihalyi, M. (1990) *Flow: the Psychology of Optimal Experience*. New York: Harper and Row.

Csikszentmihalyi, M. (1999) 'Creativity', in R. Sternberg (ed.), *Handbook of Creativity*. Cambridge: Cambridge University Press.

Csikszentmihalyi, M. and Rathunde, K. R. (1997) *Talented Teenagers: the Roots of Success and Failure*. Cambridge: Cambridge University Press.

Danner, D., Snowden, D. and Friesen, W. (2001) 'Positive Emotions Early in Life and Longevity: Findings from the Nun Study', *Journal of Personality and Social Psychology*, 80: 804–13.

David, S. (2006) 'Emotional Intelligence in Coaching for Well-being', paper presented to the 3rd European Positive Psychology Conference, Braga, Portugal.

Deiner, E. (1984) 'Subjective Well-Being', *Psychological Bulletin*, 235: 542–75.

Deiner, E. and Seligman, M. E. P. (2002) 'Very Happy People', *Psychological Science*, 13, 1: 81–4.

Delle Fave, A. and Massimini, F. (2004) 'Bringing Subjectivity into Focus: Optimal Experiences, Life Themes and Person-Centered Rehabilitation', in P. A. Linley and S. Joseph (eds), *Positive Psychology in Practice*. London: Wiley.

Fordyce, M. W. (1983) 'A Program to Increase Happiness: Further Studies', *Journal of Counseling Psychology*, 30: 483–98.

Fredrikson, B. (2002) 'Positive Emotions', in C. R. Synder and S. J. Lopez (eds), *Handbook of Positive Psychology*. New York: Oxford University Press, 120-34.

Harker, L. and Kaltner, D. (2001) 'Expressions of Positive Emotion in Women's College Year Book Photos and their Relationship to Personality and Life Outcomes across Adulthood', *Journal of Personality and Social Psychology*, 80: 112–24.

Haworth, J. (2004) 'Work, Leisure and Well-Being', in J. T. Haworth and A. J. Veal (eds), *Work and Leisure*. London: Routledge.

Henry, J. (2001) *Creativity and Perception in Management*. London: Sage.

Henry, J. (2006) 'Strategies for Achieving Well-Being', in M. Csikszentmihalyi and I. S. Csikszentmihalyi (eds), *A Life Worth Living: Contributions to Positive Psychology*. Oxford: Oxford University Press.

Jahoda, M. (1982) *Employment and Unemployment: a Social Psychological Analysis.* Cambridge: Cambridge University Press.

Kabat-Zhin, J. (1996) 'Mindfulness Meditation: What It Is and What It Isn't', in Y. Haruki., Y. Ishii and M. Suzuki (eds), *Comparative and Psychological Study in Mediation.* Netherlands: Eburon, 161–70.

Kahneman, E., Diener, E. and Schwartz, N. (eds) (1999) *Well-Being: the Foundations of Hedonic Psychology.* New York: Russell Sage.

Kaufmann, K. (2003) 'Expanding the Mood Creativity Equation', *Creativity Research Journal*, 15, 2 and 3: 131–5.

Keyes, C. (2002) 'The Mental Health Continuum from Languishing to Flourishing in Life', *Journal of Health and Social Behaviour*, 43: 207–22.

Layard, R. (2005) *Happiness: Lessons From a New Science.* New York: Penguin.

Lazarus, R. S. (2003) 'Does the Positive Psychology Movement Have Legs?' *Psychological Inquiry*, 14: 93–109.

Linley, P. A. and Joseph, S. (2004) *Positive Psychology in Practice.* Hoboken, NJ: John Wiley.

Marks, N. (2004) *A Well-Being Manifesto for a Flourishing Society: the Power of Well-Being.* London: NEF.

Maslow, A. (1970) *Towards a Psychology of Being.* Princeton, NJ: Van Nostrand.

Myers, D. G. (2000) 'The Funds, Friends and Faith of Happy People', *American Psychologist*, 55, 1: 56–67.

Peterson, C. and Seligman, M. (2004) *Character Strengths and Virtues: a Handbook and Classification.* New York: Oxford University Press.

Rubenstein, G. (1999) 'The Bright Side Isn't That Bright', paper presented to 5th CEP Conference: Imagination and Transformation, Durham.

Ryan, R. M. and Deci, E. L. (2000) 'Self-determination Theory and the Facilitation of Intrinsic Motivation and Well-Being', *American Psychologist*, 55: 68–78.

Ryff, C. D. and Keyes, C. L. M. (1995) 'The Structure of Psychological Well-Being', *Journal of Personality and Social Psychology*, 69: 719–27.

Seligman, M. (1998) *Learned Optimism: How to Change Your Mind and Your Life.* New York: Pocket Books.

Seligman, M. (2002) *Authentic Happiness.* New York: Free Press.

Seligman, M. (2004) 'Keynote Presentation to the 2nd European Positive Psychology Conference', Verbania, Italy.

Seligman, M. and Csikszentmihalyi, M. (2000) *An Introduction to Positive Psychology.*

Seligman, M., Park, N. and Peterson, C. (2005) 'Positive Psychology Progress: Empirical Validation of Interventions', *American Psychologist*, 60, 5: 411–21.

Sheldon, K. and Lyubomirsky, S. (2004) 'Achieving Sustainable New Happiness: Prospects, Practices and Prescriptions', in P. A. Linley and S. Joseph (eds), *Positive Psychology in Practice.* Hoboken, NJ: John Wiley.

Snyder, C. R. and Lopez, S. J. (eds) (2002) *Handbook of Positive Psychology.* New York: Oxford University Press.

Taylor, S. and Brown, J. D. (1994) 'Positive Illusions and Mental Well-Being Revisited: Separating Fact from Fiction', *Psychological Bulletin*, 116, 1: 21–7.

Vallaint, G. E. (1993) *The Wisdom of the Ego.* Cambridge, MA : Harvard University Press.

Van Eeden, C. et al. (2006) 'Character Strengths in South African Young Adults', paper presented to the 3rd European Positive Psychology Conference, Braga, Portugal.

Veenhoven, R. (2003) 'World Database of Happiness', www.eur.nl/fsw/research/ happiness.

Warr, P. (1999) 'Well-Being and the Workplace', in E. Kahneman, E. Diener and N. Schwartz (eds), *Well-Being: the Foundations of Hedonic Psychology*. New York: Russell Sage.

Websites

www.enpp.org

www.eur.nl/fsw/research/happiness

www.positive psychology.org

2
Individual Development and Community Empowerment: Suggestions from Studies on Optimal Experience

Antonella Delle Fave

In the social and behavioural sciences, the concepts of selection and adaptation have been fruitfully applied to the analysis of human behaviour. While most researchers agree that humans are bio-cultural entities, theoretical approaches differ in their emphasis on the role and relevance of natural selection (Barkow et al. 1992), cultural pressures, or the interaction between the two systems in influencing human behaviour (Durham 1991; Richerson and Boyd 2005). The aim of this chapter is to emphasize the role of individuals as active agents in shaping their cultural environment and in promoting its complexity. From this perspective, attention will be paid to psychological selection, that is the individual processing of bio-cultural information (Csikszentmihalyi and Massimini 1985), and to its potential in fostering personal growth and culture empowerment.

The bio-cultural inheritance system

Humans show some emergent biological features that enhance individual fitness and promote species adaptation. The most remarkable ones are the upright standing position, the hand structure with opposing thumb, the development of the neocortex and the phonatory system. Thanks to these biological features, humans evolved as cultural animals (Baumeister 2005): they started to build artefacts, to perform abstract reasoning, to set long-term goals and make plans, to develop language, to establish social ties outside kinship and proximate groups, to live in large and stable communities characterized by work and social role division, to set norms and rules, and to interpret reality according to symbolic meanings (Dunbar 1998; Jablonka and Lamb 2005).

Culture remarkably enhanced human fitness, and expanded to such an extent that it can be considered as a second inheritance system showing evolutionary features (Durham 1991; Richerson and Boyd 1978). Like biology, culture is transmitted across generations and it undergoes changes in time. However, some basic differences from biology can be detected in its replication and transmission patterns (Mundinger 1980; Richerson and Boyd 1978).

Firstly, genes are carried by individuals, and spread by means of biological reproduction. In contrast, cultural information units can be stored both in the central nervous system of individuals (*intrasomatic culture*, Cloak 1975) and in human artefacts, that represent *extrasomatic* carriers. This double storage is crucial to culture replication, in that cultural units can survive their carriers, while genes cannot. An entire human community may disappear, but its artefacts can resist the vagaries of time and nature. Secondly, genes are solely coded in DNA, while cultural information can be translated into natural languages, non-verbal behaviour, mathematics and music.

The pattern of transmission of the information accounts for a third difference between biology and culture. Genes are passed all at once during biological conception, and ontogenesis requires a fixed amount of time. In contrast, cultural information can be transmitted with variable speed and throughout the individual life span. By virtue of this, culture can spread faster than biology. One individual can transmit information to several people at the same time. Technology and industrialization enormously increased the creation of large amounts of artefacts. The amount of cultural information that we could potentially store in our brain networks largely outgrows the constraints imposed by our average life span and biological needs.

Finally, biology and culture differ as regards the main sources of change. In biology change is due to the random and unintentional event of genetic mutation. Moreover, among all the occurring mutations, only very few and rare ones enhance the fitness of their carrier. Adaptation is a very slow process. As a consequence, rapid environmental disruptions can lead even well-adapted species to quick extinction. In contrast, new cultural information prominently originates in individual minds, as ideas or solutions to problems often arising out of a long elaboration. Humans can intentionally direct and actively search for cultural changes. In this perspective, culture can adapt faster than biology to environmental demands. Moreover, individuals themselves can modify it through their voluntary effort.

Culture: advantages and pitfalls

These described differences between culture and biology highlight a remarkable feature of culture, namely its flexibility, that provided humans with extremely adaptive equipment. The ability to plan, to build artefacts, to formulate abstract theories, to quantify physical and natural phenomena enabled our species to overcome its biological constraints and to reproduce in every ecological niche. The differentiation of cultures according to the environmental demands increased the variety of survival strategies available to humans. Moreover, due to the changes introduced in the ecosystem, culture became the prominent environment for our species. The adaptation process turned into an increasingly cultural issue: in each human community, individuals have to adapt to their cultural environment, which implies the acquisition of a huge amount of information through social interactions, imitation and other forms of learning. This is supported by another uniquely human biological feature: neoteny, which is the retention of juvenile physical characteristics well into adulthood. Neoteny delays physiological and sexual maturity, thus supporting the development of attachment relations during the long period of parental care and education necessary to acquire culturally adaptive behaviours (Brune 2000).

However, besides promoting adaptation, culture can also generate obstacles to human survival. Two kinds of problems are particularly recurrent throughout history. The first one concerns the relationship with the natural environment. Whenever a human community settles down in a geographical area, it introduces changes in the ecosystem. In several circumstances, however, these changes turned out to be non-adaptive for the bio-cultural survival of the community itself: many cultures have become extinct because of their disruptive exploitation of the environmental resources (Diamond 2005). The second problem is a consequence of culture differentiation. The emergence of different languages, habits, rules and values entailed difficulties in intra-specific interaction between individuals as well as between groups. In addition, contact among cultures has often produced conflicts and dominance relationships (Mays et al. 1998) mostly based on the complexity of artefacts, rather than on the complexity and universality of values. The degree of technological development has been prominent – in influencing the chances of a culture to win a war, to spread its values, to colonize other populations. This imposed a specific evolutionary trend to human communities. Throughout history, technological societies have prevailed thanks to the efficiency of their artefacts, be they weapons, computers or industrial machines. This caused the extinction of other cultures all over the world.

Psychological selection and optimal experience

Humans beings, as open and self-organizing living systems, play the twofold role of heirs and transmitters of cultural information, actively contributing to the construction of their own environmental niche (Laland et al. 2000). Again, individuals' prominent role in shaping both the environment and their own developmental pathway is related to species-specific biological features, namely our ability to develop a theory of mind, recognizing the shared nature of mental processes and representations (Tomasello 1999), and the awareness of our internal states. Thanks to this awareness, human beings actively select and differentially replicate and cultivate in time activities, values, behaviours and relationships according to the quality of subjective experience associated with them. In this process of *psychological selection* (Csikszentmihalyi and Massimini 1985) a prominent role is played by optimal experience (Csikszentmihalyi and Csikszentmihalyi 1988). Optimal experience is a peculiarly positive state characterized by the perception of engagement, involvement, focused attention, intrinsic motivation, enjoyment and clear goals. Thanks to its rewarding features, the associated activities are likely to be preferentially cultivated, thus shaping individuals' identity, goals, values and specific skill development (Csikszentmihalyi and Beattie 1979). Psychological selection and optimal experience thus contribute to the developmental trend and the socialization pattern of each individual, the ultimate result depending upon the type of activities individuals associate with this experience, and therefore differentially reproduce in their lives. Since these activities are usually available in the daily contexts people live in, their selective replication and transmission also shed light on the evolutionary trend of the culture individuals belong to (Massimini and Delle Fave 2000).

The cross-cultural investigation of optimal experience

The hypothesized universality and relevance of optimal experience to individual and cultural functioning has to be supported through cross-cultural findings. Moreover, in order to understand the potential of optimal experience in fostering personal growth and culture empower-ment, it is important to investigate the associated activities and their meaning for the person and the culture. It can be assumed that not all opportunities for optimal experience have the same consequences on individual and group development.

To this purpose, findings obtained from a cross-cultural sample will be illustrated. Data were gathered among 1106 participants, 542 women and 564 men, aged 15–86 (average age 34), living in different countries. Non-Western cultures were represented by 456 participants (41.2 per cent of the sample) from India, Indonesia, Iran, Ivory Coast, Morocco, Philippines, Somalia and Thailand. Other participants belonged to non-Western cultures despite their Western nationality: this was true of Navajo living in Arizona and New Mexico and Rom Gypsies settled in Italy. Western cultures were represented by 650 Italian participants (58.8 per cent of the sample). The participants varied widely in their occupational status: the group comprised farmers, researchers, tailors, blue- and white-collar workers, housewives, college students, nurses, teachers and craftsmen.

Data were gathered through the Flow Questionnaire (FQ, Csikszentmihalyi 1975; Massimini et al. 1988), which investigates the occurrence of optimal experiences in participants' lives, its psychological features, and the associated activities. Participants were first asked to read three quotations that described optimal experience. Subsequently, they were invited to report whether they ever had similar experiences, and, if yes, to list the associated activities or situations (defined as optimal activities). Participants were then invited to select from their list the activity associated with the most intense and pervasive optimal experiences, and to describe the associated cognitive, affective and motivational dimensions, through 0–8 point scaled variables. The FQ also comprised other open-ended questions that will not be illustrated here. More details on the instrument are provided in Delle Fave (2004).

Optimal activities

The majority of participants (953, 86.2 per cent of the sample) reported optimal experiences in their lives, and associated them with one or more optimal activities. For sake of clarity, activities were grouped into functional categories widely used in cross-cultural studies on optimal experience (Csikszentmihalyi 1997; Delle Fave and Massimini 2004).

Table 2.1 shows the activity categories associated with the most pervasive optimal experience. Participants predominantly selected

Table 2.1: Percentage distribution of the activity categories associated with the most pervasive optimal experiences

Activity categories	% (N = 953)
Productive activities	40.9
Structured leisure	36.5
Interactions	10.5
Mass media	6.3
Thoughts, introspection	2.8
Religious practices	2.7
Other	0.3
	100.0

Note: N = number of participants (each participant selected one activity)

productive activities (work or study) and structured leisure (sports, arts and crafts, hobbies). Social and family interactions and the use of mass media followed with lower percentages. The remaining categories were quoted by a much lower number of participants. The category 'Other' comprised answers from three participants. One of them referred to sleeping (included in the category 'Personal care'), and the other two referred to shopping and buying clothes (category 'Material goods'). The fact that such an irrelevant number of participants quoted acquiring and possessing artefacts or money as an opportunity for optimal experience supports the evidence, provided by other studies (see, for example, Kasser and Ryan 1996; Myers 2000), that wealth, material goods and extrinsic rewards do not foster *per se* well-being and optimal states.

Although the activities quoted within the categories were strongly related to each participant's education level, cultural context and traditions, they shared some common features across individuals and samples. For example, as concerns work, the tasks associated with optimal experience were suited to provide opportunities for creativity, autonomy and skill development, either embedded in the activity structure itself (e.g. in handicrafts, nursing, teaching, farming, cooking, building mathematical models, tailoring, developing software, repairing electrical equipment) or connected to peculiarly engaging situations (e.g. 'when I have to deal with something new'; 'when the work requires concentration'; 'when there is a problem to solve'; 'in the project phase'). Analogously, structured leisure comprised activities characterized by well-defined rules and requiring specific competencies and skill cultivation, such as playing soccer or basketball, skiing, playing musical instruments, drawing, painting, creative writing, reading, singing and dancing.

Interactions, which accounted for 10.5 per cent of the answers, mostly referred to family and intimate relationships (64.3 per cent of the answers within the category) and to a lesser extent to socialization with friends and significant others.

Out of the 60 participants who provided answers in the mass media category (6.6 per cent of the sample), 34 (56.7 per cent in the category) quoted listening to music, while only 24 (40 per cent in the category) reported watching TV. Despite its widespread and daily use across cultures, watching TV did not emerge as a relevant opportunity for optimal experience, thus confirming previous findings (Delle Fave and Massimini, 2005b).

The features of optimal experience: constancies and variations across activities

Table 2.2 illustrates the main psychological features of optimal experience across the four major optimal activity categories. For the sake of synthesis, only the values of nine key variables are reported, which cover the affective, cognitive and motivational dimensions: focus

Table 2.2: The psychological features of optimal experience in the major selected optimal activity categories: mean values and non-parametric ANOVA comparison across categories

Variables	Productive act. (N = 386)		Struct. leisure (N = 343)		Interactions (N = 98)		Mass media (N = 60)		F	p
	M	SD	M	SD	M	SD	M	SD		
Focus of attention	6.5	1.7	6.3	2.0	6.8	1.7	6.2	2.0	2.0	n.s.
Clear feedback	7.0	1.4	6.7	1.7	7.0	1.4	6.7	1.7	2.4	n.s.
Control of situation	6.9	1.4	6.8	1.7	6.8	1.3	6.7	1.8	0.3	n.s.
Excitement	7.3	1.2	7.7	0.8	7.8	0.6	7.5	1.0	10.1	<.001
Enjoyment	6.9	1.6	7.0	1.4	7.4	1.0	6.6	1.5	4.6	<.01
Relaxation	6.1	2.3	6.7	1.9	6.3	2.4	7.4	1.3	9.5	<.001
Involvement	6.6	1.4	6.8	1.5	7.4	1.1	6.5	1.6	6.9	<.001
Wish doing the act.	6.7	1.8	7.3	1.3	7.5	1.0	7.2	1.8	12.8	<.001
Clear goals	7.3	1.3	6.9	1.7	6.8	1.7	6.5	2.1	5.1	<.01

Note: N = number of participants

of attention, clear feedback concerning one's own performance, control of the situation, excitement, enjoyment, relaxation, involvement, wish to do the activity, and perceived goals.

Optimal experience showed a recurrent structure across activity categories. All the variables scored above 6, thus highlighting the positive features of the experience. A non-parametric ANOVA comparison, however, detected significant differences across categories in the values of the affective variables (excitement, enjoyment and relaxation) and of the motivational ones (involvement, wish to do the activity and clear goals). More specifically, productive activities were associated with the lowest values of excitement, relaxation and wish to do the activity, and with the highest values of perceived goals. Conversely, interactions were associated with the highest values of excitement, enjoyment, involvement and wish to do the activity. Participants reported the lowest values of enjoyment, involvement and perceived goals in association with the use of mass media. In contrast, the cognitive variables' focus of attention, feedback and control of the situation did not show significant differences across categories.

Non-parametric pairwise comparisons of the variables' values between categories were also conducted through Wilcoxon procedure, which analyses the rank score distribution for variables rated on ordinal scales, based on a simple linear rank statistics. As Table 2.3 shows, the highest number of significant differences in the variable values were detected between productive activities and each of the other categories. Again, most differences concerned the values of affective and motivational variables, while the cognitive components of the experience showed stable values across categories, except for feedback which scored significantly higher in work than in structured leisure.

In particular, in structured leisure participants reported significantly higher excitement, relaxation, involvement and wish to do the activity than in productive activities, but significantly lower perceived goals. Similarly, interactions were associated with significantly higher excitement, enjoyment, involvement and wish to do the activity than productive activities, but with significantly lower perceived goals. Finally, participants associated mass media with significantly higher relaxation and wish to do the activity than productive tasks, but also with significantly lower values of enjoyment, involvement and perceived goals.

Wilcoxon pairwise comparisons between the other categories detected only scattered differences in the features of optimal experience. Since they did not add any relevant information for the purpose of this study, they are not reported here.

Table 2.3: The psychological features of optimal experience in the major selected optimal activity categories: Wilcoxon comparisons between categories

Variables	Productive activities / Structured leisure		Productive activities / Interactions		Productive activities / Mass media	
	Z	p	Z	p	Z	p
Focus of attention	−0.7	n.s.	1.6	n.s.	−.86	n.s.
Clear feedback	−2.4	<.05	0.6	n.s.	−.89	n.s.
Control of situation	.01	n.s.	−1.1	n.s.	−.18	n.s.
Excitement	4.6	<.001	3.6	<.001	1.2	n.s.
Enjoyment	0.7	n.s.	2.9	<.01	−2.2	<.05
Relaxation	4.0	<.001	1.1	n.s.	4.3	<.001
Involvement	2.3	<.05	4.7	<.001	−.32	n.s.
Wish to do the activity	5.0	<.001	3.9	<.001	2.6	<.01
Clear goals	−3.3	<.01	−2.9	<.01	−2.6	<.01

Optimal experience and positive development

The findings showed that optimal experience is a state of high complexity, characterized by the recruitment of affective, motivational and cognitive components towards their positive pole. This pattern fosters optimal functioning, skill enhancement and a fruitful inform-ation exchange with the environment. The findings also showed that optimal experience comprises a stable cognitive core across activity categories. On the opposite, wider variations across categories were detected in the values of affective and motivational variables. These findings support evidence obtained from other samples by means of experience sampling procedures (Bassi and Delle Fave 2004; Delle Fave and Massimini 2005a).

More specifically, as concerns the motivational components of the experience, the findings highlighted wide cross-domain variations in the values of perceived goals and wish to do the activity. In particular, while interactions and leisure were associated with high values of both variables, in productive activities the perception of goals was prominent, but the wish to do the activity scored significantly lower than in the other domains. The opposite was true of watching TV, characterized by a remarkable short-term desirability, but by the lowest perception of goals.

These results can be interpreted from both the individual and cultural perspectives. The relevance of setting and pursuing goals for individual and group functioning is undeniable. The ability to plan future actions and to anticipate long-term events characterizes humans as cultural animals, equipped with language, abstract reasoning and socially acquired meanings (Baumeister 2005; Oettingen and Gollwitzer 2001). Goals support development through the implementation of skills and competencies (Gollwitzer 1999), and shape individual identity and meaning-making (Ferrari and Mahalingam 1998; Salmela-Aro and Nurmi 1997). In addition, goals facilitate the integration of the individual into the cultural context, in that they are usually selected from a set of shared values and meanings (Oishi 2000; Stromberg and Boehnke 2001). Our findings showed that the short-term desirability of optimal activities is not necessarily related to their long-term relevance. Participants most frequently associated optimal experiences with the work and study domain, but they also distinguished between the immediate motivation to act and the meaning of the task for future achievements. This has to be taken into account in educational and organizational interventions. The focus on extrinsic motives and rewards has proved widely ineffective in promoting personal well-being and productivity in work and study domains (Hui and Luk 1997; Ranson and Martin 1996). On the contrary, findings suggest that in order to facilitate positive performances in the long run, learning and work activities should be more effectively linked both to short-term intrinsic motivation and to personal long-term meanings (Delle Fave and Massimini 2003a; Ryan et al. 1994; van Mierlo et al. 2001).

Finally, the findings shed light on the relevance of optimal activities in supporting development through creative engagement in self-selected tasks, independent from performance outcomes or social expectations. Despite the previously outlined differences across activities, optimal experience is overall characterized by high values of concentration and involvement in tasks that people wish to do and enjoy. Findings in both individualistic and collectivistic cultures highlighted the relationship between well-being and the promotion of creativity and autonomy (Chirkov and Ryan 2001; Hayamizu 1997; Ryan and Deci 2001).

Opportunities for optimal experience: the interplay between individual and culture

Previous studies showed that optimal experience is preferentially associated with highly structured tasks (Csikszentmihalyi et al. 1993; Delle

Fave and Bassi 2000). This study confirmed the cross-cultural prominent role of engaging, intrinsically organized and complex activities in fostering it, through the development of competencies both in the domains of work and leisure.

As concerns productive activities, previous investigations showed – on the other side – the negative effects of automation on the quality of experience (Delle Fave and Massimini 1991). The increasing standardization of work tasks and of their products through technology implementation entails restrictions on individual initiative, as well as a decrease in the variation of tasks and outcomes themselves. It is thus not surprising that none of the blue-collar and white-collar participants in the present study (around 200 people) associated assembly line work or routine office tasks with the most pervasive optimal experiences.

Similarly, in the domain of leisure, low-engaging activities, entailing energy and artefact consumption, presently represent worldwide easily available entertainment opportunities, often prevailing on more complex activities that could foster creativity and a more effective use of environmental resources (Oskamp 2000). As shown in the previous sections and in other studies, relaxed leisure tasks such as watching TV are only rarely associated with optimal experience (Kubey and Csikszentmihalyi 1990). In addition, our findings clearly highlighted some peculiarities in the experience reported during these activities. In comparison with other domains, participants perceived significantly lower values of enjoyment, involvement and perceived goals. From a different perspective, these results outline a specific positive role of relaxed leisure activities in daily life: they promote relaxation and relief from pressure, thus contributing to overall well-being. In particular, as concerns watching TV, various studies have shown that it prevents people from falling into unpleasant states of apathy and disengagement (Delle Fave and Bassi 2000). Problems arise, however, when relaxed leisure activities become the prominent or only opportunities for enjoyment and recreation, in that they easily lead to passiveness rather than fostering mobilization of personal resources (Iso-Ahola 1997).

Also the lack of perceived opportunities for optimal experiences in the daily context can provide information on the individual potential for development. The small sub-sample of participants in this study who did not report optimal experiences in their lives mostly included people facing hardship and maladjustment, due to both environmental and personal factors. The negative implications of disengagement and lack of perceived meaningful goals have been explored at the educational and developmental levels (Larson 2000; Delle Fave and Massimini 2005a), and in clinical studies conducted through experience sampling proced-ures among people with affective disorders (Delle Fave and Massimini 1992). Findings obtained through FQ from adolescents and adults living under difficult circumstances also showed the risks entailed in the deprivation of optimal experience. Street boys and homeless people, for example, reported only few opportunities for optimal experiences in ordinary daily life. This exposed them to the thrill and excitement provided by illegal activities (Delle Fave and Massimini 2005b). Girls entrusted to institutions for the custody of minors because of family problems reported optimal experience with lower frequency than girls raised in intact families (Delle Fave and Massimini 2000). Moreover, they prominently associated it with unstructured and low-engaging leisure activities, such as watching TV and free peer interactions.

Finally, some activities provide apparently positive experiences, but they do not support development in the long run. Drug intake, for example, is often quoted as a source of optimal experience by addicts. However, it is associated with high values of anxiety, as well as with low levels of control of the situation and perceived goals (Delle Fave and Massimini 2003b). Therefore, drug taking provides only a 'mimetic' or pseudo-optimal experience. Although desirable and enjoyable in the short term, it entails negative long-term consequences at various levels. Beside health and marginalization problems, with time addicts face the loss of the positive experiences previously associated with drug intake, a deterioration in lifestyle, a decrease in motivation to make plans and to develop competencies (Olievenstein 2000), with consequent reduction of behavioural complexity.

Conclusion

These findings suggest that regardless of their age, gender, culture and social conditions, people do clearly recognize the presence or absence of complexity and long-term meanings in their daily activities. This human ability should be taken into account more seriously in educa-tion, work and leisure policies. More specifically, the extent to which a society provides its members with long-term meaningful, intrinsic-ally rewarding and engaging activities can be indicative of a successful cultural transmission, in that it facilitates the preferential replication of such activities through psychological selection.

Individuals – in their turn – are active carriers of cultural information and agents of change, according to their personality characteristics and attitudes. They produce, elaborate and select cultural information units thanks to their ability to preferentially pursue complexity and optimal experiences, to make plans, set goals, and intentionally correct previous mistakes. This has enormous implications for the potential role of individuals in the promotion of positive changes in every human domain.

Like biological evolution, cultural evolution is a process of change in neutral terms: change, *per se*, does not necessarily mean improvement, but fitness enhancement. Like genes, cultural information is submitted to the principle of survival of the fittest, regardless of its consequences in terms of ethics or universally shared values. In order to promote individual well-being and community empowerment, the creation of new cultural information has to enhance complexity of the social system, improving the co-ordination and integration of its components, and its exchanges with the environment. Cultural fitness can be promoted by enhancing complexity, but not necessarily: it can also derive from a reduction in complexity. In contrast, empowerment can only be achieved through a progressive harmonization of the culture's needs and values with the individual and environmental ones. The devastating effects of artefacts on the ecosystem, the increasing impact of virtual needs on real life, the primacy of cultural manipulation on biology with no concern about consequences are examples of the blind fitness-centred evolution of culture. The dominant utilitarian principles in economics contributed to sharpen inequalities, instead of promoting welfare (Sen 1992). The growing dependence upon technology and artefacts made human life easier, but our species is becoming less and less able to survive without them. Earth resources are not inexhaustible, but environment exploitation seems actually inexorable.

Information on people's perception of opportunities for optimal experiences in their daily domains is essential to designing intervention programmes grounded in individual potential for empowerment, and not only focused on cultural fitness. This can facilitate an effective match between individual needs and values, on the one side, and society development and integration, on the other side.

From a broader perspective, in order to promote empowerment, the introduction of any cultural information – be it represented by an artefact, a law, a value, a philosophical outlook, an educational or organizational strategy – has to take into account its consequences for the well-being of individuals, of the ecosystem, and of other societies at the same time. This seems a daunting task, but responsible citizens and communities worldwide should face this challenge. Taking a psychological stance, the quality of subjective experience, the broadness of meanings embedded in perceived goals, and the complexity of competencies and skills at the individual level could be used as indicators of the degree of health and positive development of a culture. This runs against the present trend towards homogenization and social levelling of behaviours and aspirations, but – as human history has repeatedly showed – the authentically adaptive function of culture for the sake of mankind's survival should be the transmission of an intentionally shared set of meanings promoting co-operation, growth and balanced exchange between systems – be they natural, cultural or both.

References

Barkow, J. H., Cosmides, L. and Tooby, J. (1992) *The Adapted Mind: Evolutionary Psychology and the Generation of Culture*. New York: Oxford University Press.

Bassi, M. and Delle Fave, A. (2004) 'Adolescence and the Changing Context of Optimal Experience in Time: Italy 1986–2000', *Journal of Happiness Studies*, 5: 155–79.

Baumeister, R. F. (2005) *The Cultural Animal*. New York: Oxford University Press.

Brune, M. (2000) 'Neoteny, Psychiatric Disorders and the Social Brain: Hypotheses on Heterochrony and the Modularity of the Mind', *Anthropology & Medicine*, 7: 301–18.

Chirkov, V. I. and Ryan, R. M. (2001) 'Control versus Autonomy Support in Russia and the US: Effects on Well-Being and Academic Motivation', *Journal of Cross-Cultural Psychology*, 32: 618–35.

Cloak, F. T. (1975) 'Is a Cultural Ethology Possible?' *Human Ecology*, 3: 161–82.

Csikszentmihalyi, M. (1975) *Beyond Boredom and Anxiety*. San Francisco: Jossey Bass.

Csikszentmihalyi, M. (1997) 'Activity, Experience and Personal Growth', in J. Curtis and S. Russell (eds), *Physical Activity in Human Experience: Interdisciplinary Perspectives*. Champaign, IL: Human Kinetics.

Csikszentmihalyi, M. and Beattie, O. (1979) 'Life Themes: a Theoretical and Empirical Exploration of their Origins and Effects', *Journal of Humanistic Psychology*, 19: 677–93.

Csikszentmihalyi, M. and Csikszentmihalyi, I. (eds) (1988) *Optimal Experience*. New York: Cambridge University Press.

Csikszentmihalyi, M. and Massimini, F. (1985) 'On the Psychological Selection of Bio-cultural Information', *New Ideas in Psychology*, 3: 115–38.

Csikszentmihalyi, M., Rathunde, K. and Whalen, S. (1993) *Talented Teenagers*. New York: Cambridge University Press.

Delle Fave, A. (2004) 'A Feeling of Wellbeing in Learning and Teaching', in M. Tokoro and L. Steels (eds), *A Learning Zone of One's Own*. Amsterdam: IOS Press, 97–110.

Delle Fave, A. and Bassi, M. (2000) 'The Quality of Experience in Adolescents' Daily Lives: Developmental Perspectives', *Genetic, Social and General Psychology Monographs*, 126: 347–67.

Delle Fave, A. and Massimini, F. (1991) 'Modernization and the Quality of Daily Experience in a Southern Italy Village', in N. Bleichrodt and P. J. D. Drenth (eds), *Contemporary Issues in Cross-Cultural Psychology*. Amsterdam: Swets & Zeitlinger B. V.

Delle Fave, A. and Massimini, F. (1992) 'Experience Sampling Method and the Measurement of Clinical Change: a Case of Anxiety Disorder', in M. W. de Vries (ed.), *The Experience of Psychopathology*. New York: Cambridge University Press.

Delle Fave, A. and Massimini, F. (2000) 'Living at Home or in Institution: Adolescents' Optimal Experience and Life Theme', *Paideia*, 19: 55–66.

Delle Fave, A. and Massimini, F. (2003a) 'Optimal Experience in Work and Leisure among Teachers and Physicians: Individual and Bio-cultural Implications', *Leisure Studies*, 22: 323–42.

Delle Fave, A. and Massimini, F. (2003b) 'Drug Addiction: the Paradox of Mimetic Optimal Experience', in J. Henry (ed.), *European Positive Psychology Proceedings*. Leicester: British Psychological Society.

Delle Fave, A. and Massimini, F. (2004) 'The Cross-cultural Investigation of Optimal Experience', *Ricerche di Psicologia*, 27: 79–102.

Delle Fave, A. and Massimini, F. (2005a) 'The Investigation of Optimal Experience and Apathy: Developmental and Psychosocial Implications', *European Psychologist*, 10: 264–74.

Delle Fave, A. and Massimini, F. (2005b) 'The Relevance of Subjective Wellbeing to Social Policies: Optimal Experience and Tailored Intervention', in F. Huppert, B. Keverne and N. Baylis (eds), *The Science of Wellbeing*. Oxford: Oxford University Press.

Diamond, J. (2005) *Collapse: How Societies Choose to Fail or Succeed*. New York: Viking Books.

Dunbar, R. J. M. (1998) 'The Social Brain Hypothesis', *Evolutionary Anthropology*, 6: 178–90.

Durham, W. H. (1991) *Coevolution: Genes, Culture and Human Diversity*. Stanford, CA: Stanford University Press.

Ferrari, M. and Mahalingam, R. (1998) 'Personal Cognitive Development and its Implications for Teaching and Learning', *Educational Psychologist*, 33: 35–44.

Gollwitzer, P. M. (1999) 'Implementation Intentions: Strong Effects of Simple Plans', *American Psychologist*, 54: 493–503.

Hayamizu, T. (1997) 'Between Intrinsic and Extrinsic Motivation: Examination of Reasons for Academic Study Based on the Theory of Internalization', *Japanese Psychological Research*, 39: 98–108.

Hui, H. and Luk, C. L. (1997) 'Industrial/Organizational Psychology', in J. W. Berry. M. H. Segall and C. Kagitçibasi (eds), *Handbook of Cross-cultural Psychology*, vol. 3. Boston: Allyn and Bacon.

Iso-Ahola, S. E. (1997) 'A Psychological Analysis of Leisure and Health', in J. T. Haworth (ed.) *Work, Leisure and Well-Being*. London: Routledge.

Jablonka, E. and Lamb, M. J. (2005) *Evolution in Four Dimensions. Genetic, Epigenetic, Behavioural and Symbolic Variation in the History of Life*. Cambridge, MA: MIT Press.

Kasser, T. and Ryan, R. (1996) 'Further Examining the American Dream: Differential Correlates of Intrinsic and Extrinsic Goals', *Personality and Social Psychology Bulletin*, 22: 280–7.

Kubey, R. W. and Csikszentmihalyi, M. (1990) *Television and the Quality of Life*. New Jersey: Lawrence Erlbaum Associates.

Laland, K. N., Odling-Smee, J. and Feldman, M. W. (2000) 'Niche Construction, Biological Evolution, and Cultural Change', *Behavioral and Brain Sciences*, 23: 131–46.

Larson, R. W. (2000) 'Toward a Psychology of Positive Youth Development', *American Psychologist*, 55: 170–83.

Massimini, F., Csikszentmihalyi, M. and Delle Fave, A. (1988) 'Flow and Biocultural Evolution', in M. Csikszentmihalyi and I. Csikszentmihalyi (eds), *Optimal Experience: Psychological Studies of Flow in Consciousness*. New York: Cambridge University Press.

Massimini, F. and Delle Fave, A. (2000) 'Individual Development in a Bio-cultural Perspective', *American Psychologist*, 55: 24–33.

Mays, V. M., Bullock, M., Rosenzweig, M. R. and Wessells, M. (1998) 'Ethnic Conflict: Global Challenges and Psychological Perspectives', *American Psychologist*, 53: 737–42.

Mundinger, P. C. (1980) 'Animal Culture and a General Theory of Cultural Evolution', *Ethology and Sociobiology*, 1: 183–223.

Myers, D. G. (2000) 'The Funds, Friends and Faith of Happy People', *American Psychologist*, 55: 56–67.

Oettingen, G. and Gollwitzer, P. M. (2001) 'Goal Setting and Goal Striving', in A. Tesser and N. Schwartz (eds), *Blackwell Handbook of Social Psychology: Intraindividual Processes*. Oxford: Blackwell.

Oishi, S. (2000) 'Goals as Cornerstones of Subjective Well-Being: Linking Individuals and Cultures', in E. Diener and E. M. Suh (eds), *Culture and Subjective Well-Being*. Cambridge, MA: MIT Press.

Olievenstein, C. (2000) *La drogue, 30 ans après*. Paris: Editions Odile Jacob.

Oskamp, S. (2000) 'A Sustainable Future for Humanity?' *American Psychologist*, 55: 496–508.

Ranson, S. and Martin, J. (1996) 'Towards a Theory of Learning', *British Journal of Educational Studies*, 44: 9–26.

Richerson, P. J. and Boyd, R. (1978) 'A Dual Inheritance Model of Human Evolutionary Process: Basic Postulates and a Simple Model I', *Journal of Social and Biological Structures*, 1: 127–54.

Richerson, P. J. and Boyd, R. (2005) *Not by Genes Alone: How Culture Transformed Human Evolution*. Chicago: University of Chicago Press.

Ryan, R. M. and Deci, E. L. (2001) 'On Happiness and Human Potentials: a Review of Research on Hedonic and Eudaimonic Well-Being', *Annual Review of Psychology*, 52: 141–66.

Ryan, R., Stiller, J. and Lynch, J. (1994) 'Representations of Relationships to Teachers, Parents, and Friends as Predictors of Academic Motivation and Self-esteem', *Journal of Early Adolescence*, 14: 226–49.

Salmela-Aro, K. and Nurmi, J. E. (1997) 'Goal Contents, Well-Being, and Life Context during Transition to University: a Longitudinal Study', *International Journal of Behavioral Development*, 20: 471–91.

Sen, A. (1992) *Inequality Reexamined*. Oxford: Oxford University Press.

Stromberg, C. and Boehnke, K. (2001) 'Person/Society Value Congruence and Well-Being: the Role of Acculturation Strategies', in P. Schmuck and K. M. Sheldon (eds), *Life Goals and Well-Being*. Göttingen: Hogrefe & Huber.

Tomasello, M. (1999) *The Cultural Origins of Human Cognition*. Cambridge, MA: Harvard University Press.

van Mierlo, H., Rutte, C. R., Seinen, S. and Kompier, M. (2001) 'Autonomous Teamwork and Psychological Well-Being', *European Journal of Work and Organizational Psychology*, 10: 291–301.

3
Webs of Well-Being: the Interdependence of Personal, Relational, Organizational and Communal Well-Being

Isaac Prilleltensky and Ora Prilleltensky

Contrary to prevalent notions that well-being is a personal issue, in this chapter we argue that it is also relational, organizational and communal. If we were to define well-being strictly in terms of subjective reports, as most of the literature on the topic does, we would be hard pressed to denote organizational or communal well-being. After all, the walls of organizations or the streets of communities do not feel or report ill- or well-being. However, if we define well-being as inclusive of social indicators such as levels of unemployment, organizational climate and social capital, the story changes dramatically. Our assumption is that levels of relational, organizational and communal well-being, as measured by different methods and indicators, have a potent influence on the well-being of a particular individual.

By focusing exclusively on subjective measures of well-being, we fail to question the impact of contextual dynamics on people who report high levels of well-being despite living in very deprived community conditions. It is entirely possible that poor people experience and accurately report high levels of well-being despite poor living conditions, but it is also possible that some of them do not want to portray themselves as the object of pity. There are many reasons why self-reports are problematic ways of assessing well-being. The sources of bias are many, and social desirability is very strong (Eckersley 2000, 2001, 2005).

Subjective well-being by itself is insufficient to cover the entire experience of well-being. Indeed, at times it seems difficult to reconcile self-reports of subjective well-being with more objective perspectives that take into account other domains of well-being. As Eckersley has noted, 'there is a range of evidence that suggests a positive bias in the results of happiness and life satisfaction surveys' (2001: 63). In a careful review of measures used in assessing levels of happiness and life satisfaction, Eckersley (2000) found great inconsistencies between people's report of happiness and a number of objective measures of well-being. He found that levels of happiness reported by people, usually quite high across a number of countries and contexts, are incommensurate with rather pronounced levels of stress, mental illness, sleeping problems, depression, low self-esteem, lack of energy, worries about weight, lack of satisfaction with their economic situation, and other measures. The inconsistency between elevated reports of subjective happiness and depressed measures of physical, psychological and collective well-ness was found in studies across different countries and contexts. In summary, Eckersley writes, 'there are several aspects of measures of subjective well-being (SWB) or happiness that present a problem... These are the relative stability of SWB despite dramatic social, cultural and economic changes in recent decades; the complex, non-linear rela-tionship between objective conditions and subjective states; and the positive biases in measures of SWB' (2000: 274).

By using primarily self-reports there is a risk of over-generalizing subjective well-being and undermining objective factors in well-being, a risk reinforced by some positive psychologists who claim that happi-ness is determined largely by genetics (50 per cent) and volitional factors (40 per cent) and only moderately by circumstances (10 per cent) (Seligman 2002; Sheldon et al. 2003). Although positive psychologists claim that circumstantial factors account for only about 10 per cent of happiness and volitional factors for about 40 per cent, we should keep in mind that the psychological and behavioural variables said to account for the 40 per cent cannot be easily disentangled from the circumstances of people's lives (McGue and Bouchard 1998; Turkheimer 1998); a point acknowledged by Sheldon et al. (2003). In our view, some positive psychologists risk engaging in what Shinn and Toohey have recently called the 'context minimization error', according to which there is a 'tendency to ignore the impact of enduring neighborhood and community contexts on human behavior. The error has adverse consequences for understanding psychological processes and efforts at social change' (2003: 428). Shinn and Toohey argue that

Psychologists should pay more attention to the community contexts of human behavior. Conditions in neighborhoods and community settings are associated with residents' mental and physical health, opportunities, satisfactions, and commitments. They are associated with children's academic achievement and developmental outcomes, from behavior problems to teenage childbearing. Contexts also moderate other individual or family processes, suggesting that many psychological theories may not hold across the range of environments in which ordinary Americans live their lives. For example, optimal types of parenting may depend on levels of neighborhood risk. Further... contextual effects may masquerade as effects of individual characteristics, leading to flawed inferences. (2003: 428)

Subjective well-being is indeed only one way, among many, of studying and promoting well-being. The evidence is clear that although demographic factors such as gender and socio-economic status account only for a portion of the variance in subjective well-being (Seligman 2002), in some societies these indicators are associated with higher levels of discrimination, oppression, morbidity and mortality (Marmot 2004; Nussbaum 1999; Wilkinson 2005). Therefore, we have to face the fact that while some people may report average levels of subjective well-being, they are also enduring a higher burden of disease, exclusion, marginalization and death (Hofrichter 2003; Navarro 2000, 2004).

In previous writings (Prilleltensky and Nelson 2002; Prilleltensky and Prilleltensky 2003), we emphasized the role of relationships and collective dynamics on personal well-being, as measured by subjective reports or objective indicators, such as unemployment and disease levels. In line with our recent thinking, in this chapter we expand the web of wellness to include the role of organizational determinants (Prilleltensky and Prilleltensky, in press). Our conceptualization of well-being consists of sites, signs, sources, strategies and synergy. This 5Ss model captures the interdependence of personal, relational, organizational and communal well-being. The aim of this chapter is to introduce the model and draw implications for action.

The five Ss of well-being

We can talk about the well-being of a person, a relationship, an organization or a community. These are different *sites* where well-being takes place. We can tell if each one of these sites or places is experiencing well-being by certain *signs*. A sign of personal well-being is a sense of control over your life, something that many people have in short supply (Marmot 2004). Many decisions affecting workers' lives are made by their bosses, without a lot of input from workers themselves. Physical health is another sign of personal well-being. We can all relate to that.

Love and affection are signs of a strong relationship. Emotional support is a manifestation of caring bonds among peers, colleagues, friends or lovers (Gottman 1999; Ornish 1997). Worker participation in decision-making is a sign of organizational well-being. Good communication among workers and colleagues is another. Clear roles and productivity are also important signs of organizational well-being (Warr 1999). A clean environment, freedom from discrimination, safe neighbourhoods, good schools and employment opportunities are signs of community well-being. These are communal goods that benefit everyone (Nelson and Prilleltensky 2005).

The next S stands for *sources*. Personal, relational, organizational and community well-being derive from a variety of sources. Experiences of mastery and success contribute to self-esteem and personal well-being (Thomas and Chess 1977), while nurturance and early positive experiences of attachment enhance relational well-being (Hazan and Shaver 1987, 2004; Mikulincer 2004). Participatory structures, clear roles and efficient practices bring about organizational wellness (Bolman and Deal 2003). Community well-being, in turn, derives from multiple sources such as a sense of cohesion, belonging, equality, universal access to healthcare and democratic traditions (Nelson and Prilleltensky 2005).

The fourth S is for *strategies*. To promote well-being in each one of the sites of interest – persons, relationships, organizations and communities – we need a plan of action. *Synergy*, the fifth S, comes about when we combine an understanding of sources and strategies. In accord with the concept of webs, the best results for any one site of wellness come about when we work on all fronts at the same time. Personal solutions often include organizational solutions. Organizational solutions, in turn, are supported by collective norms of respect for the well-being of workers, and by communal expectations of ethical practice. When collective norms weaken, corporations and public institutions cease to be responsive to community needs. Personal, relational, organizational and community solutions are closely linked. We create synergy among various solutions when we address a problem on multiple fronts at the same time.

If you work in the helping professions, you know the experience of working with clients on a strategy, only to see it diminished by overwhelming social forces. How far can you go in helping a teenager feel safer when he goes back to a crime-infested neighbourhood? How effectively can we curb violence against women when the media and the culture are full of it? Collective problems require collective solutions.

Although there are things we can do to help people individually, such as fitness plans, assertiveness training or communication skills, many of these problems are organizational and communal, and as a result they demand organizational and communal solutions. This chapter is about ways to tackle personal, relational, organizational and communal issues at the same time. We have tried doing one at a time, and it hasn't worked very well (Prilleltensky and Nelson 2002). It surely hasn't worked for many of the problems that health and human service workers face; problems such as child abuse, addictions, poverty, diabetes, crime, teenage pregnancy, gang violence, poor parenting, educational under-achievement, obesity and unemployment (Nelson and Prilleltensky 2005). The time has come to address problems comprehensively and synergistically. Research has shown that the mere act of working with others on collective problems can improve self-esteem, self-efficacy, social support and empowerment. It is not only the outcome that matters, but the process itself (Nelson et al. 2001).

To promote well-being we need an understanding of its main constituents. To recap, well-being consists of (a) sites, (b) signs, (c) sources, (d) strategies and (e) synergy. There are four primary sites of well-being (personal, relational, organizational and collective), each of which has specific signs or manifestations, sources or determinants, and strategies. Once we understand what well-being is all about, we can identify the most promising approaches to its maximization.

Various traditions within the health and social sciences have concentrated on either personal or collective correlates as manifestations of well-being. Whereas psychology has focused on subjective reports of happiness, well-being and psychological wellness (Seligman 2002), sociology and public health have focused on collective and objective measures such as longevity and infant mortality (Marmot 2004; Marmot and Wilkinson 1999; Wilkinson 2005). A group of medical sociologists and investigators has also concentrated on the importance of relationships, an important part of personal and organizational well-being (Berkman 1995). Our claim is that well-being is not one or the other, but rather the combination of personal, relational, organizational and collective sites, signs, sources and strategies of well-being (Nelson and Prilleltensky 2005). In other words, well-being is not either personal, relational, organizational or collective, but rather the integration of them all. For any one of these spheres – personal, relational, organizational or collective – to experience well-being, the other three need to be in equally good shape.

In our view, well-being is a positive state of affairs, brought about by the synergistic satisfaction of personal, relational, organizational and collective needs of individuals, relationships, organizations and communities alike. There cannot be well-being but in the combined presence of personal, relational, organizational and collective wellness (Prilleltensky and Nelson 2002; Prilleltensky and Prilleltensky, in press).

Sites of well-being

Sites, as noted, refer to the location of well-being. Here we concern ourselves with 'where' well-being is situated. We maintain that there are four primary sites of well-being: individual persons, relationships, organizations and communities. Even though we can distinguish the well-being of a person, a relationship, an organization or a community, they are interdependent. Each one of these entities is unique and dependent on the others at the same time. None can be subsumed under the others, nor can they exist in isolation. They are distinguishable sites, but inseparable entities all the same.

There is empirical evidence to suggest that the well-being of relationships in informal and formal organizations like families and work, respectively (relationships where there is caring, compassion, and formal and informal supports), has beneficial effects on persons (Gottman 1999; Ornish 1997). Likewise, there is a wealth of research documenting the deleterious or advantageous consequences of deprived or prosperous communities on individuals, as the case might be (Hofrichter 2003).

Communities as sites of well-being embody characteristics such as affordable housing, clean air, accessible transportation, and high quality healthcare and education. All these factors take place in the physical space of communities. Organizations, in turn, are sites where exchanges of material (money, physical help) and psychological (affection, caring, nurturance) resources and goods occur. People work for money, but not only for money. Exchanges of affirmation and appreciation, in both informal and formal relationships, are a vital part of healthy relationships. Persons, finally, are sites where feelings, cognitions and phenomenological experiences of well-being reside. Interpersonal or relational well-being is the glue that connects personal, organizational and community wellness.

We have to be able to honour the uniqueness of the four sites of well-being and their interdependence at the same time. We can have a community endowed with excellent jobs, schools, parks and hospitals where many people feel miserable because relationships in the community are acrimonious or alienating. If we only thought of well-being in terms of community, we would miss the experiential component of personal well-being and the influential role of organizations and relationships in advancing personal satisfaction. Conversely, we can have a select group of people who, despite poor community conditions, experience high levels of well-being because of privilege. In this case, exclusive focus on the well-being of these people might miss the need to heal, repair and transform the community conditions (poverty, discrimination, epidemics) that are diminishing the well-being of those who cannot protect themselves.

From this general level of geographical and physical location of well-being, we can proceed to ask more specific questions about signs of well-being in each one of the three different sites. While interconnected, we will see that each site has distinct signs of well-being.

Signs of well-being

By signs we refer to manifestations or expressions of well-being at the different sites we explored earlier. Signs answer the question 'How do I know that this site is experiencing well-being?' At the personal level, signs of well-being are identified by looking at correlates, by asking people to share what they feel and think when they are happy, satisfied, or experience high quality of life. A variety of research methods have been used to look at personal signs of well-being, including surveys, interviews, observations and comparative analyses (Snyder and Lopez 2002). Similarly, multiple approaches have been used to find out the signs, characteristics or correlates of well or healthy relationships, communities and organizations (Eckersley et al. 2002; Gottman 1999).

Based on multiple sources of evidence, a few signs of personal well-being come to the fore: self-determination and a sense of control, self-efficacy, physical and mental health, optimism, meaning and spirituality. Signs of relational well-being include caring, respect for diversity, reciprocity, nurturance and affection, support, collaboration and democratic participation in decision-making processes. John Gottman (1999), a researcher and family therapist at the University of Washington in Seattle, conducts observational studies with couples who agree to spend a weekend in a simulated university apartment. The couples spend a typical weekend at the university retreat and are videotaped, observed and monitored for the majority of their waking hours. Within the first five minutes of observing a couple interact, Gottman can predict with a disturbingly high level of accuracy which couples will stay together and which are headed for divorce. Troubled relationships are marked by harsh start-ups of argument; interactions that are marked by criticism, contempt and defensiveness; physiological reactions of fight-or-flight in times of conflict; and failed attempts to de-escalate tension. On the other hand, happy couples share a deep friendship and stay emotionally connected even as they deal with conflict. They know each other intimately and can easily answer questions about their partner's likes, dislikes, hopes and dreams. They also know about important people, events and circumstances that have shaped their partner's life and are aware of key players and events affecting their partner in the present.

Gottman claims that what makes for a happy marriage is surprisingly simple. Happy couples have a wealth of positive thoughts and feelings towards one another. This positivity and connectedness is reflected in their daily interactions and serves to protect them in times of conflict. All partners periodically experience negative thoughts and feelings about each other. In the case of happily married couples, these are overridden by the wealth of mutual affection and positivity that characterizes the relationship. Gottman equates this to the set weight theory of weight loss. 'Once your marriage gets "set" at a certain degree of positivity, it will take far more negativity to harm your relationship than if your "set point" were lower. And if your relationship becomes overwhelmingly negative, it will be more difficult to repair it' (Gottman 1999: 21).

From the relational we move to the organizational. Signs of organizational well-being include respect for diversity, democratic participation, collaborative relationships, clarity of roles, engagement and learning opportunities. Expressions of collective well-being, in turn, include a fair and equitable allocation of bargaining powers, resources and obligations in society, gender and race equality, universal access to high quality educational, health and recreational facilities, affordable housing, employment opportunities, access to nutritious foods at reasonable prices, safety, public transportation, a clean environment and peace (Sen 1999a, 1999b). Though not exhaustive by any means, these lists are representative of the research on well-being at the four levels (Goleman 1998; Maton and Salem 1995; Totikidis and Prilleltensky 2006).

Each one of the signs noted above is intrinsically beneficial to the well-being of a particular site and extrinsically beneficial to the well-being of the other two sites. Supportive organizations foster self-determination of their members while just communities contribute to personal growth through a fair allocation of opportunities in society. An interesting study shows the connections between organizational climate and personal health. Chronic high levels of stress compromise our immune system and increases the likelihood of suffering ill health. A recent investigation with nurses found that having latitude in making work-related decisions was an important factor in mitigating their stress. Stress among nurses was measured by the level of cortisol (the stress hormone) secreted by their endocrine glands. Cortisol levels did not vary based on objective measures of the nurses' workload. On the other hand, the degree to which they believed they could exert control over their work environments was highly correlated with their level of stress. The greatest increase in cortisol levels was found among nurses with the highest workload coupled with the least amount of control (Ganster et al. 2001). These examples point to the interaction between environmental (workload and amount of control) and personal (belief in ability to control environment) factors. It is never one or another. Personal and environmental signs of well-being are co-determined.

A propitious work climate enables its workers to exercise voice and choice, which, in turn, can be used to modify the surroundings to make them more conducive to personal well-being. The emotional and productive state of workers depends not only on internal drives and motivators, but also on the cultural norms of the environment. Organizational practices, in turn, depend on the actions of individual employees and workers. When organizational climate is hostile, the place becomes negatively infective. When the climate is accepting, the setting is positively infective, generating energy and engagement for workers and clients in the community (Harter et al. 2003).

The organization as a whole, through its structures, procedures, regularities and habits, can foster positive climates. Workers need to be rewarded for supporting enabling structures, and structures have to be user-friendly and participatory. When the place is internally together, signs of organizational well-being start to be reflected in the community. Positive climates are intrinsically beneficial for workers and the community that the organization serves. Without personal contributions, the organization doesn't function, and without enabling structures there is nothing to support and institutionalize good intentions.

Sources of well-being

Each one of the sites of well-being and their corresponding signs has particular sources or groups of determinants. Self-determination, for example, derives from prior opportunities to exercise control, voice and choice. In the relational domain, expressions of caring and compassion derive from positive experiences of trust, nurturance and affection. In the organizational sphere, participation and collaboration derive from traditions of inclusion, learning and horizontal structures.

If a cohesive and supportive work environment is conducive to personal well-being, so is one that provides many opportunities for growth, engagement and self-determination. Warr (1999) has compiled a list of key features of work that are correlated with personal well-being. First on the list are opportunities for personal control where employees have decision latitude, autonomy and freedom of choice, coupled with the absence of close supervision.

The combination of very high demands on the job, along with little opportunities for control is particularly damaging to worker well-being (Warr 1999), and by extension, to organizational well-being. Like a tightly controlled classroom whose teacher unexpectedly leaves the room, workers who are not trusted and are micromanaged by their supervisor will lower their productivity when the supervisor is not present. Those who have other options will choose to leave the job, and those who have no choice will grow increasingly resentful and less productive. Disgruntled employees who are on the outlook for an opportunity to leave their job will often reduce their productivity as they explore other options. Most important to personal well-being, little control is associated with high levels of stress and stressed individuals are more prone to a host of physical and psychological ailments (Halpern 2005).

But it wasn't until Sir Michael Marmot published the Whitehall studies that health and social scientists could really appreciate the impact of control on personal wellness (Marmot 1999, 2004; Marmot and Feeney, 1996). The British scientist, who was knighted for his ground-breaking research in England, studied the lives of thousands of British civil servants. He followed up the lives of government employees for over 25 years. After he eliminated all other possible sources of health and illness, he realized that those workers who experienced little control over their jobs were two, three, and even four times more likely to die than those who experienced a lot of control over their jobs.

Marmot divided the civil servants into four groups: managers, professionals, clerical and others. Managers had the most amount of control over their jobs whereas the group called 'other' had the least. Professionals were second and clerical staff third. Compared to managers, professionals were twice as likely to die, clerical staff three times as likely, and the group called other, which included people with few skills, four times more likely to die. If anyone had doubts about the role of control on personal wellness, Marmot erased them.

Having autonomy and self-determination is not enough, however. Workers also strive for environments that will enable them to utilize valued skills and abilities and provide interest, variety and opportunities for growth and engagement. Various studies have shown that personal well-being varies as a function of changing job conditions. In one study summarized by Warr (1999), the overall job satisfaction of clerical workers significantly increased after their jobs were restructured to increase skill utilization and knowledge demands. There is an optimal level of challenge conducive to well-being. Not enough or too much challenge is associated with either boredom or high levels of stress (Warr 1999).

'Roles influence group members' happiness and well-being in significant ways. By taking on a role in a group, individuals secure their connection to their fellow members, building the interdependence that is essential for group cohesion and productivity' (Forsyth 2006: 183). Gallup polls conducted by the Gallup Management Journal (GMJ) categorized respondents according to their level of engagement at work. As a group, engaged workers are passionate about their work and have a strong sense of connection to the organization and to their fellow workers (27 per cent of respondents). Non-engaged workers (59 per cent of respondents) simply go through the motions at work with little passion for what they do. In turn, those classified as actively disengaged (14 per cent of respondents) act out their unhappiness by undermining the work of their co-workers (Gallup 2006).

As opposed to non-engaged and actively disengaged workers, many engaged workers reported that their interactions with their co-workers are always or mostly positive; that they are often challenged but rarely frustrated on the job; and that their supervisor mainly focuses on their strengths. Furthermore, engaged workers were much more likely to report feeling happy while on the job (86 per cent); indicate their work as an important source of happiness for them; and report much higher levels of overall life satisfaction (Gallup 2006).

Of course, correlation does not equal causation and a multitude of constitutional, familial and environmental factors likely contribute to the difference between engaged and non-engaged workers. Nevertheless, there is little doubt that a work environment that actively promotes worker engagement and where supervisors focus on building strengths rather than accentuating faults, is more likely to promote personal and organizational well-being.

The main premise of this chapter is that what happens in any domain of well-being – collective, organizational, relational or personal – affects the others. Multiple sources support this hypothesis. Economic down-turns resulting in unemployment have an impact in organizational climate. When job security is threatened, tensions rise in the office, workers feel anxious, families react to the stress, and risk of disease increases. We can take any of the social determinants of health reviewed by Marmot and Wilkinson (1999) and follow their health enhancing or inhibiting effects. To take but one more example, neighbourhoods that are high on psychological sense of community help members to feel supported, enhance coping, and breed trust among its members. Supported individuals, in turn, are more likely to have fun, share their pleasures and sorrows, and infuse a joyous attitude at work. The trick is always to see the connections, for good or bad. Negative and positive chain reactions happen all the time, and if we see only isolated events, as opposed to chained events, we risk misdiagnosing the sources of problems and missing the bright lights.

Strategies for well-being

The key to successful strategies is that they must be specific enough to address each one of the sites, signs and respective sources of well-being at the same time. In other words, they must simultaneously address multiple sources, signs and sites of well-being. Interventions that concentrate strictly on personal sites neglect the many resources that organizations and communities contribute to personal well-being. Paradoxically, strategies that concentrate exclusively on personal well-being undermine well-being because they do not support the infra-structure that enhances well-being itself. This has been a major gap in previous efforts to sustain individual well-being through strictly psychological means such as cognitive reframing, positive thinking, information sharing and skill building. Individuals cannot significantly alter their level of well-being in the absence of concordant environ-mental changes (Smedley and Syme 2000). Conversely, any strategy that promotes well-being by environmental changes alone is bound to be limited. There is ample evidence to suggest that the most prom-ising approaches combine strategies for personal, organizational and collective change (Stokols 2000). It is not one or the other, but the combination of them all that is the best avenue to seek higher levels of well-being in the three sites of our interest.

Take for example the powerful influence of social support on health. Support for the soul can increase or restore health and wellness in two ways. First, social support can enhance wellness through bonding, attachment, appreciation and affirming messages. The more support I have the better I feel, the better I feel the more likely I am to withstand adversity and develop resilience. According to our model, interpersonal wellness leads to personal wellness.

The second mechanism through which social support enhances wellness is by providing emotional and instrumental support in times of crises. The stressful reactions associated with divorce, moves, transitions or loss may be buffered by the presence of helpful and supportive others.

Compared with people with lower levels of supports, those who enjoy more support from relatives or friends live longer, recover faster from illnesses, report better health, and cope better with adversities (Cohen 2004). Studies have shown that women with advanced breast cancer have better chances of survival when they participate in support groups. After a follow up of 48 months, Spiegel and colleagues reported in 1989 that all the women in the control group had died, whereas a third of those who received group support were still alive. The average survival for the women in the support group was 36 months, compared to 19 months in the control sample who had not received group support. Their study, reported in the prestigious British journal *Lancet* made medical history (Spiegel et al. 1989).

One year later, Richardson and colleagues made similar claims on a sample of patients with blood malignancies. Their study, published in the *Journal of Clinical Oncology*, claimed that, 'the use of special educational and supportive programs ... are associated with significant prolongation of patient survival' (Richardson et al. 1990: 356). Finally, Fawzy and colleagues reported in 1993 that patients with malignant melanoma were more likely to die or experience recurrence of the disease if they did not receive the group intervention that the experimental group received. Out of 34 patients in each group, of those who received group support, only 7 had experienced recurrence and 3 had died at the five-year follow-up, compared with 13 who experienced recurrence and 10 who had died in the control group. Altogether, these three teams of researchers found that social support can enhance health and longevity in the face of deadly diseases (Fawzy et al. 1993).

One way to make sure that we maximize the benefits of social support is by enhancing sense of community and the availability of support throughout the life cycle, and not just in times of need. There is a role here for the community at large, and for public institutions in promoting belonging, affection and mutual help. We need to think of public institutions as promoters of well-being and not only as restorers of well-being when our physical or emotional integrity is compromised by illness or crises.

In *Better Together: Restoring the American Community* (2003), Putnam and Feldstein survey the United States for projects that promote social capital, from libraries in Chicago to Dudley Street neighbourhood in Boston, to Portland to Saddleback Church in Lake Forest, California, back to Boston where they studied Harvard's Union of Clerical Workers. In total, they studied twelve initiatives throughout the country where social capital has served to improve literacy, build cohesion, advance businesses, bridge across ethnic groups, and otherwise foster community well-being. The projects ranged from the ameliorative to the more transformative and political, but they all had something in common. They all used networking, small groups and face-to-face meetings to create bonding within homogeneous groups and bridging among diverse groups. All the projects involved a measure of personal, relational, organizational and community change. What they learned was that linking these four domains is fundamental. They also learned that for meaningful dialogue to take place, groups should not exceed ten people. In fact, small is good. When you are part of a small group, you cannot fade into the background and let others do the work, nor can you be easily ignored.

Some groups studied by Putnam and Feldstein, like the Harvard Union of Clerical Workers, were highly political in their aspiration. Others were more interested in the arts. However, they all engaged people in ways that affected their core identity. In all cases, members of these little cells were touched by a vision and a mission. The power of solidarity and teamwork is what links personal, organizational and community change. It is the relational aspect of community well-being that binds and sustains people in a just cause. Teaming for a good cause is not only good for the community, but it is also very good for those who team up. It is the stories people tell each other and the narratives they create in common that foster a sense of community. When people act in concert and when their voices are heard, new possibilities emerge. As Smith observed:

> Well-being is fundamentally individual, but is also social. Direct participation in one's immediate community, and indirect participation in the larger society, can affect well-being. At the basic village, neighbourhood, or township level, to escape from poverty you must have a voice within your community that is taken seriously when you have a legitimate concern. Your community, or communities, however

humble, must be informed, empowered to stand up for their interests, and able to defend their rights. (Smith 2005: 43)

Putnam and Feldstein claim that 'organizing is about transforming private aches and pains into a shared vision of collective action' (2003: 282). This is precisely the way to move from mere amelioration of suffering to social transformation.

Synergy of sites, signs, sources and strategies

We can integrate sites, signs, sources and strategies in the following formulation: The well-being of a *site* is reflected in a particular *sign*, which derives from a particular *source* and is promoted by a certain *strategy*. To wit, personal well-being is reflected in control, which derives from opportunities to exercise voice and choice, and is promoted by empowerment. In this case, the site is personal wellness, the sign is control, the source is opportunities to experience voice and choice and the strategy is empowerment.

In the organizational domain we can integrate the four Ss as follows: Organizational well-being is reflected in the presence of supportive relationships among workers, which derive from a culture of trust and reciprocity, and is promoted by empathy and opportunities to give and receive caring, compassion and constructive feedback. In the collective domain we can claim that collective well-being is reflected in universal access to health care, which derives from policies of social justice, and is promoted by social movements that strive to create, maintain and improve institutions that deliver services to all citizens, irrespective of means.

In synthesis, then, the well-being of site q is reflected in sign x, which derives from source y, and is promoted by strategy z. By using this simple formulation, we can integrate a vast amount of research in operational and actionable terms. An example of synergy is the beneficial effects that accrue from community cohesion. Individuals, organizations and communities all gain when high participation and reciprocity are the social norm.

References

Berkman, L. (1995) 'The Role of Social Relationships in Health Promotion', *Psychosomatic Research*, 57: 245–54.

Bolman, L. and Deal, T. (2003) *Reframing Organizations*. San Francisco: Jossey Bass.

Bruton, H. (2001) *On the Search for Well-Being*. Ann Arbor, MI: University of Michigan Press.

Cohen, S. (2004) 'Social Relationships and Health', *American Psychologist*, 59: 676–84.

Eckersley, R. (2000) 'The Mixed Blessing of Material Progress: Diminishing Returns in the Pursuit of Progress', *Journal of Happiness Studies*, 1: 267–92.

Eckersley, R. (2002) 'Culture, Health and Well-Being', in R. Eckersley, J. Dixon and B. Douglas (eds), *The Social Origins of Health and Well-Being*. New York: Cambridge University Press.

Eckersley, R. (2005) *Well and Good: Morality, Meaning and Happiness*. Melbourne: Text Publishing.

Eckersley, R., Dixon, J. and Douglas B. (eds) (2002) *The Social Origins of Health and Well-Being*. New York: Cambridge University Press.

Fawzy, F. I., Fawzy, N. W., Hyun, C. S., Elashoff, R., Guthrie, D., Fahey, J. L. and Morton, D. L. (1993) 'Malignant Melanoma: Effects of an Early Structured Psychiatric Intervention, Coping, and Affective State on Recurrence and Survival 6 Years Later', *Archives of General Psychiatry*, 50: 681–9.

Forsyth, D. (2006) *Group Dynamics* (4th edition). New York: Brooks/Cole.

Fryer, D. (1998) 'Editor's Preface: Special Issue on Unemployment', *Journal of Community and Applied Social Psychology*, 8: 75–88.

Gallup (2006) 'Gallup Study: Feeling Good Matters in the Workplace'. Retrieved on 4 February 2006 from http://gmj.gallup.com/content/default.asp?ci=2077.

Ganster, D. C., Fox, M. L. and Dwyer, D. J. (2001) 'Explaining Employees' Health Care Costs: a Prospective Examination of Stressful Job Demands, Personal Control, and Physiological Reactivity', *Journal of Applied Psychology*, 86: 954–64.

Goleman, D. (1998) *Working with Emotional Intelligence*. New York: Bantam.

Gottman, J. (1999) *The Seven Principles for Making Marriage Work*. New York: Three Rivers Press.

Halpern, D. F. (2005) 'Psychology at the Intersection of Work and Family: Recommendations for Employers, Working Families, and Policymakers', *American Psychologist*, 60(5): 397–409.

Harter, J., Schmidt, F. and Keyes, C. (2003) 'Well-Being in the Workplace and its Relationship to Business Outcomes: a review of the Gallup Studies', in C. Keyes and J. Haidt (eds), *Flourishing: Positive Psychology and the Life Well-lived*. Washington, DC: American Psychological Association.

Hazan, C. and Shaver, P. (1987) 'Romantic Love Conceptualized as an Attachment Process', *Journal of Personality and Social Psychology*, 52: 511–24.

Hazan, C. and Shaver, P. (2004) 'Attachment as an Organizational Framework for Research on Close Relationships', in H. Reis and C. Rusbult (eds), *Close Relationships*. New York: Psychology Press.

Hofrichter, R. (ed.) (2003) *Health and Social Justice*. San Francisco: Jossey Bass.

Marmot, M. (1999) 'Introduction', in M. Marmot and R. Wilkinson (eds), *Social Determinants of Health*. New York: Oxford University Press.

Marmot, M. (2004) *The Status Syndrome: How Social Standing Affects Our Health and Longevity*. New York: Times Books.

Marmot, M., and Feeney, A. (1996) 'Work and Health: Implications for Individuals and Society', in D. Blane, E. Bruner and R. Wilkinson (eds), *Health and Social Organization*. London: Routledge.

Marmot, M. and Wilkinson, R. (eds) (1999) *Social Determinants of Health*. New York: Oxford University Press.

Maton, K. I. and Salem, D. A. (1995) 'Organizational Characteristics of Empowering Community Settings: a Multiple Case Study Approach', *American Journal of Community Psychology*, 23: 631–56.

McGue, M. and Bouchard, T. J. (1998) 'Genetic and Environmental Influences on Human Behavioural Differences', *Annual Review of Neuroscience*, 21: 1–24.

Mikulincer, M. (2004) 'Attachment Working Models and the Sense of Trust: an Exploration of Interaction Goals and Affect Regulation', in H. Reis and C. Rusbult (eds), *Close Relationships*. New York: Psychology Press.

Narayan, D., Chambers, R., Shah, M. and Petesch, P. (1999) *Global Synthesis: Consultations with the Poor*. Poverty Group, World Bank. Available online at: www.worldbank.org/poverty/voices/synthes.pdf.

Navarro, V. (ed.) (2000) *The Political Economy of Social Inequalities: Consequences for Health and Quality of Life*. Amityville, NY: Baywood.

Navarro, V. (ed.) (2004) *The Political and Social Contexts of Health*. Amityville, NY: Baywood.

Nelson, G., Lord, J. and Ochocka, J. (2001) *Shifting the Paradigm in Community Mental Health: Towards Empowerment and Community*. Toronto: University of Toronto Press.

Nelson, G. and Prilleltensky, I. (2005) (eds) *Community Psychology: In Pursuit of Liberation and Well-Being*. New York: Palgrave Macmillan.

Nussbaum, M. (1999) *Sex and Social Justice*. Oxford: Oxford University Press.

Ornish, D. (1997) *Love and Survival: the Scientific Basis for the Healing Power of Intimacy*. New York: HarperCollins.

Prilleltensky, I. and Nelson, G. (2002) *Doing Psychology Critically: Making a Difference in Diverse Settings*. New York: Palgrave Macmillan.

Prilleltensky, I. and Prilleltensky. O. (2003) 'Towards a Critical Health Psychology Practice', *Journal of Health Psychology*, 8: 197–210.

Prilleltensky, I. and Prilleltensky, O. (2006) *Promoting Well-Being: Linking Personal, Organizational, and Community Change*. Hoboken. NJ: Wiley.

Putnam, R. and Feldstein, L. (2003) *Better Together: Restoring the American Community*. New York: Simon & Schuster.

Richardson, J., Sheldon, D., Krailo, M. and Levine, A. (1990) 'The Effect of Compliance with Treatment on Survival among Patients with Hematologic Malignancies', *Journal of Clinical Oncology*, 18: 356–64.

Seligman, M. E. P. (2002) *Authentic Happiness*. New York: Free Press.

Sen, A. (1999a) *Beyond the Crisis: Development Strategies in Asia*. Singapore: Institute of Southeast Asian Studies.

Sen, A. (1999b) *Development as Freedom*. New York: Anchor Books.

Sheldon, K., Lyubomirsky, S. and Schkade, D. (2003) *Pursuing Happiness: the Architecture of Sustainable Change*. Submitted for publication.

Shinn, M. and Toohey, S. M. (2003) 'Community Contexts of Human Welfare', *Annual Review of Psychology*, 54: 427–59.

Smedley, B. D. and Syme, S. L. (eds) (2000) *Promoting Health: Intervention Strategies from Social and Behavioural Research*. Washington, DC: National Academy Press.

Smith, S. (2005) *Ending Global Poverty: a Guide to What Works*. New York: Palgrave Macmillan.

Snyder, C. and Lopez, S. (eds) (2002) *Handbook of Positive Psychology*. New York: Oxford University Press.

Spiegel, D., Bloom, J. R. and Kraemer, H. C. (1989) 'Effect of Psychosocial Treatment on Survival of Patients with Metastatic Breast Cancer', *The Lancet*, 2: 888–91.

Stokols, D. (2000) 'The Social Ecological Paradigm of Wellness Promotion', in M. Jamner and D. Stokols (eds), *Promoting Human Wellness*. Los Angeles: University of California Press.

Thomas, A. and Chess, S. (1977) *Temperament and Development*. New York: Brunner/Mazel.

Totikidis, V. and Prilleltensky, I. (2006) 'Engaging Community in a Cycle of Praxis: Multicultural Perspectives on Personal, Relational, and Collective Wellness', *Community, Work and Family*, 9: 47–67.

Turkheimer, E. (1998) 'Heritability and Biological Explanation', *Psychological Review*, 105: 782–91.

Warr, P. (1999) 'Well-Being in the Workplace', in D. Kahneman, E. Diener and N. Schwarz (eds), *Well-Being: the Foundations of Hedonic Psychology*. New York: Russell Sage Foundation.

Wilkinson, R. G. (1996) *Unhealthy Societies: the Afflictions of Inequality*. London: Routledge.

Wilkinson, R. G. (2005) *The Impact of Inequality: How to Make Sick Societies Healthier*. New York: New Press.

4
Health, Well-Being and Social Capital

Judith Sixsmith and Margaret Boneham

The concept of social capital is examined in this chapter, focusing on the key components of participation, trust and reciprocity, and social networks of bonding, bridging and linking ties. This is set in the context of recent critical debates. The value of social capital in understanding individual and community health and well-being is then explored, taking into account recent qualitative and quantitative research. Finally, the implications of social capital for policy development are considered and recommendations made for the promotion of health-enhancing communities.

The concept of social capital

The concept of social capital, it can be argued, originates in the ideas of Durkheim and Adam Smith (Halpern 2005). The application of the concept was first seen at the beginning of the twentieth century (Hanifan 1916). More recently it has re-emerged in the work of Pierre Bourdieu (1986), James Coleman (1988) and Robert Putnam (1993, 1995, 2000). Their different perspectives have contributed to a concept which is somewhat ambiguous and elastic, with Bourdieu's emphasis on social networks and their connections, exchanges and obligations, and Coleman's immersion in social exchange theory (Morgan and Swann 2004). The notion of social capital which has gained most in popularity was identified by Putnam and has attracted considerable academic and political attention in recent years (Halpern 2005). Within Putnam's work, social capital has been defined as the: 'features of social organisa-tion, such as networks, norms, and trust, that facilitate co-ordination and co-operation for mutual benefit' (Putnam 1995: 67).

A community or neighbourhood which is rich in social capital has been described as a socially cohesive, co-operative and caring community in which people work together for mutual benefit. Accordingly, social capital has been seen as 'both a glue that bonds society together and a lubricant that permits the smooth running of society's interactions (both interpersonal and among people, groups, and organisations)' (Smith 1997: 170).

Conversely, a community poor in social capital might be described as one where people become isolated, suspicious of others and reluctant to participate in social, economic and political life. Indeed, a community lacking in social capital is said to be characterized by the breakdown of the social fabric that binds people together within their communities (Cooper et al. 1999).

The breakdown in social fabric may well have a very negative impact on the lives of individual people living within the community. It is in this sense that social capital can also exist at an individual level. Accordingly, Brehm and Rahn (1997) have pointed to the importance of psychosocial variables, particularly the tight reciprocal relationship between civic engagement and interpersonal trust. More often, social capital at the individual level has been measured by the extent and quality of a person's social networks. Putnam (2000) has focused his attention on four key areas which exist at the interface between individual and community and underpin social capital: civic engagement and participation; notions of trust; shared norms of reciprocity; and social networking.

Civic participation

Putnam (2000) suggests that individual participation in formal groups is not only a barometer of civic involvement but also constitutes one important way in which people can develop supportive social networks. Group participation is thus a focus for the sharing of behavioural and attitudinal norms. Putnam prioritizes involvement in formal groups (such as community-based, church-based and work-based voluntary organizations) as a cornerstone of social capital. Here, participation integrally involves people getting together, generating ideas for action and becoming highly involved in joint ventures, revolving around social and community change, i.e. changing community life for the mutual benefit of community members. In psychosocial terms, participation in formal groups, activities and campaigns is often linked to the development of a sense of personal and social empowerment (Sixsmith and

Boneham 2002a), although the everyday hassles of taking responsibility for community life can also prove to be distressing for some people (Sixsmith and Boneham 2003).

Putnam has less to say concerning the development of social capital within more informal community networks, i.e. those beyond 'card parties and bowling leagues, bar cliques and ball games, picnics and parties' (Putnam 2000: 27). Recent work in deconstructing the notion of social capital has indicated that participation in informal groups and networks (Campbell et al. 1999) can be particularly important in more disadvantaged communities where the personal, social and financial resources required for formal participation are in short supply. This means that a fuller understanding of social capital must consider participation amongst more marginalized groups in society.

Trust and reciprocity

Trust according to Putnam acts to lubricate social life (Putnam 1993). However, numerous definitions of trust abound in the literature. Farrel and Knight (2003: 540), for example, define trust as 'a set of expectations held by one party that another party or parties will behave in an appropriate manner with regard to a specific issue'. On the other hand Kawachi et al. (1997:44) argue that trust is the 'belief in the good will and benign intent of others [and] differs from context to context, dependent on whether or not the person to be trusted is known personally to the respondent'. In this sense, trust cannot be conceptualized as a unitary concept (Scott 1980). Indeed, Putnam (2000) distinguishes between thick and thin trust. Thick trust is that found within enduring family and friendship relationships. Putnam is less clear about the meaning of thin trust which he suggests is evident in contacts with acquaintances, i.e. the relatively unknown generalized other. Thick and thin trust, Putnam suggests:

> represent the ends of a continuum, for thick-trust, refers to trust with a short radius, encompassing only others who are close to the truster, sociologically speaking, and 'thin-trust' refers to trust with a long radius, encompassing people at a greater social distance from the truster. (Putnam 2000: 466)

In Fukuyama's (1995: 26) terms, trust emerges from 'the expectation that arises within a community of regular, honest and co-operative behaviour, based on commonly shared norms'. Common to these definitions, trust involves positively valued expectations about the future behaviour of well-known and generalized others.

Trust may act as a foundation for reciprocal helping found in family, friendship and community relationships. Campbell et al. suggest that reciprocity is defined as 'an obligation to help others; [in the] confidence that others will help oneself' (1999: 7). In terms of social capital, generalized reciprocity (a term emphasized by Woolcock 2001) refers to the notion that individuals will help others and do favours, etc. without anticipating a return and perhaps even without knowing the individual(s) involved. Putnam contends that the norm of generalized reciprocity is bolstered by highly dense networks of social exchange. Here members of tight-knit communities are more likely to help each other out because they will encounter each other in current and future everyday life.

Social networks

In addition to notions of participation, trust and reciprocity, Putnam also considers the meaning of social networks in relation to social capital:

> Of all the dimensions along which forms of social capital vary, perhaps the most important is the distinction between *bridging* . . . and *bonding* . . . Some forms of capital are, by choice or necessity, inward looking and tend to reinforce exclusive identities and homogeneous groups . . . bonding social capital is good for undergirding specific reciprocity and mobilising solidarity. (Putnam 2000: 22)

As such, bonding capital involves exclusive and strong ties found in close kinship and friendship relationships characterized by thick trust. Alternatively, bridging capital involves weaker ties and thinner trust with representatives of organizations, groups and others beyond the intimate circle of family and friends. According to Putnam:

> Other networks are outward looking and encompass people across diverse social cleavages. Examples of bridging social capital include the civil rights movement, many youth service groups, and ecumenical religious organisations . . . bridging networks are better for linkage to external assets and for information diffusion. (Putnam 2000: 22)

Putnam implies that both bonding and bridging ties are integrally involved in the creation, maintenance and use of social capital.

However, it is not clear which networks are more beneficial to the individual. On the one hand, it is argued that, 'the most fundamental form of social capital is the family' (Putnam 1995: 73), thus suggesting bonding capital is of fundamental importance. On the other hand, Putnam points to the benefits of bridging ties generally found in relationships between acquaintances and individuals outside of one's intimate social networks, thereby suggesting that they are more effective at generating social capital (Putnam 1993; Winter 2000). However, research has indicated that bridging capital declines more quickly than bonding capital (Burt 2002). Moreover, bonding and bridging ties may have different spheres of influence. Whereas bonding ties may be extremely supportive in times of stress and ill health, bridging ties may be more helpful when seeking a new job, as suggested by Granovetter's (1973) work, 'The Strength of Weak Ties'. The fact that middle-class people tend to have more access to bridging capital brings more advantages to them in terms of work-related and social advancement (Halpern 2005). Thus, social capital is seen as an available resource emerging from both tight-knit community networks and those broader based and more distant relationships.

A further dimension of social capital has been suggested by Woolcock (2001), namely 'linking social capital'. Woolcock distinguishes linking from bridging capital on the basis that 'bridging (capital) is essentially a horizontal metaphor ... implying connections between people who share broadly similar demographic characteristics' (2001: 13). He argues that for those who are disadvantaged, it is desirable that their activities not only 'reach out' but are 'scaled up':

> Hence linking social capital may be provisionally viewed as a special form of bridging social capital that specifically concerns power – it is a vertical bridge across asymmetrical power and resources. (Halpern 2005: 25)

As Woolcock maintains, 'the capacity to leverage resources, ideas and information from formal institutions beyond the community is a key function of linking social capital' (Woolcock 2001: 13). Woolcock highlights the institutional context within which social networks are embedded, the power relations which constitute them and the role of the state and the effect that its institutions have on community life. Linking social capital, therefore, incorporates relations developed between people and representatives of public and professional institutions (such as NGOs, banks).

Recent critical debates

As suggested above, there are several ambiguities concerning the notion of social capital (Halpern 2005; Anhier and Kendall 2002; Nuissl 2002) and critique of the concept is evident in recent debate. In particular, social capital has been described as too vague, slippery and poorly specified (Baum 1999) to be useful in terms of measurement as well as attempting to tie together too broad a range of different social and psychological concepts. Such criticism may have overplayed an apparent weakness which, from a different perspective, can be seen as a strength. Moscovici (1984) has argued that a concept which is too tightly defined may well prevent investigations beyond its boundaries and therefore act as a blinker preventing truly innovative research. In summarizing the promise of social capital, Schuller et al. (2000) conclude that whilst there are problems of definition and measurement, social capital has many merits as a heuristic tool. They argue that it challenges current modes of thinking, shifting analysis from the individual 'to the patterns of relationships between agents, social units and institutions' (Schuller et al. 2000: 35).

The ways in which social capital has been operationalized in survey research has varied considerably (Blaxter and Poland 2002; Blaxter 2004) with each survey emphasizing different aspects of the concept. Durlauf (2002) and Fine (2001) have argued that lack of precision in operationalization has rendered the concept meaningless. Moreover, its specificity to the (primarily) American context calls into question transferability of the concept into the UK and elsewhere. Further investigations and more qualitative research (Devine and Roberts 2003) are required in order to clarify the mechanisms and processes through which social capital works as well as elaborating its value within very different social-cultural contexts.

Social capital, as Putnam defines it, tends to assume that all people are similar. These assumptions can be contested in terms of gender, age and ethnicity. Empirical research has begun to disentangle genderized social capital (Sixsmith et al. 2001; Molinas 1998) as well as the role of age (Morrow 2000; Cattell and Herring 2002; Sixsmith and Boneham 2002a) and ethnicity (Campbell and McLean 2002) in understanding the ways in which social capital is manifest in community living.

The notion of social capital has often been romanticized. It is assumed that communities with high stocks of social capital have highly positive outcomes, are pleasant to live in and can be characterized as secure and cohesive. However, the apparent negative aspects of social capital are rarely explicated. For instance, social capital, based on shared norms, may bond people together in tight-knit communities, which then become extremely difficult to escape from. Here, social capital is both exclusionary to outsiders and inhibitive to insiders. Putnam (2000) and others (for example, Portes and Landolt 1996) have begun to acknow-ledge the 'dark side' to social capital, but there is still a tendency in the literature for social capital to equate with positive community living.

Perhaps a key critique question is whether or not social capital is about 'capital' at all as Bankston and Zhou (2002) have argued. Borrowing from the economic world, the word 'capital' has connotations of a concrete reality whereby social relations can be metaphorically stored and trans-ferred with value equivalents for health and well-being. However, it is vital to stop referring to social capital within the narrow confines of an economic term and to reap the richer rewards of exploring the social processes in which it operates and can be enhanced to improve health and well-being.

Social capital, health and well-being

It has been argued that social capital has the potential to impact posit-ively (and negatively) upon people's mental and physical health and well-being through the medium of social networks and the quality of social relationships (Putnam 2000; Halpern 2005; Veenstra 2000; Kawachi et al. 1997). Such arguments might be expected in view of the close links which social capital has to social networking and the wealth of research pointing to improvements in health brought about by community, family and friendships networks (Cohen and Wills 1985; Berkman et al. 2000). Putnam's (2000) thesis in this respect maintains that plentiful social capital is clearly linked to good health and high levels of happiness. He draws on recent research into US public health, confirming the beneficial health effects of involvement with different social networks. This work shows that the more socially integrated an individual is, the less likely they are to suffer from a range of condi-tions such as heart attacks, cancer, premature death of many kinds and even colds and minor ailments. Moreover, he claims social integration not only prevents disease but also aids recovery from illness. Among the reasons for this are the potential for practical assistance that social networks bring and the absence of the damaging effects of social isola-tion (shown to accelerate the ageing process due to negative chemical effects on the body). Putnam also emphasizes the therapeutic advant-ages of social capital in inhibiting depression. He concludes that life satisfaction and happiness are strongly linked to the extent of an individual's social connectivity and participation in group activity. Indeed research has shown that married people are happier than single people (Donavan and Halpern 2003) and that friendship and membership in groups such as church and voluntary organizations increased well-being (Argyle 1987).

At the level of the individual, empirical work on health and social capital can reveal the mechanisms and processes which link health to social capital. For example, Rose (2000) has found that the more socially integrated a person is, the better their emotional health. One possible explanation is that social support acts as a source of buffering (see Cohen and Wills 1985) against stressful events, 'facilitating possible adaptive coping' (Gielen et al. 2001: 321). Furthermore, there are potentially more practical, social and psychological resources to alleviate health-related problems as well as health benefits that derive from the sense of belonging to social support networks which help the individual feel competent and efficacious (Campbell et al. 1999: 23). Social support can promote good physical health in that it encourages healthy behaviour whereas a lack of social support can encourage unhealthy behaviours (Staha et al. 2001). However, social support is not a unitary concept, as by its relational nature it is multidimensional and represents different things to different sections of the community (Rose et al. 2000). Moreover, it is unclear whether social networks actually promote good health and well-being or conversely whether good health creates opportunities for strong networking.

At the community level, links between community health, well-being and social capital have been studied. Survey research into social capital by Kawachi et al. (1997) and by Smith (1997) suggests that communities which are poor in social capital tend to be economically deprived with higher levels of morbidity and mortality. In this respect, Kawachi's work highlights that while socio-economic inequality is important in understanding health outcomes, social connectivity also needs to be considered. Indeed, it is not the richest countries that have the best health, but those with the smallest income disparity. Wilkinson (1996, 1997) has found in his work that the 'psychosocial effects of social position accounted for the largest part of health inequalities' (Wilkinson 1997: 2) and that community health is dependent on the development of social capital alongside economic development. It may be that the positive process of network enhancement promotes health enabling social and community structures (Gillies 1996).

Moreover, Kawachi et al. (1997) have suggested that it is theoretically possible for an isolated person (in terms of interpersonal relationships, bridging and bonding capital) to live within a community which is rich in social capital and subsequently benefit from the available resources the community has to offer. In this respect, bridging, bonding and linking capital may be important in promoting individual and community health as well as participation in community activities. Research efforts need to disentangle the relative contributions of different forms of social capital for health and well-being. As Campbell et al. (1999: 33) have pointed out, social capital may be constructed differently within the UK and 'certain dimensions of social capital might be more relevant to health than others'.

What is not yet clear is what sort of participation in networks, levels of individual or community trust and reciprocity is health enhancing, especially within different cultural contexts. It still seems unclear which 'type' of social network is most beneficial to the health of both the community and the individual. In Campbell et al.'s (1999) qualitative study, types of social networks differed in their potential to be health enabling. Campbell concludes that inward-looking narrowly focused bonding networks were less effective than diverse outward-looking bridging networks. However, Sixsmith et al.'s (2001) work points to the differential value of both bonding and bridging networks. The link between bonding ties and individual well-being was clear from their studies, where an increase in close networks had health benefits for most community members. In their study of the relationship between social capital, health and gender in a disadvantaged community, intimate social bonds offered important opportunities for social support, paralleling Kagan et al.'s (2000: 2) conclusions that, 'The poor neighbourhood may have weak and inward looking networks, which nevertheless offer strong support in adversity.' However, the relationship between bridging capital and individual well-being was more complex, with advantages for the community as a whole in the establishment of bridging ties to professional help but less benefit for individual community leaders whose expectations were poorly aligned to professional methods of communication. The lack of accessible bridging and linking capital to professional advice meant that more inventive ways of perceiving health and illness were not aired (Sixsmith and Boneham 2003).

Furthermore, Arber and Ginn (1995) and Sixsmith and Boneham's (2002a, 2002b) work suggests that an understanding of the relationships between social capital, health and well-being must involve an appreciation of issues of gender. In the latter study, women experienced social capital in terms of strong bonding ties underpinned by thick trust (developed through shared community and life events) and mutual reciprocal relations. For women, social identities of motherhood and parenting engendered shared neighbourliness and concerns of family support. In times of poor health and high stress, women relied on family, friends and neighbours to help them through difficult life transitions such as drug abuse and divorce (Sixsmith and Boneham 2002a). In contrast, men's social capital was less based on community and neighbourliness and more on work-based relationships in which reciprocity and trust were less prominent. When men faced ill health and high stress, they were more likely to turn to alcohol and drugs than to draw on available stocks of social capital. This sometimes led to a spiral of self-destruction whereby men's health and family life deteriorated (Sixsmith and Boneham 2002a).

Exploring issues of gender, Sixsmith and Boneham (2004) also revealed the ways gender and place interact and the implications this had for social capital and health, very much reflecting Morrow's (2002, 2003) work with children. Community space was conceived of as women's terrain. It was in the streets and community centres, the school gates and shops that women forged social relationships and widened the scope of their social networks. They linked their own sense of positive well-being to such encounters which were an antidote to home-based isolation. Men, on the other hand, often felt uncomfortable in such places, characterizing them as feminized space to be avoided. This meant that men spent less time in public places such as shops, school gates, parks and community centres and tended to be more socially isolated within their wider communities. Men, in general, used community facilities and services less than women, an important finding given Cattell and Herring's work which has shown such community resources to be vital for the generation of social capital (Cattell and Herring 2002). The few men who were active in community participation took on specific work-related roles and so did not develop the sorts of social relationships which provide supportive social capital in times of need.

Research has shown that women and men differentially access health services (Usscher 2000; Mackenbach and Bakker 2002; Carroll 1992). This may be explained in part by women's greater expertise in health and medical matters, derived from caring family roles. They were more liable than men to visit the doctor at the outset of health problems, and to engage in health talk, sharing knowledge and opinions with each other. On the whole, women critically appraised medical advice and thus were involved more integrally in their own and their families' health (Boneham and Sixsmith 2006). As men were less active in seeking medical help, they relied on their female family members to negotiate their health concerns, diagnosis and treatment. Health talk, for them, was felt to be too personal, risking ridicule or condemnation as 'real men' (Sixsmith 2004). Once again, men's reluctance to use their bonding and bridging ties was detrimental to their general physical health status (Sixsmith and Boneham 2002b).

Qualitative research into the concept of social capital and its relationship to health and well-being has highlighted the need to understand the significance of age and intergenerational connections (Cattell and Herring 2002; Sixsmith and Boneham 2002b; Boneham and Sixsmith 2006). In terms of age and intergeneration, Cattell and Herring (2002: 62) found that younger people 'were more individualistic than previous generations, but individualism could coexist with reciprocity, and both were associated with well-being'. They further suggest that younger people's tolerance can prove useful 'for the creation of more inclusive social capital' (2002: 62). Sixsmith and Boneham (2004) and Boneham and Sixsmith (2006) paint a rather complex picture in which older people perceived the community to be dangerous at night and were consequently isolated in their homes with little opportunity to build social relationships. On the other hand, younger people, especially the men, congregated in street groups and eschewed organized community activity. This restricted their development to bonding forms of social capital with 'others like them'. Without access to bridging capital, they were not able to benefit from social advantages (employment, education etc.) that wider networks provide. This was not the case amongst younger women, who were better able to integrate with a variety of community members across different generations and so gained from a richer social context.

It is important to note that social capital may operate in different ways, reflecting heterogeneous community groups. Campbell and McLean (2002) have explored how social capital is created and maintained within multiethnic communities. They concluded that, in terms of social capital and its impact on health, geographical community ties were less important than ethnic groupings across physical space. Within such marginalized ethnic communities, obstacles to participation were evident and social exclusions from the majority population restricted their access to the benefits of social capital. This means that any analysis of social capital needs to pay attention to marginalized groups and how everyday lives are lived in diverse community contexts.

This qualitative body of work has begun to unpack the very different ways in which social capital in terms of bonding, bridging and linking ties, trust, reciprocity and participation interact with gender and place to construct different opportunities and constraints on the relationship between social capital, health and well-being.

Conclusions

Theoretical implications

Critics of social capital have highlighted its ambiguous nature and rarely emphasized its heuristic value. By bringing together diverse concepts of networking, shared norms, reciprocity, trust and participation, social capital offers researchers and policy-makers alike a way of thinking about the interrelatedness of community living and its relationship to health. Dismissing social capital at this early stage in its theoretical and empirical development runs the risk of losing a complex and holistic approach to understanding social relations in real-life contexts. The sort of qualitative work reviewed in this chapter has begun to map out the different processes and mechanisms through which social capital is fundamental to an understanding of community relations and has implications for health and well-being.

If a cornerstone of social capital is to be found in the notion of formal group participation as Putnam suggests (e.g. religious groups), then its relative absence in disadvantaged communities constitutes a threat to present and future community and social cohesion. However, the disadvantaged communities studied in the UK were rich in informal participation (e.g. street-corner groups and mother and toddler groups) and, as such, enjoyed the health and well-being benefits of participatory social capital.

This review has also indicated that both trust and reciprocity are multi-faceted and interlinked concepts rather than static resources. Moreover, both are situationally specific and issues of generalized mistrust were as evident as generalized trust in the disadvantaged communities. General unease, stress and anxiety were all part of community living for many people. As such, trust and reciprocity were under constant renegotiation between people and groups, suggesting that future research needs to explore the ever-changing dynamics of social capital rather than concentrate on social capital as an immutable, unchanging given.

Past work has indicated a tendency towards romanticization and the emphasis on social capital as inevitably a benign force for good, ignoring the negative aspects to social capital (Winter 2000). For instance, qualitative studies suggest that bonding capital in working-class communities reveals strong intimate ties but people in such situations are also constrained in terms of what they can do and what they can think. Bridging and linking ties, which have currency in middle-class areas, are largely absent in working-class communities. This has implications for health and well-being if disadvantaged people do not have access to the opportunities that come with such ties. Future research into social capital in working-class communities needs to concentrate on exploring the bridging ties that do exist to see how they can be further enhanced as a resource for social benefits.

Quantitative work on social capital has often assumed homogeneity of people and place. However, it is apparent through qualitative research that social capital is a highly complex, multidimensional concept and is fundamentally affected by issues of gender, place and ethnicity. Being a man or a woman, and living in a particular place, present both opportunities and constraints on the sorts of social capital available. In this respect, it makes little sense to characterize whole communities as being 'high' or 'low' in social capital as this neglects addressing gendered, age and ethnic diversity and difference which clearly influence the relationship between social capital health and well-being. This cautionary note has implications for theoretical development and methodological application since:

> a healthy and effective community needs a blend of different types of social capital, just as a person needs a blend of different vitamins in their diet to be physically healthy. (Halpern 2005: 35)

Consequently, there needs to be much greater attention to fine-grained analyses of real people in real settings, and how they negotiate their everyday lives and relationships, health and well-being.

Social policy implications

Halpern (2005) argues that there is a strong case for governmental intervention to promote social capital as a positive 'public good'. This is especially so given that it is associated with nearly all the main policy objectives of modern societies and without state intervention the advantages of social capital will be unequally distributed in a population. There is a need to avoid past mistakes in policy whereby social capital was destroyed following slum clearance schemes in the 1960s. He suggests instead a range of policy innovations, which might bring people access to a variety of all types of social capital: bonding, bridging and linking. Such measures might include Sure Start projects to stimulate family bonding and interaction, neighbours sharing email networks and a system of transferable credits for voluntary carers of older people whereby rewards for tasks undertaken can be made use of in different parts of the country or later in life. However, as yet, the concept of social capital may be a little too underdeveloped to be translated directly into social policy.

The promotion of social capital in an area has been seen by policymakers as advantageous for health (White 2002) and often solutions are devised to the stipulations of outside professionals and without reference to local involvement (Sixsmith et al. 2001). In such cases, the absence of social capital can be construed as the fault of the community in failing to participate in community activities. There is a genuine danger here of 'victim blaming' in that those who find themselves economically and socially disadvantaged are blamed for their plight, despite being at the 'mercy of forces over which they have little control' (Blackshaw and Long 2005: 239). Whilst poverty, discrimination and deprivation may exert their negative influence through undermining stocks of social capital, simply bolstering communities' stocks of social capital is no panacea. Indeed, it could be argued that:

> emphasis on the role of social capital in enhancing health might divert attention away from the more urgent need to improve health through reducing income inequalities. Government or policy-makers might use the concept of social capital as a justification for retreating from relatively costly welfare measures. (Campbell et al. 1999: 27)

If the government is serious about reducing health inequalities and improving people's quality of life, there needs to be a genuine three-way partnership between people, local communities and the government (DoH, 1999). Social structures that cater for individual and social well-being and which empower people and local communities in the face of an increasingly centralising government agenda need to be strengthened. It is only when people, communities and the government work equally together that social policy can make a real positive change in people's health and well-being:

> Good health is fundamental to all of our lives. We all treasure our own health and the health of our families and friends. Good health

is the bedrock on which we build strong health, strong communities and a strong country. (DoH 1999: 1.9)

References

Anhier, H. and Kendall, J. (2002) 'Interpersonal Trust and Voluntary Associations: Examining Three Approaches'. *British Journal of Sociology*, 53(3): 343–63.

Arber, S. and Ginn, J. (eds) (1995) *Connecting Gender and Ageing: a Sociological Approach*. Buckingham: Open University Press.

Argyle, M. (1987) *The Psychology of Happiness*. London: Methuen.

Bankston, C. L. and Zhou, M. (2002) 'Social Capital as a Process: the Meanings and Problems of a Theoretical Metaphor', *Sociological Inquiry*, 72(2): 285–317.

Baum, F. (1999) 'Social Capital: Is It Good for Your Health? Issues for a Public Health Agenda', *Journal of Epidemiology and Community Health*, 53: 195–6.

Berkman, L., Glass, T., Brissette, I. and Seeman, T. (2000) 'From Social Integration to Health: Durkheim in the New Millennium', *Social Science & Medicine*, 51: 843–57.

Blackshaw, T. and Long, J. (2005) 'What's the Big Idea? A Critical Exploration of the Concept of Social Capital', *Leisure Studies*, 20(3): 239–58.

Blaxter, M. (2004) 'Questions and their Meanings in Social Capital Surveys', in A. Morgan and C. Swann (eds), *Social Capital for Health: Issues of Definition, Measurement and Links to Health*. London: Health Development Agency.

Blaxter, M. and Poland, F. (2002) 'Moving Beyond the Survey in Measuring Social Capital and Health', in C. Swann and A. Morgan (eds), *Social Capital for Health: Insights from Qualitative Research*. London: Health Development Agency.

Boneham, M. and Sixsmith, J. (2006) 'The Voices of Older Women in a Disadvantaged Community: Issues of Health and Social Capital', *Social Science & Medicine*, 62(2): 269–79.

Bourdieu, P. (1986) 'The Forms of Capital', in J. Richardson (ed.), *Handbook of Theory and Research for the Sociology of Education*. New York: Macmillan.

Brehm, J. and Rahn, W. (1997) 'Individual-level Evidence for the Causes and Consequences of Social Capital', *American Journal of Political Science*, 41(3): 999–1023.

Burt, R. (2002) 'Bridge Decay', *Social Networks*, 24(4): 333–63.

Campbell, C. and McClean, C. (2002) 'Social Capital, Exclusion and Health Factors Shaping African–Caribbean Participation in Local Community Networks', in C. Swann and A. Morgan (eds), *Social Capital for Health: Insights from Qualitative Research*. London: Health Development Agency.

Campbell, C., Wood, R. and Kelly, M. (1999) *Social Capital and Health*. London: Health Development Agency.

Carroll, D. (1992) *Health Psychology: Stress, Behaviour and Disease*. London: Falmer Press.

Cattell, V. and Herring, R. (2002) 'Social Capital, Generations and Health in East London', in C. Swann and A. Morgan (eds), *Social Capital for Health: Insights from Qualitative Research*. London: Health Development Agency.

Cohen, S. and Wills, T. (1985) 'Stress, Social Support and the Buffering Hypothesis', *Psychological Bulletin*, 98: 310–57.

Coleman, J. (1988) 'Social Capital in the Creation of Human Capital', *American Journal of Sociology*, 94: 95–120.

Cooper, H., Arber, S., Fee, L. and Ginn, J. (1999) *The Influence of Social Support and Social Capital on Health*. London: Health Development Agency.

Devine, F. and Roberts, J. M. (2003) 'Alternative Approaches to Researching Social Capital : a Comment on van Dethae's *Measuring Social Capital'*, *International Journal of Social Research Methodology*, 6(1): 93–100.

DoH (1999) *Saving Lives: Our Healthier Nation* (CM4386). London: Stationery Office.

Donavan, N. and Halpern, D. S. (2003) *Life Satisfaction: the State of Knowledge and Implications for Government*. Prime Minister's Strategy Unit. www.pm.gov.uk.

Durlauf, S. N. (2002) *'Bowling Alone*: a Review Essay', *Journal of Economic Behaviour and Organisation*, 47(3): 259–73.

Farrel, G. and Knight, J. (2003) 'Trust, Institutions and Institutional Change: Industrial Districts and the Social Capital Hypothesis', *Politics and Society*, 4(31): 537–66.

Fine, B. (2001) *Social Capital Theory versus Social Theory: Political Economy and Social Science at the Turn of the Millennium*. London: Routledge.

Fukuyama, F. (1995) 'Social Capital and the Global Economy', *Foreign Affairs*, 74(5): 89–103.

Gielen, A. C., McDonnell, K. A., Wu, A. W. and Faden, R. (2001) 'Quality of Life among Women living with HIV: the Importance of Violence, Social Support, and Self-care Behaviours', *Social Science and Medicine*, 52: 315–22.

Gillies, P. (1996) 'The Effectiveness of Alliance and Partnerships for Health Promotion', *Health Promotion International*, 13: 1–21.

Granovetter, M. (1973) 'The Strength of Weak Ties', *American Journal of Sociology*, 78: 1360–80.

Halpern, D. (2005) *Social Capital*. Cambridge: Polity Press.

Hanifan, L. J. (1916) 'The Rural School Community Centre' (*Annals of the American Academy of Political and Social Science*, 67: 130–8).

Kagan, C., Lawthom, R., Knowles, K. and Burton, M. (2000) Community Activism, Participation and Social Capital on a Peripheral Housing Estate', paper presented to European Community Psychology Conference, Bergen, Norway.

Kawachi, I., Kennedy, B., Lochner, K. and Prothrow-Stith, D. (1997) 'Social Capital, Income Inequality, and Mortality', *American Journal of Public Health*, 87(9): 1491–8.

Mackenbach, J. and Bakker, M. (eds) (2002) *Reducing Inequalities in Health: a European Perspective*. London: Routledge.

Molinas, J. R. (1998) 'The Impact of Inequality, Gender, External Assistance and Social Capital on Local-Level Cooperation', *World Development*, 26(3): 413–26.

Morgan, A. and Swann, C. (2004) *Social Capital for Health: Issues of Definition, Measurement and Links to Health*. London: Health Development Agency.

Morrow, V. (2000). ' "Dirty Looks" and "Trampy Places" in Young People's Accounts of Community and Neighbourhood', *Journal of Critical Public Health*, 10(2).

Morrow, V. (2002) 'Children's Experiences of "Community": Implications of Social Capital Discourses', in C. Swann and A. Morgan (eds), *Social Capital for Health: Insights from Qualitative Research*. London: Health Development Agency.

Morrow, V. (2003) 'Networks and Neighbourhoods: Children's Accounts of Friendship, Family and Place', in C. Phillipson, G. Allan and D. Morgan (eds),

Social Networks and Social Exclusion: Sociological and Policy Issues. Aldershot: Ashgate.

Moscovici, S. (1984) 'The Phenomenon of Social Representations', in R. Farr and S. Moscovici (eds), *Social Representations*. Cambridge: Cambridge University Press.

Nuissl, H. (2002) 'Elements of Trust: an Analysis of Trust – Concepts', *Berliner Journal für Sociology*, 12(1): 87–98.

Ong, B. (2000) 'Policy and Participation in the New NHS (12–15)', in *Improving Health through Community Participation*. London: Health Development Agency.

Portes, A. and Landolt, P. (1996) 'The Downside of Social Capital', *The American Prospect*, 26, May–June: 18–21.

Putnam, R. (1993) *Making Democracy Work: Civic Traditions in Modern Italy*. Princeton: Princeton University Press.

Putnam, R. (1995) 'Bowling Alone; America's Declining Social Capital', *Journal of Democracy*, 6(1): 65–79.

Putnam, R. (2000) *Bowling Alone*. New York: Simon & Schuster.

Rose, L. E., Campbell, J. and Kub, J. (2000) 'The Role of Social Support and Family Relationships in Women's Responses to Battering', *Health Care for Women International*, 21: 27–39.

Rose, R. (2000) 'How Much Does Social Capital Add to Individual Health? A Survey Study of Russians', *Social Science and Medicine*, 52: 1421–35.

Schuller, T., Baron, S. and Field, J. (2000) 'Social Capital: a Review and Critique', in S. Baron, J. Field and T. Schuller (eds), *Social Capital: Critical Perspectives*. Oxford: Oxford University Press: 1–38.

Scott, A. and Wenger, G. (1995) 'Gender and Social Support Networks in Later Life', in S. Arber and J. Ginn (eds), *Connecting Gender and Ageing*. Buckingham: Open University Press.

Scott, C. (1980) 'Interpersonal Trust: a Comparison of Attitudinal and Situational Factors', *Human Relations*, 11: 805–12.

Sixsmith, J. (2004) 'Young Men's Health and Group Participation: Participatory Research Gone Wrong?' *Clinical Psychology*, 43: 13–18.

Sixsmith, J. and Boneham, M. (2002a) 'Exploring Social Capital in Narrative Accounts of Life Transitions', *Auto/Biography*, 10(1&2): 123–30.

Sixsmith, J. and Boneham, M. (2002b) 'Men and Masculinities: Accounts of Health and Social Capital', in *Social Capital for Health: Insights into Qualitative Research*. London: Health Development Agency.

Sixsmith, J. and Boneham, M. (2003) 'Social Capital and the Voluntary Sector: the Case of Volunteering', *Voluntary Action*, 5(3): 47–60.

Sixsmith J. and Boneham M. (2004) 'Older Men's Participation in Community Life: Notions of Social Capital, Health and Empowerment', *Ageing International*, 28(4): 101–31.

Sixsmith, J., Boneham, M. and Goldring J. (2001) 'Accessing the Community: Gaining Insider Perspectives from the Outside', *Qualitative Health Research*, 1(3:4): 578–89.

Smith, T. (1997) 'Factors Relating to Misanthropy in Contemporary American Society', *Social Science Research*, 26: 170–96.

Staha, T., Rutten, A., Nutbeam, D., Bauman, A., Kannas, L., Abel, T., Luschen, G., Diaz, J. A., Rodriquez, J., Vinck, J. and van der Zee, J. (2001) 'The Importance of the Social Environment for Physically Active Lifestyle – Results from an International Study', *Social Science and Medicine*, 52: 1–10.

Usscher, J. (ed.) (2000) *Women's Health: Contemporary International Perspectives.* Leicester: BPS.

Veenstra, G. (2000) 'Social Capital, SES and Health: an Individual Level Analysis', *Social Science and Medicine*, 50: 619–29.

White, L. (2002) 'Connection Matters: Exploring the Implications of Social Capital and Social Networks for Social Policy', *Systems Research and Behavioural Science*, 19: 255–69.

Wilkinson, R. (1996) *Unhealthy Societies: the Afflictions of Inequality.* London: Routledge.

Wilkinson, R.G. (1997) 'Socioeconomic Determinants of Health: Health Inequalities: Relative or Absolute Material Standards?' *British Medical Journal*, 314: 591–4.

Winter, I. (2000) *Towards a Theorised Understanding of Family Life and Social Capital.* Working Paper No. 21. http://www.aifs.org.au/institute/pubs/WP21.html.

Woolcock, M. (2001) 'The Place of Social Capital in Understanding Economic and Social Outcomes', *Canadian Journal of Policy Research*, 2(1): 11–17.

5
Psychology in the Community

Carolyn Kagan and Amanda Kilroy

This chapter will outline the key principles of community psychology, look at how community well-being is understood, and explore the role of boundary critique as a means of developing critical awareness about community interventions designed to enhance well-being. A specific example of the evaluation of participatory arts projects will be used to examine one part of the process which was designed to examine boundaries between artists and researchers in order for the evaluation to proceed smoothly. The value of the concept of boundary critique will be considered as a means of examining ethical dilemmas when working to enhance well-being in the community.

Community psychology

Community psychology is a value-based practice that focuses its attention on those most marginalized by the social system (Burton and Kagan 2005). Leonard (1984: 180) defines social marginality as 'being outside the mainstream of productive activity and/or social reproductive activity'. This includes two groups: firstly, a relatively small group of people who are voluntarily marginal to the social order – new age travellers, certain religious sects, commune members, some artists, for instance; secondly, a much larger group: those who are involuntarily socially marginal. For the purposes of this chapter, it is the second group that we will be concerned with, particularly those who live in areas of multiple deprivation.

Kagan et al. (2005) summarize the underlying principles of a radical community psychological praxis as being: articulation of an explicit value base; use of ecological metaphor; adoption of a whole systems perspective; interdisciplinary working; understanding and working with

Table 5.1: Elements of a radical community psychological praxis (from Kagan and Burton 2001)

Element	Implication for community psychological praxis
A just society and its underpinning values	A just society is one that is underpinned by shared values of justice, stewardship and community, and these same values should underpin our community psychological practice
Ecological metaphor	Community psychology looks outside the individual for explanations of social experience and sometimes for solutions, whilst at the same time viewing people as agentic, purposeful beings
Whole systems perspectives	Community psychology, so long as it recognizes the contradictions inherent in systems perspectives, has the potential for enhancing the supportive features of some (elements) of the systems in the interests of the people and for identifying the causes of oppression.
Interdisciplinary	A radical community psychology practice would seek interdisciplinary understanding about how oppression is caused and maintained, and use this understanding as a guide to appropriate action
Dialectical relationship between people and systems	Community psychological praxis may provide opportunities for enhancing the creative, determining potential of people
People's consciousness	Community psychology must work as near to the people as possible, and in participation with them in order to challenge the status quo and achieve social change

the dialectical relationship between people and systems; and practices enhancing people's critical consciousness. Table 5.1 summarizes these principles and their implications for practice.

Well-being in and of community

Edge et al. (2004) suggest that, for some people, living poverty has continued for generations. For others, though, rapid economic change throws people into poverty and social marginalization. With social marginalization, identity and being are threatened. Charlesworth (2000) wrote a moving phenomenological account of working-class life in a former steel-manufacturing town in England that had, over a short space of time, undergone mill closures and consequent mass unemployment and loss of income. One of the local people in his book describes the hopelessness that such marginalization engenders:

> Ah get up some times an' it's just too much fo' mi, yer know, it creeps over yer, it just gets too much an' tha can't tek no mo'ore [...] It's heart breakin', it's just a strain all time an' tha just wants t' not live, tha just can't see n' point in thi' life. (Charlesworth 2000: 160)

Such hopelessness and despair clearly undermine well-being.

What is community well-being?

The concept of well-being *in* the community, and *of* the community is multifaceted. It variously includes those environmental factors that contribute to good standards of living, such as clean water, clean air and so on; demographic issues such as population decline or changes in divorce rates; economic issues such as poverty, loss of employment or income, or rapid social change leading to the development of new jobs; the provision and/or retrenchment of public services; educational opportunities and achievements; levels of crime and fear of crime; alcohol and drug use; significant life events; diet, food poverty and levels of obesity; perceived happiness, depression, stress and sense of fun.

Given the number of different aspects of well-being, it is not surprising that there are also numerous different means of assessing well-being in and of communities. Broadly, indicators of well-being focus on both objective and subjective assessments and use both quantitative and qualitative sources of information (Marks et al. 2004). They tap into material, social, economic, political, cultural and personal aspects of living. Figure 5.1 illustrates how different indicators map onto objectivity–subjectivity and qualitative–quantitative dimensions. The concept of community well-being is focused on understanding the contribution of a community in maintaining itself and fulfilling the various needs of local residents. This applies equally to well-being *in* and *of* the community. In the UK, recent legislation lays responsibility for community well-being at the feet of local authorities.

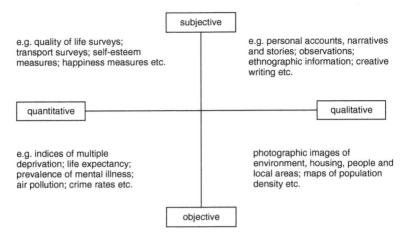

Figure 5.1: Dimensions of well-being in and of the community indicators

UK policy context for community well-being

In the UK, an Act of Parliament, the Local Government Act, 2000 (Part I) provided local authorities in England and Wales with a new power of 'well-being', which entitles them to do anything that might achieve:

- the promotion or improvement of the economic well-being of their area;
- the promotion or improvement of the social well-being of their area;
- the promotion or improvement of the environmental well-being of their area.

As a result, each authority has a *Community Strategy* outlining ways in which they will move to improve the economic, social and environmental well-being of their areas and contributing to the achievement of sustainable development in the UK. Indeed, the World Wildlife Fund (WWF) (2004: 2) suggest that, in the context of this power to promote or improve well-being, ' "Community well-being" is increasingly becoming synonymous with the term "sustainable development"'. This overlapping use of the two terms has led to an emphasis on environmental and economic factors, with the 'social' factors referring to the more objective aspects of cost-effective service delivery and objective indicators such as life expectancy and levels of crime. The role of perceived life satisfaction, sense of autonomy and purpose, happiness, stress and so on remains relatively under-developed, as is the link between objective indicators and subjective ones. Yet, it is *people* who are both the beneficiaries of and the means to achieving well-being, and it is essential to understand the complex relationship between other forms of development and personal and social development.

This is particularly so for people living in areas of (objective) multiple deprivation. The UK government produces Indices of Deprivation (ODPM 2004). Thus it is possible to uncover the relative, objective deprivation of local authorities, wards and parts of wards within these authorities. Yet, the subjective experience of living in areas with either high or low objective deprivation will often be different. Raschini et al. (2005:17) draw attention to this issue when they put objective indicators of deprivation alongside subjective assessment of quality of life (linked to, but not the same as well-being):

> Sometimes, residents seem to not be aware of the deprived conditions and their level as well as their effects on their lives. This lack of awareness may come from a lack of experience of different conditions. This may limit expectation and aspirations of the residents. After living for a long time in such areas, residents seem to not notice the signs and symptoms of deprivation existing in their areas and as a result they do not aim for better conditions of life. The national indices say that residents of those deprived areas die 10 years earlier than people living in other parts of the country although they report that their health is quite good. A high level of crime affects their neighbourhood but they say they are happy about it. They seem to be used to those conditions and to consider them normal. This attitude towards their reality probably influences the residents' attitude towards changing it. The involvement in the area's administrative decisions is consequently perceived as impossible or useless.

The relatively high perceived satisfaction in the midst of objective deprivation may be due to lack of comparisons with elsewhere, limiting ideas of what could be and thus of what is. Alternatively it might be that there is a real separation of subjective well-being from objective conditions of living. Thus there may be a need to help people develop a sense of collective identity and understanding of the social conditions in which they live; and for studies of well-being to include explorations of this. However, Shah and Peck (2005: 2) remind us, 'there is much more to life than satisfaction: people also want to be leading rich and fulfilling lives – developing their capabilities and fulfilling their potential'. They propose two dimensions of personal well-being:

- people's satisfaction with their lives, which is generally measured by indicators which capture satisfaction, pleasure and enjoyment;
- people's personal development, which includes being engaged in life, curiosity, 'flow', personal development and growth, autonomy, fulfilling potential, having a purpose in life and feeling that life has meaning.

For people to lead truly flourishing lives they need to feel they are personally satisfied and developing.

For Shah and Peck, then, eudaimonic well-being (personal development and fulfilment) is as important as hedonic well-being (satisfaction and happiness) (see Ryan and Deci 2001 for a discussion of the two approaches). Indeed this two-dimensional approach to personal well-being forms the core of an influential *well-being manifesto for a flourishing society* (Shah and Marks 2004).

A community psychological perspective, however, would suggest that both the hedonic and eudaimonic well-being of people who are socially excluded, are inseparable from not only their economic position, the environmental conditions in which they live and the political and ideological messages that confine them to poverty whilst enjoining them to break free and better themselves, but also from the human services that exist to both assist and to regulate them. (See Burton and Kagan 2006 for discussion of how human service policy plays this paradoxical role in relation to learning disability services.) In other words, well-being in and of communities must be viewed in terms of human systems, not just as individual responses to circumstances.

Experience of poverty, social deprivation, health inequality and restricted life chances in the UK are seen, in policy terms, as part of analyses of social exclusion. The current administration (Blair's government) established early in its first term a Social Exclusion Unit which oversees different strategies and interventions designed to reduce exclusion and increase inclusion (mostly in the labour market, but also in terms of participation in civil society). Few attempts have been made to explore the interconnections between these programmes and hedonic and eudaimonic well-being, and those that have, are not encouraging (Huxley et al. 2004).

The arts have been identified as one important determinant of well-being, with the potential to contribute to greater health, well-being and social inclusion for marginalized people, particularly those with enduring and common mental health problems (see, for example, Huxley and Thornicroft 2003; SEU 2004, White 2004; HDA 2000; Long et al. 2002). We have been exploring the impact of participation in the arts on health and well-being from a community psychological perspective (Sixsmith and Kagan 2005). We have, therefore, adopted an ecological approach, viewing individual hedonic and eudaimonic well-being as part of a wider, more complex social system. We have drawn on critical systems thinking (CST) in our work on evaluation (Boyd et al. 2001) and will discuss one aspect of this, namely boundary critique.

Evaluation of participatory arts and well-being

Eleven different kinds of arts projects which included people from children to elders at risk of social exclusion through poor mental health and well-being, involving nine different artists, were evaluated. The brief was to examine how participation in arts projects leads to changes in well-being and mental health and to make recommendations for project improvement. The evaluations were to involve close collaboration between the artists and researchers.[1] Early on, a number of boundary disputes became clear:

- artists and researchers disagreed about the risk posed to participants if they were to be involved in the evaluation participatively;
- artists and researchers (and project managers and commissioners) disagreed about the need for and purpose of evaluation, contributing to a reluctance to collaborate;
- artists and researchers had different agendas for the evaluation, leading to mistrust and conflict;
- artists and researchers had different ways of understanding well-being, which led to an inability to agree how best to conceptualize well-being and describe it within the evaluation;
- artists and researchers placed different values on the importance of mental health and its amelioration within the projects, which meant that agreement could not be reached about how to assess the impact of the arts work on mental health as well as well-being;
- artists and researchers disagreed about the relative importance of the aesthetic product and the processes of creation and creativity

used within the projects, which meant that agreement could not be reached about a relevant evaluation framework;
- artists and researchers had different understanding of the relative merits of different kinds of data and the best ways of collecting them, leading to a paralysis of the research process;
- the need to proceed quickly as the projects were already in operation when the evaluation began meant that there were limited opportunities to build capacity of the artists for data collection and trust within the research team, affecting mutual understanding and trust.

As the artists were all freelance, the time available to work through these issues with researchers was limited. Although we had tried to explore the issues through meetings, it was clear that the very nature of the boundary disputes meant that just talking about them strengthened the impasse we were in. Unless we were able to do something about the situation, we would not be in a position to examine how participation in the arts projects affected well-being, and we would not be in a position to undertake the evaluation with any sense of well-being within the team.

At this stage it was decided to use a process specifically to make explicit and negotiate boundary issues between researchers and artists, prior to proceeding. Before any further data were collected, an appreciative inquiry (AI) (Cooperrider 1995) workshop was held, involving artists and researchers, along with some facilitators external to this specific evaluation. An AI approach was chosen to encourage from the outset of the inquiry a deeper and more meaningful means of communication.

Appreciative inquiry workshop

Appreciative inquiry (AI) describes the co-evolutionary search for the best in people, their organizations, and the relevant world around them. It involves systematic discovery of what gives 'life' to a living system, in this case the collaborative evaluation. Its aim is to ask questions that strengthen a system's capacity to apprehend, anticipate and heighten positive potential, and the process deliberately seeks to work from accounts of this 'positive change core' (Cooperrider and Whitney 1999). AI seeks to discover people's exceptionality – their unique gifts, strengths and qualities and it is based on principles of equality of voice – everyone is asked to speak about their vision of the true, the good and the possible (Cooperrider 2001).

AI has four clear stages:

- Discovery – Discovering shared values and exploring experience
- Dream – Envisioning the future
- Design – Designing what needs to be done
- Destiny – Clarity about goals and aspirations

The workshop participants began the discovery process by conducting in-depth interviews about experience of art and participative work, initially in artist–researcher pairs. This encouraged each person to gain a different view of their partner, outside of their professional role, through a positive lens, as the conversations largely sought to engage and reveal the passions and core values of the individuals involved.

Following the AI process of discovery, each participant shared a story from their interview record, and other members of the group made a note of what was important to them about the account. The collective group then organized the resultant themes into clusters which served to indicate areas of interest, conflict or aspects of the vision of the way forward (dream stage). After further facilitated discussion around specific and practical issues for the evaluation (design stage), the work-shop ended with mixed groups of researchers and artists using props and materials to devise a way of symbolizing the evaluation of arts and well-being creatively. Thus as the workshop began with artists using researcher tools, it ended with researchers using artists' tools to further collaborative and critical understanding.

The emergent themes were useful in highlighting the different inherent values, assumptions and knowledge held by artists and researchers, largely around the nature of well-being and how to identify and assess it. The themes included: control and commitment; roles; visions; and values.

Control and commitment

From the start there was a natural inclination and preference to want to use the process to air grievances and to look at 'negative experiences' to 'provide insight as to what needed to be worked on'. Clearly there were issues in the group that challenged the success of the evaluation. There was some confusion about 'what to take on board', and the group shared concerns about the level of commitment to the evaluation that each party had or should have.

Fears were expressed about the degree to which artists should remain in control of the evaluation, and that doing the artwork, trying to remain creative in the face of focusing on evaluation, often felt like being in two different head spaces. There was a sense that being fully involved was 'too much responsibility'. There was also a sense that boundaries between artists and researchers were blurring and that this created a lack of clarity about who was supposed to do what, which in turn generated anxiety and resistance. In addition, the perceived weight of expectation from both funders and evaluators created an experience of pressure for the artists in the group, who felt they had to 'be like magicians' and 'do all things well'. This response was surprising to the researchers who had intended their presence and the process to be perceived as supportive, participatory and empowering, enhancing the well-being of all concerned.

Roles

The purpose and roles of each party in the evaluation and the nature of the boundaries between those roles emerged as a central theme. There were discussions around the perceptions of 'elitism' from both artists and researchers, and also the need to 'make elite activities accessible'. Accessibility seemed to involve having a deeper appreciation of the role of the other and the degree to which each would move into the world of the other, to know the language, values and assumptions of that role and to understand it. The assumptions that the researchers would be detached, 'clinical' evaluators, and that artists were not open to learning were surfaced and shifts to becoming more involved on behalf of the researchers and more enquiring on behalf of the artists were identified.

The discomfort with shifting roles and responsibilities brought up difficulties around how best to do this, with a common focus on well-being, and concerns that doing this might erode each person's 'real' role and purpose. This in turn brought up questions around the relationships between the two groups, and the nature of their relationships with the project participants. Discussion revolved around whether the participants were to be considered as participants or artists, and questions arose as to what that difference meant. Artists saw participants as fellow artists, whereas researchers saw them more as beneficiaries (in terms of enhanced mental health and well-being) of the participatory arts process.

As the AI process progressed, each group moved closer towards shifting their position and perspectives as greater appreciation of the respective roles grew. This shift emerged as much from the incorporation of creative activities, which brought about a great deal of bonding within creative effort. Making connections and sharing experiences between artists and evaluators was seen as a potent tool for change, and helped them all develop a clearer idea of what well-being might mean in the context of evaluation of participatory arts practice. Bringing together artists and researchers also led to agreement that the practical and administrative aspects of each project were important and that evaluation could, indeed, proceed within a culture of learning (eudaimonic well-being) and enjoyment.[2]

Shared vision

The workshop led to agreement about what the team meant by well-being and how it could, perhaps, be operationalized within the projects. What the team wanted to do was to learn how to 'show the power of art to change' and to demonstrate benefits such as the sense 'that people are stronger within' as a result of participation. It was agreed that change 'needs to come from the person themselves', who could be 'encouraged to set their own start and end points in their process and the potential outcomes', where change was to be clearly recognizable and perhaps measurable. Change arose where the person 'felt free to be themselves' which brought a 'sense of belonging' and where they could 'have fun' with the process.

Components of change and enhanced well-being that were agreed upon included: sharing of experiences; increases in self-worth; feeling able to make life decisions; gains in confidence; examples of people taking control of their situations leading them to being more motivated and positive, and enabling them to do things like finding a job, going to school or planning education. What was clear was that in order to make that happen for the participants the group needed to find that *within* and *for* themselves.

Shared values

As a result of the process, from starting as individuals with fixed and in some cases fearful viewpoints, the collective group were able to identify their common values and move towards a shared vision, thus realizing individual, relational and collective well being. The emergent vision arising from the new atmosphere of co-operation and appreciation, was for generating a safe space where each individual could come together within a shared framework to explore what was happening. This space was described as housing a thriving culture – central to which was a strong team that held a shared perspective and had shared values. Core values were expressed as being those of trust, empowerment and openness, thus generating a culture of collective learning and commitment. The safe environment of the workshop had enabled both artists and researchers to identify their passion for the work. As a result of engaging with that passion they would be more inclined to produce something meaningful through evaluation that would communicate well-being in a way that would touch people (and not just provide information) so that the resulting awareness could shift people to a different level.

The workshop enabled the concept of well-being to be explored and understood, both in terms of the projects themselves and their effects and the evaluation. Within the workshop, the process of boundary critique had been employed as a vehicle for arriving at this consensual position.

Concept of boundary and boundary critique

Ulrich (2000, 2003) offers a detailed challenge to the idea that the boundaries of any system are given and linked to 'social reality'. Instead, he argues that boundaries are social or personal constructs, defining the limits of knowledge relevant to any particular analysis. He argues that a critical stance on everyday social practices, including specific interventions (such as the arts projects) poses basic boundary problems that are linked to motivation (whose interests are/ought to be served, what is/ought to be the purpose of the intervention, how is/ought improvement in well-being to be measured); sources of power (who is/ought to be able to decide how well-being is to be measured and what resources do these decision-makers hold); sources of knowledge (who is/ought to be considered to be the expert and what is/ought to be their expertise, who is/ought to be the person to ensure recommendations are implemented); sources of legitimation (who is/ought to be reflecting the interests of those who do and may benefit in the future from the project in the future; what is/ought to be the overall vision for improvement for those affected by the project). Of central concern early on in our project were questions of definition and measurement of mental health and well-being; predictions of what might change and why; how changes might be measured; how success would be defined. Thus the boundary dilemmas were in the main in the areas of motivation, power and knowledge. Artists, researchers, project commissioners, health service staff all had different views on these matters. Before the project could proceed, some exploration of the a priori assumptions both artists and researchers were making was necessary. Had we failed to address our divergences, any evaluation and associated recommendations would have been rejected. Indeed, it would probably not have been possible to work collaboratively with the artists at all. As Ulrich says:

> The facts we observe, and the way we evaluate them, depend on how we bound the system of concern. Different value judgements can make us change boundary judgements, which in turn makes the facts look different. Knowledge of new facts can equally make us change boundary judgements, which in turn makes previous evaluations look different, etc. (1998: 6)

In the practice of boundary critique, Ulrich (2000) distinguishes between three arenas of critique within action projects:

1. Self-reflective boundary questioning requires us to ask *What are my boundary judgements?*
2. Dialogical boundary questioning requires us to ask *Can we agree on our boundary judgements?*
3. Controversial boundary questioning requires us to ask *Don't you claim too much?*

The AI workshops enabled all three arenas to be addressed.

Beyond Ulrich's notion of boundary judgements, Churchman (1970) argues that what is to be included or excluded for any analysis of a situation is a vital consideration. Something that appears to be relevant to overall project improvement (Churchman's definition of intervention) given a narrowly defined boundary, may not be seen as relevant at all if the boundaries are pushed out. Thus the outcome of the boundary explorations through the AI process may have been different if actual or potential participants, or commissioners of projects, had been involved. We did, in fact, want participants to be present, but this idea was premature. At this point in time, there was insufficient trust of the researchers by the artists, and insufficient understanding on the part of researchers for the boundary to be extended or renegotiated. Nevertheless, the possibility remains that the workshop would have resulted in different outcomes had different participants been there.

Conclusions

The upshot of resolving boundary dilemmas through an AI workshop in this project, led to a particular way of viewing well-being.

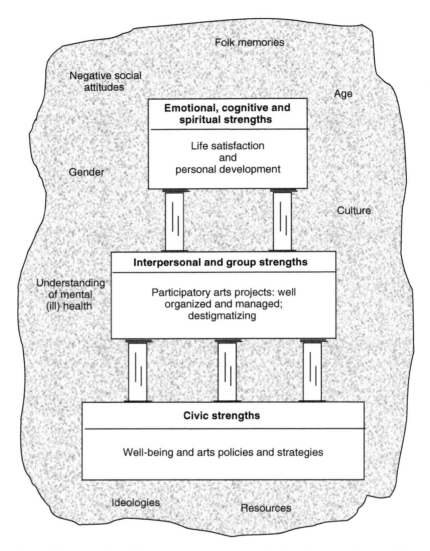

Figure 5.2: Personal well-being supported by participation in arts projects within a wider social context

Figure 5.2 illustrates how personal well-being is supported through participation in arts. Well-being was understood as personal well-being, but within a social context of relationships, personal agency and personal development. However, the role of social attitudes and destigmatizing practices (particularly in the form of a public exhibition arising from the work in the projects) was recognized as an important part of the context. Resources available to the project and overall management of the projects were also identified as having indirect impacts on personal well-being. The particular boundary judgements made excluded detailed consideration of a wider social context to people's well-being in terms of wider policies and ideological forces affecting the health system of which the projects were a part. Most importantly within this wider context is the focus on the individual as the agent of her or his own well-being. Nevertheless, within community settings, we assert the importance of understanding both hedonic and eudomonic well-being within a complex social system at individual, relational and collective levels, always saturated by different boundary judgements which have the potential to be explored, and thereby enabling us to maintain a stance of critical awareness (Midgley et al. 1998: 467).

Notes

1. The research team was brought in well after the projects had begun. Whilst the preference of the research team was to involve fully participants in the design and execution of the evaluation, artists argued convincingly that this would be inappropriate, thus establishing a clear collaboration boundary, limiting from the outset the possibilities for the evaluation (see Churchman 1970 for further discussion).
2. It was clear that lack of time for planning at the outset of the project had meant that there had not been the time to develop relationships, explore and agree boundaries and frameworks for practice, and that this had led to an environment and culture of diminished individual, relational and collective well-being.

References

Boyd, A., Geerling, T., Gregory, W., Midgley, G., Murray, P., Walsh, M. and Kagan, C. (2001) *Capacity Building for Evaluation: Report to the Manchester, Salford and Trafford Health Action Zone.* Hull: University of Hull.

Burton, M. and Kagan, C. (2005) 'Marginalization', in G. Nelson and I. Prilleltensky (eds), *Community Psychology: In Pursuit of Liberation and Well-Being.* London: Palgrave Macmillan: 293–308.

Burton, M. and Kagan, C. (2006) 'Decoding "Valuing People"', *Disability and Society*, 21, 4: 299–313.

Charlesworth, S. J. (2000) *A Phenomenology of Working Class Experience.* Cambridge: Cambridge University Press.

Churchman, W. (1970) 'Operations Research as a Profession', *Management Science*, 17: B37–53.

Cooperrider, D. L. (1995) 'Introduction to Appreciative Inquiry', in W. French and C. Bell (eds), *Organization Development* (5th edn). Englewood Cliffs, NJ: Prentice Hall.

Cooperrider, D. L. (2001) 'Why Appreciative Inquiry?', in S. A. Hammond and C. Royal (eds), *Lessons from the Field: Applying Appreciative Inquiry*. Plano, TX: Thin Book Publishing.

Cooperrrider, D. L. and Whitney, D. (1999) 'Appreciative Inquiry: a Positive Revolution in Change', in P. Holman and T. Devane (eds), *The Change Handbook: Group Methods for Shaping the Future*. San Francisco: Berrett-Koehler.

Edge, I., Kagan, C. and Stewart, A. (2004) 'Living Poverty: Surviving on the Edge', *Clinical Psychology*, 38: 28–31.

HDA (2000) *Art for Health: a Review of Good Practice in Community-based Arts Projects and Initiatives which Impact on Health and Well-Being*. London: Health Development Agency.

Huxley P., Evans, S., Leese, M., Gately, C., Rogers, A., Thomas, R., and Robson, B. (2004) 'Urban Regeneration and Mental Health', *Social Psychiatry Psychiatric Epidemiology*, 39(4): 280–5.

Huxley, P., and Thornicroft, G. (2003), 'Social Inclusion, Social Quality and Mental Illness', *British Journal of Psychiatry*, 182: 289–90.

Kagan, C. and Burton, M. (2001) *Critical Community Psychological Practice for the 21st Century*. Manchester: IOD Research Group.

Kagan, C., Duckett, P., Lawthom, R. and Burton, M. (2005) 'Community Psychology and Disabled People', in D. Goodley and R. Lawthom (eds), *Disability and Psychology: Critical Introductions and Reflections*. Basingstoke: Palgrave Macmillan.

Leonard, P. (1984) *Ideology and Personality: Towards a Materialist Understanding of the Individual*. Basingstoke: Macmillan.

Long, J., Welch, M., Bramham, P., Butterfield, J., Hylton, K. and Lloyd, E. (2002) *Count Me In: the Dimensions of Social Inclusion through Culture and Sport*. Leeds: Leeds Metropolitan University.

Marks, N., Shah, H. and Westall, A. (2004) *The Power and Potential of Well-Being Indicators: Measuring Young People's Well-Being in Nottingham*. London: New Economics Foundation. http://www.neweconomics.org/gen/well-being. Retrieved 10 October 2005.

Midgley, G., Munro, I. and Brown, M. (1998) 'The Theory and Practice of Boundary Critique: Developing Housing Services for Older People', *Journal of the Operational Research Society*, 49: 467–78.

ODPM (2004) Indices of Deprivation. Office Deputy Prime Minister, UK government. http://www.odpm.gov.uk/index.asp?id=1128439. Retrieved 22 January 2006.

Raschini, S., Stewart, A. and Kagan, C. (2005) *Community Activists' Accounts of Their Activism*. Manchester: RIHSC.

Ryan, R. M. and Deci, E. L. (2001) 'On Happiness and Human Potentials: a Review of Research on Hedonic and Eudaimonic Well-Being', *Annual Review of Psychology*, 52: 141–66.

SEU (2004) *Mental Health and Social Exclusion*. London: ODPM, Social Exclusion Unit.

Shah, H. and Marks, N. (2004) *A Well-Being Manifesto for a Flourishing Society*. London, New Economics Foundation. http://www.neweconomics.org. Retrieved 12 January 2006.

Shah, H. and Peck, J. (2005) *Well-Being and the Environment: Achieving One Planet Living and Quality of Life*. London, New Economics Foundation. http://www. neweconomics.org/gen/z_sys_publicationdetail.aspx?pid=214. Retrieved 22 January 2006.

Sixsmith, J. and Kagan, C. (2005) 'Art makes me feel I have resources, otherwise untapped'. *Final Pathways Evaluation Report*. Manchester: RIHSC.

Ulrich, W. (1998) *Systems Thinking as if People Mattered: Critical Systems Thinking for Citizens and Managers. Working Paper No. 23*. Lincoln: Lincoln School of Management.

Ulrich, W. (2000) 'Reflective Practice in the Civil Society: the Contribution of Critically Systemic Thinking', *Reflective Practice*, 1(2): 247–68. Pre-publication version of W. Ulrich, *Critical Heuristics for Social Planning: a New Approach to Practical Philosophy*. Berne: Haupt.

Ulrich, W. (2003) *Pragmatizing Critical Systems Thinking for Professionals and Citizens*. www.geocities.com/csh_home/cst_pragmatizing.html. Retrieved 16 August 2004.

White, M. (2004) 'Arts in Mental Health for Social Inclusion: Towards a Framework for Programme Evaluation', in J. Cowling (ed.), *For Arts Sake: Society and the Arts in the 21st Century*. London: IPPR.

WWF (World Wildlife Fund) (2004) *Why Sustainable Development is Important for Local Authorities and their Partners*. London: WWF-UK. http://sites.wwflearning. co.uk. Retrieved 22 January 2006.

6
Art, Health and Well-Being

This chapter consists of two parts, by different authors, each invited to contribute independently to a chapter on 'Art, Health and Well-Being'. David Haley in Part 1 argues that an expanded dynamic notion of art could provide the creative dialogue needed to value disparate readings of well-being. Peter Senior in Part 2 summarizes the important part played to date by the arts for health in the UK and elsewhere.

Part 1: Is well-being worth dying for?
David Haley

A conclusion

In the foyer of Manchester's imposing neo-Gothic Town Hall there is a monumental plaque dedicated to the men and women from the Greater Manchester area who fought against fascism in Spain:

> Mothers! Women! When the years pass by and the wounds of war are staunched, when the cloudy memory of the sorrowful, bloody days returns in a present of freedom, love and well-being, when the feelings of rancour dying away and when pride in a free country is felt equally by all Spaniards then speak to your children. Tell them of the International Brigades. Tell them how coming over seas and mountains, crossing frontiers bristling with bayonets, and watched for by ravening dogs thirsty to tear at their flesh, these

men reached our country as crusaders for freedom. They gave up everything, their homes, their country, home and fortune, fathers and mothers, wives, brothers, sisters and children and they came and told us: we are here, your cause, Spain's cause, is ours. It is the cause of all advanced and progressive mankind. Today they are going away. Many of them, thousands of them, are staying here with the Spanish earth for their shroud, and all Spaniards remember them with the deepest feeling .... We shall not forget you and when the olive tree of peace puts forth its leaves again mingled with the laurels of the Spanish Republic's victory, come back!

La Pasionaria
Barcelona
November 15th 1938

It is interesting to note the phrase, '...in a present of freedom, love and well-being...' – first, the assumption in 1938 that at some point in the future freedom, love and well-being would together prevail and secondly, that these were values worth dying for and indeed represent, 'the cause of all advanced and progressive mankind'. Time has told us the way these utopian ideals were played out in the concentration camps, on the battlefields and the killing fields of history. It is also worth noting that the Spanish Civil War generated two of the most enduring, iconic images of the twentieth century – Pablo Picasso's *Guernica* and Robert Capa's photograph of a shot Spanish soldier, falling, rifle held high. The arts seem to be the only means of making the particular archetypal, and thereby conveying the horrors of war meaningfully.

But most Westerners would argue that things have got better since then. The general standard of living has certainly improved since 1938 – most people, it seems, are more concerned with cheap holidays and managing their credit facilities than malnutrition and affording a pair of shoes. People are living longer, child mortalities have dropped dramatically and the big diseases like smallpox, polio, diphtheria, whooping cough and tuberculosis are relatively rare. And as for art, well, each year we hear of another major gallery, museum or theatre opening, and each year these venues announce record attendances.

So, art, health and well-being appear to be doing well. Or are they? Nearly sixty years after the Spanish Civil War, the United Nations claims to uphold the virtues and the moral right of each human being to be able to attain them. Yet, as Nelson Mandela pointed out in the World

Health Organization's publication, *The Right to Water* (2003), such ideals may be considered by some to be a luxury, rather than a necessity: 'Freedom alone is not enough without light to read at night, without time or access to water to irrigate your farm, without the ability to catch fish to feed your family.'[1]

Article 25 of the Universal Declaration of Human Rights (1948) states: 'Everyone has the right to a standard of living adequate for the health and well-being of himself and his family.'[2] The UN Millennium Development Goals[3] add specific, utilitarian values to otherwise general and idealized notions of well-being:

1. Eradicate extreme poverty and hunger
2. Achieve universal primary education
3. Promote gender equality and empower women
4. Reduce child mortality
5. Improve maternal health
6. Combat HIV/AIDS, malaria and other diseases
7. Ensure environmental sustainability
8. Develop a global partnership for development

This may seem like an unusual place to start a discussion on the relation between art, health and well-being, but it is necessary to establish the context in which this combination may exist. Few would challenge health and well-being as essential elements to include in any list of quality of life indicators. But if art is excluded from the equation, we run the risk of making a similar mistake to the 1992 Rio Summit when it established the 'three pillars' of sustainable development: social, economic and environmental. So (to continue the metaphor), if we consider the function of a lintel linking those pillars, this would be 'culture' – the connecting agent necessary to deliver the other factors for environmental sustainability and well-being. And indeed, it may be argued that an expanded dynamic notion of art could provide the creative dialogue needed to value disparate readings of well-being.

But according to the philosopher W. B. Gallie (1956), art, freedom and democracy mean different things to different people and are 'essentially contested'.[4] These and other concepts, such as well-being and health, cannot therefore be defined in terms of formal, analytical philosophy. George Lakoff and Mark Johnson, in *Philosophy in the Flesh: the Embodied Mind and its Challenge to Western Thought* (1999), however, argue 'for an experientially responsible philosophy, one that incorporates results concerning the embodiment of mind, the cognitive unconscious, and metaphysical thought'.[5] The following text will, therefore, explore some aspects of art, health and well-being to try to understand how they may resonate with each other to generate understandings of what a 'better quality of life' might be.

Notions of art as well-being

The UK government increasingly uses the term 'well-being' in catch-all phrases like 'contributing to enjoyment, general well-being, as well as to education and health', to express a kind of generally benevolent set of values. But while there are departments dealing with Health, Education, Art and even 'enjoyment' (Culture, Media and Sport), there is none that deals directly with 'well-being'. Similar to the terms 'sustainable development', 'partnerships' and 'social inclusion', the term 'well-being' has become an amorphous, meaningless phrase, yet, as a part of common language it contributes to our normative frames of reference.

For the past forty years or so, societies in the developed world have been preoccupied with myopic concepts of regeneration, and a public art associated with corporate branding. Meaningful planning, like sustainable development and 'art in the public interest',[6] seems to be largely lost to cynicism. Now, perhaps as a synthesis of the concepts of 'new genre public art',[7] artists are developing practices to engage society and ecology at the scale and with the strategies of spatial planning. This may provoke a paradigm shift from dystopia and contribute to a deeper societal well-being.

So, if the original meaning of the word art ('rt' from the *Rg Vedas*) was the continuing creation of the cosmos, virtuously, then we may understand the potential for the arts to practise things other than the production of commodities for a niche, value added, consumer market. The word *rt* retains its meaning in modern Hindi, but as it passed into ancient Greek (*arête*) the use diversified and became the etymological root of words like architecture, arithmetic, rite, ritual, right, write as well as art – virtuous ways of making and understanding the world, and creating beautifully if you will. This moral imperative refers to a dynamic cosmic correctness, an order and process integral to art, health and well-being. We may even recognize the embodied need for all organisms to engage with their evolutionary development and participate in creative processes.

In human terms these needs are articulated through the arts to provide diverse forms that facilitate the many narratives and understandings of the many strategies that maintain our evolutionary interconnectedness.

Denial of this embodied ecology and these therapeutic activities can be experienced as chronic forms of personal, community and societal neuroses – an intrinsic lack of well-being.

Metaphorically, well-being may be restored in the form of a river, dissolving the conflicts between nature and culture in dialogical processes, where the many may participate in the making of their society – an ecocentric culture, immune system or 'social sculpture'.

Unpacking some problems with well-being

Western societies continue to be dominated by industrial and economic value systems. These systems not only affect the material aspects of our lives, they pervade our language, philosophy and belief systems – what we consider to be normal, moral and real. The situation is compounded by the evolutionary folk myth, 'survival of the fittest', that gives credence to the dominant culture – 'it's got to be right and good, because we say it's right and good, and if you don't agree, then you are wrong and bad'.

A further way in which this culture dominates is of course through education and in particular, rationally justifiable, deterministic, 'problem-based learning' (PBL). Problem-based learning is designed to empower experts to analyse and solve, diagnose and heal. The world and well-being are reduced to cause and effect 'problematics'.

Here the problem starts with the assumed ability and right to go into the world to solve other people's problems – it's an extension of cultural imperialism, as the premise starts with the assumption that 'we who are good and right must solve what is bad and wrong'. Of course, the lack of any real problem renders our abilities redundant, so problems must be identified in anything that does not fit our norms and morals – thus applying a rational approach to what is an irrational situation. Regarding morality and rationality, Lakoff and Johnson state that:

> Real human reason is embodied, mostly imaginative and metaphorical, largely unconscious, and emotionally engaged. It is often about human well-being and about ends determined by human well-being. Since morality concerns well-being and since our conceptions of morality arise from our models of well-being, morality enters into human reason most of the time. It not only affects the choice of ends, but also the kinds of reasoning done in achieving those ends. Rationality almost always has a major moral dimension. The idea that human rationality is purely mechanical, disengaged, and separable

from moral issues is a myth, a myth that is harmful when we live our lives according to it.[8]

An alternative to this PBL scenario might be something called 'question-based learning'. Here the premise is that we don't know, and that we have to listen and learn from a situation before acting. This approach informs a constantly evolving notion of well-being, achieved as a dynamic creative process. But what are the benefits of engaging the world in this way? First, the development of a 'transformative reflective practice' – something more akin to art than engineering or science. And secondly, an expanded, diverse notion of well-being.

So how may this paradigm shift be achieved? David Bohm, the celebrated quantum physicist, proposed that:

> a form of free dialogue may well be one of the most effective ways of investigating the crisis which faces society, and indeed the whole of human nature and consciousness today. Moreover, it may turn out that such a form of free exchange of ideas and information is of fundamental relevance for transforming culture and freeing it of destructive misinformation, so that creativity can be liberated.[9]

Indeed, that creativity is what the pre-eminent ecological artists Helen Mayer Harrison and Newton Harrison refer to when they talk of 'creating the conditions for improvisation and invention'.[10] While referencing society's inability to accept uncertainty in a quantum world, they consider the potential for art to be a strategy for surviving climate change, 'gracefully'.[11]

Embodied ecology and 'biofilia'

We may, therefore, develop opportunities for people to participate in art that also engages ecology – creating relationships between organisms – within their environment. Our immune system promotes well-being by facilitating dynamic relationships with other diverse organisms, thereby maintaining our integrated connection to our environment – that environment is therefore perceived to be harmonious and beneficial – a form of symbiosis that dissolves ego in the need for interdependence. Lakoff and Johnson bring these ideas together very eloquently:

> The environment is not an 'other' to us. It is not a collection of things that we encounter. Rather, it's part of our being. It is the locus

of our being and identity. We cannot and do not exist apart from it. It is through empathetic projection that we come to know our environment, understand how we are part of it and how it is part of us. This is the bodily mechanism by which we can participate in nature, not just as hikers or climbers or swimmers, but as part of nature itself, part of a larger, all-encompassing whole. A mindful embodied spirituality is thus an ecological spirituality.

An embodied spirituality requires an aesthetic attitude to the world that is central to self-nurturance, to the nurturance of others, and the nurturance of the world itself. Embodied spirituality requires an understanding that nature is not inanimate and less than human, but animated and more than human. It requires pleasure, joy in the bodily connection with earth and air, sea and sky, plants and animals – and the recognition that they are all more than human, more than any human beings could ever achieve. Embodied spirituality is more than experience. It is an ethical relationship to the physical world.

But emphatic connection to the world is only one dimension of spirituality that the body makes possible. It is the body that makes spiritual existence passionate, that brings to it intense desire and pleasure, pain, delight, and remorse. Without all these things, spirituality is bland. In the world's spiritual transitions, sex and art and music and dance and the taste of food have been for millennia forms of spiritual experience just as much as ritual practice, meditation and prayer.[12]

So too, our engagement with 'nature'.

In November 2005, the *British Medical Journal* published findings of the first randomized, single blind, controlled trial of animal facilitated therapy with dolphins, for people suffering from depression. The authors wrote in their study findings, 'The natural setting itself is also an important factor that has to be considered in the treatment of emotional disorders. This is confirmed by other studies.' The effects exerted by the animals were significantly greater than those of just the natural setting, they added. 'The echolocation system, the aesthetic value, and the emotions raised by the interaction with dolphins may explain the mammals' healing properties.'[13]

The researchers, from the division of clinical psychiatry at the University of Leicester Medical School, noted that the study supports the theory of 'biophilia', which contends that human health and well-being is dependent on the human connection with the natural world. Marine biologist Commodore Jacques Cousteau expresses his love for water and the profound sense of well-being it can evoke:

> My body floated weightlessly through space, the water took possession of my skin, the clear outlines of marine creatures had something almost provocative, and economy of movement acquired moral significance. Gravity – I saw it in a flash – was the original sin, committed by the first living beings who left the sea. Redemption could come only when we returned to the ocean as already the sea mammals have done.[14]

Arts, mental health and well-being

Contemporary Western art has its own problems, not least the claims of art for art's sake, the perpetuation of the genius myth and art as value added commodity. However, many Eastern cultures and 'undeveloped' peoples still maintain 'art as everyday life'. Here art is integral to the way everything is done and is not separated from religion, work, food production and rites of passage.

One of the criteria our society might use to define people from an 'ethnic' culture would be the popular practice of 'folk arts' – arts participation as integral to daily life. To disconnect these people from their 'art', or to make them self-conscious and precious about these activities is to undermine their normal pattern of behaviour and separate them from a 'language' that connects them to 'natural' phenomena and processes. This culture shock is experienced by a number of immigrants living in developed Western countries. Most people who are born into Western culture adapt to the normative effects of not living embodied arts or ecological lives; however, some do not and they experience various mental and physical health problems as a result. I am not a clinician, so I do not have the diagnostic language to categorize such complaints – language itself can exacerbate these problems, as it is often unable to express such understanding. Here we may return to education and the difference between the art therapist (designer) and the artist. The former is usually trained in problem solving (diagnosis) and is taught a variety of solutions that may be applied. The latter (not always) is taught from an enquiry basis and trained to make or 'form' questions – problems may then be identified and solutions developed with the person in question as an ongoing 'arts' process, not a cure.

Well-being and the destiny of species

Familiar to most of us, the Yin/Yang symbol depicts the dynamic balance that represents our potential well-being with the world and Feng Shui (wind water) puts this into daily living – not conflicting opposites, but the dynamic unity of opposites. However, well-being in the Western tradition has often been seen as the pursuit of self-interest, the rational maximization of pleasure and the avoidance of pain. This is carried over to the common folk theory that evolution is a competitive struggle to survive and reproduce, at the expense of others. Now, it is realized that this conviction may be held at the expense of the planet. In her evaluation report of 'Climate Change Explorer' (an arts-led project with children about the science of global warming) by Helix Arts, Wallace Heim writes:

> What runs off the pages, is their apprehension for the future, and disbelief that it could be allowed to happen, and continue – dimensions of knowledge and emotional knowledge that get missed all too often.[15]

Or, as Jared Diamond in his excellent book *Collapse* explains, knowing our limits will not only be the antidote to dystopia and the way to well-being, it will be fundamental to our survival as a species. So, our interpretation of well-being may well determine if it is worth dying for.

Notes

1. *The Right to Water* (2003), World Health Organization, France, p. 22.
2. Article 25, Universal Declaration of Human Rights (1948) quoted in *The Right to Water*, World Health Organization, France. p. 7.
3. United Nations Millennium Goals (http://www.un.org/millenniumgoals/goals.html).
4. W. B. Gallie, 'Essentially Contested Concepts', *Proceedings of the Aristotelian Society*, 56: 167–98.
5. G. Lakoff and M. Johnson (1999) *Philosophy in the Flesh: the Embodied Mind and its Challenge to Western Thought*. New York: Basic Books (1999), p. 512.
6. A. Raven, *Art in the Public Interest*. Cambridge, MA: Da Capo Press (1993).
7. S. Lacy, *Mapping the Terrain: New Genre Public Art*. Seattle: Bay Press (1995), Introduction.
8. Lakoff and Johnson, *Philosophy in the Flesh*, p. 536.
9. D. Bohm, *Bohm Dialogue* (www.david-bohm.net/dialogue/).
10. H. Mayer Harrison and N. Harrison (2006), *Greenhouse Britain*, unpublished lecture series, UK.

11. H. Mayer Harrison and N. Harrison (1985), *The Lagoon Cycle*, Herbert F. Jouhnson Museum of Art. Ithaca: Cornell University Press, p. 96.
12. Lakoff and Johnson, *Philosophy in the Flesh*, pp. 566–7.
13. C. Antonioli and M. Reveley, 'Randomised Controlled Trial of Animal Facilitated Therapy with Dolphins in the Treatment of Depression', *British Medical Journal*, 331: 1231 (26 November 2005) (doi: 10.1136/bmj.331.7527.1231).
14. T. Schwenk and J. Y. Cousteau, *Sensitive Chaos: the Creation of Flowing Forms in Water and Air*. London: Rudolf Steiner Press (1996), p. 7.
15. W. Heim (2006), unpublished report.

Part 2: Art and well-being
Peter Senior

> May all be happy,
> May all be without disease,
> May all creatures have well-being,
> And none should be in misery of any sort.

This ancient prayer of the wise expresses the essence of arts for health. Just over thirty years ago I set about establishing, in practice, an idea that the arts could complement the work of healthcare professionals by raising the spirits of patients and staff. Throughout the centuries man has often used some aspect of the arts to improve the state of his mind and heart. Health is a balance of body, mind and spirit.

The idea that the built environment plays a role in the healing and caring process is by no means a new one. In ancient Greece the arts played an important part in the healing sanctuary at Epidaurus, and in Renaissance Europe religious communities endeavoured to provide the best possible care for orphans and the victims of disease and plague in healing sanctuaries. These buildings were often designed with a view to promoting the spiritual life alongside the patient's physical well-being. Sensitive care-providers have always known that the environment in which care is given may assist that care by its beneficial effect on the patient. Marsilio Ficino, philosopher, physician, priest and musician, the intellectual and spiritual inspiration of the Renaissance, recognized that the arts, and in particular fine music, nourished the soul. Dr Thomas Sydenham, a seventeenth-century physician, is reputed to have said, 'The arrival of a good clown exercises more beneficial influence upon the health of a town than twenty asses laden with drugs.'

If we are to move nearer towards a holistic view of healthy living we need to rediscover the cultural and artistic principles which will help us

The arts today can bring many benefits to the healing environment. They assist recovery by encouraging feelings of well-being and alleviating stress. They can improve the quality of healthcare environments by linking art, architecture and interior design. Through their involve-ment in the arts the lives of patients, visitors and staff can be enriched. Closer links between the health services and the community can be developed through arts and cultural activities.

A wide range of arts activities in Britain's health service is now provided by partnerships between the health service and arts organiza-tions from the state and voluntary sectors, and between artists, health-care staff and local communities. Activities include performances of music, theatre, puppetry, poetry, environmental and decorative arts schemes, and participatory arts projects for patients, staff and public.

The partnership between the arts and the National Health Service is now well established and leads the world in using these resources creat-ively. It is not a one-way process, with the arts benefiting the healing environment alone. It is clear that artists benefit from the experience of working within a framework which challenges their skill and profession-alism. Unwittingly the National Health Service has become an important patron of the arts over the past thirty years and it now possesses a huge collection of contemporary art. It is estimated that there are well over 300 arts in healthcare projects employing around 600 people in a full- or part-time capacity. A national survey is long overdue – such a survey would reveal programmes for all ages and all conditions, involving visual, literary and performing arts. It would show that money spent on commis-sioning art for hospitals, hospices and health centres has resulted in many opportunities for artists of all disciplines working with and for the public.

How did this movement develop and the partnership between the arts and health begin?

In 1973 I worked as 'artist in residence' at St Mary's Hospital Manchester, and in the following year established the Hospital Arts Team there. This was the first time that contemporary artists were employed solely to work in and for the health service. This initiative grew over a period of ten years into a multidisciplinary team of eight artists working throughout Manchester's hospitals and health centres. Their work inspired people in other areas of the country to follow suit. A scheme to loan artists' works to hospitals, called 'Paintings in Hospitals' had been operating in the London area since 1959. Other organizations with a remit to bring the arts into healthcare were to follow in the late 1970s: the Shape/Artlink network, the King's Fund Scheme to commission art for London Hospitals, the Council for Music in Hospitals, Live Music Now, the National Network for the Arts in Health, the Centre for Arts and Humanities in Health and Medicine, and many others.

In 1988 Arts for Health was established as a national centre, located in the Faculty of Art and Design at the Manchester Metropolitan University. Its aim was to unite artists, designers and health authorities in establishing arts for health projects as an integral part of the nation's healthcare culture.

Concerned with developing models of good practice for trusts throughout the UK, Arts for Health now leads the way in developing studies and research to evaluate the efficacy of this work. To this end the centre collaborates with the Department of Health, the Department of Culture, Media and Sport, the Arts Council of England, King's Fund, the British Council, the Nuffield Trust and other similar organizations and benefactors. The illustration in Figure 6.1 gives a flavour of the results of artists and healthcare professionals working in partnership throughout the UK to provide environments that are truly 'a prescription for recovery'.

The partnership between arts and health is not exclusive to this country; it is now a worldwide concept with artists, designers and health providers eager to join in and share the rich diversity of ways in which the arts contribute to healing. To capitalize on this enthusiasm, Arts for Health hosted a World Symposium, 'Culture, Health and the Arts', in 1999. Over 600 delegates from twenty-three countries were represented. In 2006, the Arts Council of Ireland hosted the second. European Forum, 'Art & Culture in Hospitals and Healthcare', in Dublin. Over the last few years I have been privileged to work with initiatives in America, Australia, Ireland, Japan, Jersey, Lebanon, Russia, Singapore and Malaysia. A continuing dialogue with the French Ministry of Culture provides opportunities for European collaborations and exchanges between French and British arts in health projects.

The need is enormous, with opportunities for creative collaborations in all areas of health, which could occupy artists for many years to come. Providing uplifting environments is not the only aim. Just as the purpose of medicine is to restore the human being to a state of well-being, so the aim of art within healthcare should be to reflect beauty, harmony and delight in ways that echo that purpose.

Commissioning artists and arts activities on a regular basis to assist healthcare carries with it a responsibility of 'doing the patient no harm' (the Hippocratic oath). Admission to hospital can be a fearful experience, which lowers the spirit, and the arts should always aim to be uplifting. With wide variations in approaches and aims of contemporary artists, arts in health co-ordinators need to be very discriminating.

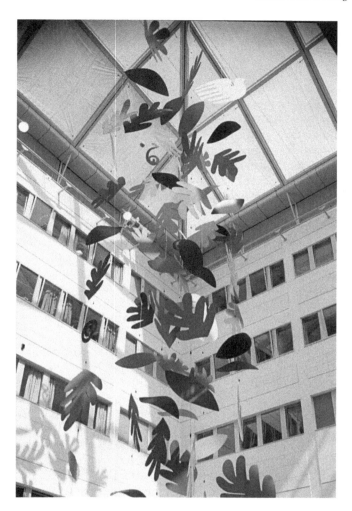

Figure 6.1: *Falling leaves*

The effectiveness of the arts may be difficult to measure in some research terms, whereas 'smiles' and 'enjoyment' are obvious. Existing projects need to be evaluated and this information and experience shared to increase understanding and inform practice. Any evaluation of the arts in healthcare needs to consider the context. A presentation by a local drama group, bringing delight to children in hospital, may not receive accolades from critics but the effect on its audience may be invaluable. This does not mean that second-best will do. We should always try to present the finest work – for example the Royal Ballet and the Royal Shakespeare Company have both undertaken programmes in hospitals.

Arts for Health aims to provide guidelines by which projects can be assessed. How to measure subjective arts experiences is a difficult question. Through qualitative research we are trying to measure the effects objectively. The Centre holds a national archive of arts in healthcare projects, which is continually being developed, and studies in this field are encouraged. For example, one study, *Patient Focused Architecture for Healthcare* (Scher 1996), looks at healthcare, architecture and design from the patient's viewpoint and has been acknowledged as an invaluable manual for architects and health managers. Culture and creativity are now very high on the modern health manager's agenda. Hospitals appreciate the need to create good first impressions, and in many cases the arts project has become the public face of the hospital.

Another important area of development is the training of artists and designers for work in the health field. Arts for Health has initiated several useful collaborations between the health services and university students. These broaden the students' artistic experience and bring vitality and new ideas into healthcare.

There is much more to this concept than just pictures on the wall. Sir Kenneth Calman, as Chief Medical Officer, said at a conference entitled 'Arts on Prescription' organized by the Nuffield Trust in 1998:

> There is an increasing interest in the use of the arts and the humanities in medicine and health. Humanities in this context are defined broadly to include literature, the visual arts, drama, ethics and philosophy. They bring a different dimension to clinical practice, that of the art of healing, and are complementary to the science base. The objective of including the humanities is to assist in improving the quality of life of patients and the communities in which they live and work... The healing powers of dance, music, literature, painting and drama, and their capacity to enhance the quality of life in Britain's multicultural, multiethnic society, has yet to be fully exploited within the NHS and beyond. The wider use of the arts in healthcare will reduce dependence on anti-depressant prescription drugs and help combat social exclusion.

There are many factors that contribute to the stress associated with a visit to hospital. In addition to the anxiety associated with ill health, there may be difficulty in parking, finding the way to your destination or department as a result of confusing signs and notices, wondering which door to go through in often dismal and forbidding surroundings. There is often a lack of stimulation, natural light, fresh air and a view of nature, no quiet room in which to pray, cry, meditate or just be still.

Experience and research have confirmed that the arts enrich the day-to-day life of patients, visitors and staff. They assist recovery, alleviate stress and foster feelings of well-being. They enable staff and patients to contribute to their healthcare environment, generating a greater sense of ownership and pride, generally promoting a sense of quality and an identity which increases the admiration and respect of all. All this plays its part in retention of staff and the valuable skills they bring. Not least, the arts have contributed to way-finding systems, by providing familiar landmarks in the form of memorable art works and signposting using attractive visual symbols.

Artists and cultural projects in healthcare assume many forms. Painters, performers, writers, dancers, musicians and clowns etc. may be commissioned to work in and with the hospital community. They may be commissioned to create site-specific works in healthcare buildings, or lead a community-based health project. They include artists whose work stems from or is focused on therapeutic values, or is motivated by specific health issues. Some patients and many members of staff rediscover interest in art and their artistic abilities.

Funding is an ever-present problem. Although millions of pounds have been raised to finance arts and health projects over the years, it has always been a hand-to-mouth operation with arts co-ordinators spending valuable time fundraising when their time could be used more creatively. Evaluation of existing projects is helping to persuade funding bodies – business sponsors, government departments, regional arts councils, and hospital endowment funds – to be more supportive.

Recently, Arts for Health was awarded a substantial grant from the Treasury for a significant arts in health initiative in the Northwest Health Region. In a new partnership between the Department of Health Public Health Team Northwest, the Arts Council England Northwest and Manchester Metropolitan University, this £385,000 project will work to improve arts services to the NHS in the Northwest Region. Arts for Health will promote and assist artists and arts organizations within the region and organize support and training for artists and healthcare staff. A key aspect of the project will be to monitor and evaluate the impact and the effectiveness of the arts on the delivery of healthcare. By such things as helping healthcare staff to be more imaginative in their approach to work, assisting them to present difficult health issues creatively and by providing a more stimulating working environment, we hope to improve the recruitment and retention of staff.

A recent European 'Music and Health' exchange project has provided convincing proof that the effect of sounds and music on human beings can be most profound. Witnessing the beneficial effect of skilled musicians working at the bedside of patients just a few days old and as old as 102 years, reinforces the age-old belief in the power of sound, including the spoken word, to reach parts of the human psyche that other sense elements cannot. This raises the question about the amount of detrimental sound, which commonly occurs, particularly in hospitals and places of healthcare. Certainly unwanted sound must be a major factor in dis-ease and a negative contributor to well-being.

It is remarkable what the intervention of artists of all kinds working in health settings has done to raise awareness of the effect of the physical and social environment on staff, public and patients. Studies by Ulrich (1991), Scher and Senior (2000) and Staricoff (2004), demonstrate this phenomenon. Arts and health projects of all kinds increasingly recognize the value of linking research to their work, and although in its infancy it is clear that in conjunction with other health professionals and experienced researchers some remarkable insights are possible into the effect of arts and cultural activities on the human condition.

As this international field of activity grows, Arts for Health at Manchester Metropolitan University will continue to foster research into a greater understanding of the fundamental relationship of the arts and culture to human well-being.

References

Scher, P. (1996) *Patient Focused Architecture for Healthcare*. Manchester Metropolitan University.

Scher, P. and Senior P. (2000) 'Research and Evaluation of the Exeter Health Care Arts Project', *Journal of Medical Ethics: Medical Humanities*, 26: 71–8.

Staricoff, R. L. (2004) *Arts in Health: a Review of the Medical Literature*. UK: Arts Council.

Ulrich, R. (1991) 'Effects of Interior Design on Wellness: Theory and Recent Research', *Journal of Healthcare Interior Design*, 3: 97–109.

For further information, publications etc., visit the Arts for Health website (www.mmu.ac.uk/artsforhealth/).

7
Sense and Solidarities: Politics and Human Well-Being
Perri 6

Introduction: - a neo-Durkheimian institutional theory of well-being and its implications for public policy

Aspirations for politics in the West have recently moved from focusing mainly on deterring invasion, promoting economic growth, alleviating sickness and destitution and containing class conflict, to wider concerns often called 'well-being'. Governments are expected to care not just about the standard of living, but the quality of life in work, careers, retirement, residential communities, health, and in the experience of public services.

Well-being encompasses a wide range of subjective and objective measures, including self-reported happiness, the projected state of health in the final years, qualities of friendship and relationships with children, as well as concerns with the material standard of living. Typically, it is treated as a variable to be optimized. Many studies correlate social phenomena with high scores in cross-sectional, self-reported happiness or contentment and urge policy-makers to act to reinforce those features (Frey and Stutzer 2001; Diener and Suh 2000; Prescott-Allen 2001). This chapter will argue that this understanding of well-being is misguided, and it will propose an alternative account.

Well-being is a much more demanding ideal than health or employability, material security and self-reported happiness. Rather, it is about what people will recognize, under particular institutions, as shared life well lived and worth living together over the life course.

Well-being is achieved as much by the ways in which people, under different institutions, *make sense* (Douglas and Isherwood 1979; Douglas 1992a; Weick 1995, 2001; Louis 1980; 6 2004a) of their lives and their social world, as by securing income, wealth, health, environment, or property or persons. Well-being turns upon being able to sustain narratives, myths (in the anthropological sense, not meaning falsehoods or tall tales, but rather guiding tropes that structure sense-making, and shared life), everyday rituals (Goffman 1967) that support memory and aspirations, and by bonds to institutions and other individuals.

Moreover, all the good things do not go together to add up to some unitary phenomenon to be 'optimized' by technical policy design. Well-being is a set of practices, not a state. Indeed, a measure of ill-being may be necessary to well-being, understood as a richer process than mere contentment. For in the individual life, the integration of disappointment is essential to learning and to narrative sense-making, while, collectively, conflict is not merely unavoidable but vital to the viability of the very settlements that seek to contain it. This is no justification for misery, but a recognition that simply improving one's material lot is not sufficient for well-being and that relatively modest standards of living can support well-being, if other things that support appropriate sense-making are also in place.

Many of the capabilities for well-being inhere in social relations and social organization, not in the individual, and still less in individually owned resources. *Well-being is something that we do together, not something that we each possess.* It follows that an adequate account of well-being will require a theory of the kind presented here, of the range of basic institutions of social organization, within which people can make viable sense of their lives. This chapter uses a neo-Durkheimian institutional approach, derived from the anthropologist Mary Douglas (1982a, 1982b, 1992a, 1992b, 1996; Fardon 1999) and her school (Thompson 1982, 1992, 1996; Thompson et al. 1990, 1999; Mars 1982; Rayner 1992; Adams 1995; Wildavsky 1998; Hood 1998; 6 2002, 2004a; 6 et al. 2002, 2006), derived ultimately from Evans-Pritchard (1976, 1940), Durkheim (1951, 1984) and from the sociology of knowledge tradition (Merton 1996; Fleck 1979; Mannheim 1936; Zerubavel 1997). It argues, contrary to postmodern conceptions, that the forms of social organization – and hence of well-being – are not indefinitely various. Rather, there is a limited plurality of basic institutional forms, which support several hybrids or coalitions. In each form, quite distinct styles of sense-making and therefore of well-being, are to be found. These basic forms of social organization are in perpetual conflict with each other. Each springs up in response to the others. None can be eliminated from any viable society: attempts to do so will result in the return of the suppressed form, often in corrupt, illicit or violent forms.

The central challenge for policy and politics of well-being, then, is to find ways in which the basic commitments of each of the forms can be articulated in an overarching settlement. This is best understood by recasting Durkheim's concept of 'organic solidarity'. The chapter presents the theory before briefly exploring the approach to public policy implied in the use of this theoretical apparatus. A case is examined to illustrate the practical uses of the approach – the debate about so-called 'social capital'.

Well-being and sense-making by solidarities

Durkheim (1951) argued that forms of social organization vary along two central dimensions, namely, *social regulation* – the extent to which social life is governed by role, or alternatively by the outcome of voluntarily entered relations, and *social integration* – the extent to which individual persons are held accountable to larger collectivities (cf. Durkheim 1961). After Durkheim wrongly treated them as having nothing much to do with each other, it took 75 years before Douglas (1970) cross-tabulated them, showing that the resulting four combinations are robust. Table 7.1 shows the four elementary forms of social institution defined by their signature forms of power and network structures.

Table 7.2 summarizes these key differences in basic conceptions of well-being in the basic solidarities, showing aspects pursued as a priority, style of sense-making for well-being, worldview, style of memory and of future time horizon of well-being focused upon, social basis of experiencing well-being and typical ritual form and mythic trope for life in

Table 7.1: The basic forms of social organization

Social regulation	Social integration
Isolate	**Hierarchy**
Basis of power: Domination	*Basis of power*: Status, authorization
Network: Sparse, only liminally structured social ties	*Network*: Dense social ties at top; sparse, mainly bilateral and vertical ties at the bottom
Individualism	**Enclave**
Basis of power: Personal control of resources	*Basis of power*: Personal commitment to collective principle, constant collective reaffirmation (e.g. through rituals to produce collective effervescence: Durkheim 1995 [1912])
Network: Sparse social ties, spanned by brokers	*Network*: Dense social ties

Table 7.2: Commitments to styles of well-being differ by the institutional form of social organization

Social regulation	Social integration
Isolate	**Hierarchy**
Priority: Material prospering	*Priority:* Psychosocial prospering, especially whole life, institutional evaluations
Well-being as: Successful survival of crisis and threats	*Well-being as:* Achievement of satisfaction through appropriate and skilled performance of ascribed or achieved place in social order
Time horizon: Short term, individual or at most familial	*Time horizon:* Long term, collective
Basis: Response to immediate needs	*Basis:* Individual fulfilment of collectively recognized status, defined role, acquired capability
Ideology of well-being: Both stoic endurance and ironic laughter help one to cope with reversals of fortune	*Ideology of well-being:* Conformity with the disciplines of the community will bring status, understanding, dignity
Memory: Not greatly valued	*Memory:* Continuity of great tradition
Type of rhetoric: Ironic	*Type of rhetoric:* Deliberative, display (epideictic)
Myth: Survival or loss in the lottery: the wheel of fortune, the blind Fates	*Myth:* Glory of ordered cosmos and dangers of disorder: Olympian victory over Titans; emptiness of individual assertion: Pygmalion, Midas
Ritual style: carnival ('The world turned upside down')	*Ritual style:* procession
Capabilities: Institutionalized capabilities for surviving through volatilities in economic and health status, e.g. capacity to limit personal exposure during hard times; capability to cope with setback by reducing expectations to avoid disappointment	*Capabilities:* Institutionalized capabilities for sustaining systems of authority and status rewards necessary for large-scale collective action, and for cultivating motivation around compliance with norms, e.g. capacity to sustain highly ramified division of labour; capability to cope with setback by managing it as occasion for collective problem-solving through the deepening of competence in formal disciplines

Individualism

Priority: Material prospering

Well-being as: Successful individual pursuit and achievement of personal objectives over the course of the life

Time horizon: Long term, individual

Basis: Strategic organization of individual desire

Ideology of well-being: Individual effort and merit will be rewarded

Memory: Mainly embodied in material accounts of transactions and resources, or in case studies of heroic example and 'best practice'

Type of rhetoric: Litigious/display (epideictic)

Myth: Power of individual assertion: Prometheus, Theseus, individual creative virtuoso

Ritual style: fair

Capabilities: Institutionalized capabilities for creating material incentives and cultivating responsiveness to incentive, e.g. capability to elicit action through cultivating practices of 'rational' instrumentality and 'self-interest'; capability to cope with setback by managing it as an occasion for learning, for innovation, for change of direction

Enclave

Priority: Psychosocial prospering, especially episodic, evaluations of significant others

Well-being as: Committed enactment of shared principles in community

Time horizon: Short term, collective

Basis: Shared commitments to respond to claims to be controlled and limited by enforcement of universal principles against pressures from the social order to violate those principles

Ideology of well-being: Fidelity to the shared principle will result in an admirable life, uncorrupted and exemplary, until the day when all can live in collective harmony

Memory: Long recall of past betrayals and intimations of coming revelation

Type of rhetoric: Demagogic and confrontative outside the enclave, supportive within

Myth: Apocalypse, eschatology: Book of Revelations, *Götterdämmerung*

Ritual style: *charvari* (the ridiculing of the cuckold)

Capabilities: Institutionalized capabilities for eliciting moral commitment and cultivating dense mutual support, e.g. capacity to mobilize moral conscious and fervour and use internally egalitarian structure to draw on fellow-feeling and external enemies to motivate collective action through sense of threat; capability to cope with setback by managing it as occasion for collective action and resistance, by reassertion of moral order against a disappointment that can be seen as a violation each institutional form. Although the examples given in the table are literary in character, the organizational sociology literature using the theory gives contemporary examples of structurally identical cultural forms from the developed and developing worlds (e.g. Mars 1982; Rayner 1982; Coyle and Ellis 1993; Richards 1996; Peck and 6 2006). Also shown are the distinct set of capabilities for well-being supported in each basic form.

There are certain important elective affinities along the diagonals (Douglas 1996; Wildavsky 1998). On the positive diagonal from individualism to hierarchy, we find well-being in affirmation of the sanctioned social order, whereas on the negative diagonal from isolate to enclave, we see well-being as performance of resistance to or survival of challenges presented by that sanctioned social order.

The hypothesis that there can only be a limited number of ways of organizing, and hence of making sense of and pursuing well-being, and that these are defined by the four provisionally stable points in the space created by the cross-tabulation of social integration and social regulation, is known as the 'impossibility theorem' of neo-Durkheimian institutional theory (Thompson et al. 1990).

Each of the basic forms of social organization is a 'mechanical solidarity' in Durkheim's (1984) sense. That is to say, in each, people are institutionally classified and held accountable as relevantly similar under institutions that treat all as individualists, isolates, members of a hierarchy or enclave.

Each exhibits peculiar weaknesses and limitations sustaining particular kinds of ill-being, not least by producing distinct kinds of social exclusion, or at least distinct causal pathways to social exclusion. Moreover, each solidarity tends, if not checked by the others, to go through positive feedback processes of self-reinforcement, in which its characteristics become more pronounced and more extreme, eroding capabilities for well-being and sense-making, to the point of social disorganization and ill-being. This is shown in Figure 7.1, using the forms of suicide and the pathological forms of division of labour as examples of the elementary forms of ill-being; the diagonal arrows represent the direction of positive feedback.

Well-being is only possible to the extent that each of the four is sufficiently articulated that it can provide enough negative feedback to prevent each of the others from running to disorganizing extremes. Certain kinds of four-way settlement are forms of 'organic solidarity', enabling peaceable relations between people who are defined under the prevailing institutions as being relevantly different from others, not

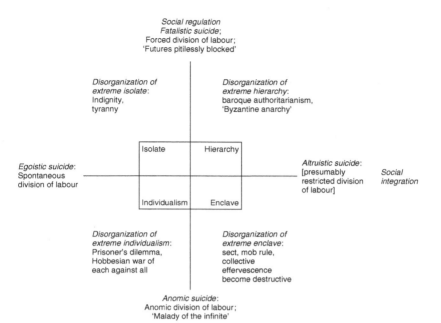

Figure 7.1: Forms of social disorganization that undermine well-being, and produce ill-being

forcing people to behave in similar ways or to adopt the same identity (Durkheim 1984: 85).

There can be more than one kind of organic solidarity, although this implication of the argument was briefly and implicit recognized but not developed by Durkheim. Perri 6 (2003b, 2006) argues that there can be four types of organic solidarity, each sustaining distinct styles of relationship between the four mechanical solidarities, defined as follows:

1. *Toleration of a specific institution or sphere* in which the commitments of each are given some recognition, or at least the commitments of none are violated.
2. *Separation* involves the establishment of institutions that allow more or less distinct *sectors* within which each of the four solidarities can operate, more or less with a local hegemony.
3. *Exchange* involves efforts for the institutionalization of key *reciprocal support* – for example, hierarchical enforcement of property rights in

order to sustain individualistic economic life, and the hierarchical forbearance from heavy regulation and high rates of taxation upon economically successful people in order to sustain sufficient wealth-creation to allow hierarchical institutions to be afforded.

4. *Compromise* involves the acceptance of restraint in the making of claims – for example, the willingness of enclave environmental social movements to refrain from resisting programmes of tradable pollution rights, even though this delivers less than they might want, but in return the business sector concedes that it will not press for absolute *laissez-faire*.

Just as no single mechanical solidarity is unambiguously superior to all others in capacity to sustain well-being, none of the forms of organic solidarity will always sustain well-being more effectively than all other organic solidarities. Rather, which can be achieved and sustained will be highly contingent upon the prior institutional situation and inheritance, the depth and intensity of the conflict between the elementary mechanical institutional forms. However, the theory proposes that *on balance, on the average, in the medium run, any form of organic solidarity will create superior conditions for well-being than will any two- or three-way coalition of mechanical solidarities.* For what organic solidarity as requisite variety can sustain is *social viability*, by preventing the kinds of disorganization and unqualified, un-integratable, senseless ill-being produced in the extreme forms of mechanical solidarity: viability is the basic condition in which each of the capabilities for well-being as sense-making can be maintained (6 2003b, 2006).

Well-being and public policy

Well-being is, then, plural, complex, even unstable. Therefore the pursuit of well-being by policy-makers can never be a matter of optimizing a variable under constraints as conventional economic analysis, linear programming and the engineering approach to policy recommend. Social science can provide understanding of the institutional framework within which policy-makers must work. But it cannot promise, and policy-makers should not demand, any universally valid, apolitical prescriptions. Because well-being results from people making accommodations between rival institutions and their ways of sense-making, only the practice and institutions of politics can elicit the kinds of information required for that settlement-making. It does not follow that the theory of organic solidarity is of no practical use to policy-makers. Social science can offer frameworks, maxims, styles of appreciation, hints, evidence – in short, some of the grist, but not the mill and certainly not the loaf. It can provide invaluable tools with which to support – but never substitute for – political judgement (6 2004a) and it can identify some pitfalls. It can provide policy-makers with, at the very least:

- a discipline of *how* to argue, and *what* to argue *about* in analysing policy problems and developing policy solutions, which can be at least as useful as specific proposals about what to recommend at the end of an argument;
- a framework with which to think about and identify the relevant range of potential claims;
- a framework with which to identify the range of risks to the robustness of any proposed settlement; and
- directions for attention when considering the kinds of indicators and instruments required for developing soundly based appreciations (Vickers 1995) of policy problems; such indicators and instruments will not be 'dials' that point conclusively to specific courses of action: they will always be 'tin openers for cans of worms' (Carter et al. 1993), and their use in policy analysis and intellectual work to support policy development will always be of an advocacy nature (Majone 1989; Fischer and Forester 1993).

One general maxim for policy-makers – at once more specific than a general framework and much less specific than a policy 'solution' – also flows from this argument. Where all good things do not go together, where complex trade-offs must be struck between the four institutional orders that yield different value systems and capabilities for well-being, each with its own weaknesses and risks, one can reasonably suggest that policy-makers ought to focus on the control of harms – accepting that there are always trade-offs between different harms – as a general priority before pursuing benefits.

For the theory suggests that one of the most important risks to be avoided is the situation where one solidarity can reinforce its control and radicalize its commitments to the point of social disorganization. Secondly, it proposes that we should avoid the risk that the solidarities become so polarized that four-way settlements are all but impossible, for these two risks threaten the viability of social organization in which settlements for well-being are possible. Liberty, equality and community order – the core values to individualism, enclave and hierarchy respectively – each has its place. The hope is not to arrest the dynamic disequilibrium process, but to curtail the violence of its oscillations.

The maxim of reducing harms does not, especially where one has to choose which of two or more harms one is prepared to risk, necessarily result in very distinctive policies. Rather, it cultivates a certain kind of political sensibility that over time may lead to less hubristic policy: again, it tells the policy-makers what to think about and how to think about those things, rather than telling them what to think (Allen 2001).

'Social capital', for example

To see how the framework might be put to practical use by policy-makers in these ways, I offer a brief example. I specifically avoid attempting spuriously to derive particular policy designs, but instead show the value in using the approach. Despite the brevity and generality of what follows, I hope that it will serve to show how the theory might be of both procedural and substantive value to policy-makers even without delivering a single one-size-fits-all 'solution'.

There has been an extensive debate about the concept of 'social capital', and increasingly about the extent to which it should be the goal of public policy to promote social capital (e.g. Putnam et al. 1993; Putnam 1995, 2000; Fukuyama 1995, 1999; Baron et al. 2000). Indeed, in the UK, the Prime Minister's Strategy Unit published a paper on public policy and social capital (Aldridge et al. 2002). A vast empirical literature spanning many disciplines purports to show that social capital is beneficial for a huge variety of dimensions of human thriving, from exit from unemployment through educational attainment and labour market attainment, to health status on many measures to happiness (for reviews, see Baron et al. 2000; Lin 2001; 6 2002).

The theory presented here would suggest that in fact the 'social capital' argument has misread and misconstrued the empirical literature. Putnam (2000) and Halpern (2005) believe it possible to identify a set of forms of social capital which will be distinct, self-consistent social phenomena that are generally beneficial, subtracting those that are not benign – exclusive 'old school tie' networks, the social bonds of the Mafia, etc. Effectively, this lumps together all the forms of social organization other than the isolate form. It implies that people can simultaneously and frictionlessly develop 'bonding' (ties between people who are similar to each other on ascribed characteristics) where appropriate and 'bridging' social capital (ties between people who are dissimilar to each other on ascribed characteristics) where appropriate. Woolcock (1998) has added the concept of 'linking' social capital (ties between people with different levels of power, resources, status, or ties to others).

The distinction between bonding, bridging and linking is inadequate. Bonding runs together the two strongly socially integrated solidarities; bridging might describe individualism or the tie sets of higher status individuals in hierarchies; linking might be found in any of the solidarities save for enclave.

Rather, the concept of social capital should be broken up into the four mechanical solidarities (6 2004b), recognizing that each has strengths and weaknesses in respect of different outcomes that matter for well-being. We therefore need more finely grained empirical studies before attempting confidently to identify the forms that conduce most effectively to outcomes; studies should also examine how far some forms of social capital undermine others.

Unfortunately, we lack a sound base of evidence upon which we might make robust assessments of the efficacy of interventions separately, and the balance of intended and unintended consequences, in terms of the network forms of the mechanical solidarities and the institutional structures that underpin them (6 2004b). Worse than this, we lack, to an even greater degree, evidence about the interaction effects of deploying combinations of these policies and programmes towards geographical communities or more widely dispersed communities of interest. Nor do we have rich understandings of how we might measure what counted as a rough balance of input and effort between categories of tools. This makes it very difficult for policy-makers to think through, with any rigour, the ways in which they might design combinations that might reflect or support different kinds of organic solidarity. Yet the weight of the evidence about the importance of different configurations of social networks for different kinds of thriving makes it important that policy can be evaluated and designed in the register of its impacts upon social structure.

Therefore, policy-makers must grope incrementally. Both policy-makers and those responsible for local implementation must follow what designers regard as good design practice in crafting partial strategies (see the rich ethnographic account in Schön 1987: especially ch. 3). However, unlike most architects and product designers, they must do this *iteratively* over the whole life cycle of policy formulation, intervention, implementation, evaluation and re-crafting, and it must be done at every level in the policy process. Designers at each level must begin with some rough scheme of aspirations, based on priority harms to be corrected (for example, in some circumstances, combating, as a priority, social isolation and fostering greater individualism for those in the labour market in greatest need of weak ties, while at the same time combating isolation through more enclave forms for elderly people at greatest risk of vulnerability). Nor should they assume that isolate life is always and everywhere harmful, still less that any other solidarity is unambiguously harmless. Then they must be prepared to break up the overall priorities by accommodating other priorities locally, and by building in detection systems on how people actually respond to what is provided – for example, the possibility of *indirect* effects such as enclave-oriented policies actually being only temporary positions for those upon whom they are targeted, who then use the resources gained to move to other solidarities.

On this view of the tools of public policy, then, attention to the *detectors* – those tools that gather intelligence – is if anything of even greater importance than attention to the *effectors* – the tools for intervening to bring about substantive change by direct means (Hood 1983). In conditions of such ignorance and uncertainty, the key challenge is to design into the programmes some systems of intelligence gathering that might enable those charged with implementation to identify the imperatives and the opportunities for, and also the barriers to, the key relationships between the policies that matter for the different kinds of organic solidarity – separation, defined spheres of provisional toleration, interdependency through exchange, and comprise or mixing of forms.

In this field, it is vital to avoid the hubris of grand social engineering (6 2004b). Most importantly from the point of view of considering social network effects upon well-being and not merely upon material utility or outcomes, policies will, the present argument requires, have to craft and re-craft into their programmes instruments that gather intelligence about the sense-making of those upon whom policies and programmes are targeted. That is to say, we need to know much more about the lay classifications of the experience of receiving services or being affected by regulatory activity, and how people fit these recognitions into their conceptions of the course of their lives more generally. This requires much more than conventional attitudinal research on public acceptance of and satisfaction with programmes.

Conclusion: public policy and well-being – the nature of policy argument

Well-being is neither a state nor a condition. It is a process, a practice, and a way of organizing, and a deeply, irreducibly *political* one at that.

Far from its elements being mutually consistent, they are rivalrous and in conflict, so that only politics can strike settlements between them: no technical or technocratic exercise of analysis can do this, because there is no 'optimal' settlement or 'mix' that can be defined in advance of the political process. For only the political process – including its continuation into the implementation of policies and their scrutiny by the media and by politicians and interest groups – can gather the kind of intelligence required to make those settlements. For what makes aspects of health, employment and so on actually *matter* for well-being is that they are organized, refracted, filtered, selected, articulated and even mobilized through sense-making, and the only way to develop rich and rounded appreciations of how people make sense of their lives that are robust enough for making policy with, is actually to engage in politics (Crick 1964; Gamble 2000). Once that is understood, then the idea has to be rejected that public policy consists in the deployment of a set of tools that have the same consequences and meanings irrespective of the shape of the social organization within which they are received or used, and that policy-making consists in designing a set of institutions, which once done, leaves all the work of distributing well-being to individual genetics, psychological make-up, natural merit and simple luck.

The focus on harm reduction is often sensible enough (6 2002). However, it is both provisional and formal. Firstly, the goal of combating all harms can never be internally consistent. For combating one kind of harm ineluctably runs the risk of creating another. The very things that one does to stimulate more weakly tied relations between people will undermine strong or medium strength ties elsewhere, and so on. If all good things do not go together, then equally, there is no greater coherence in reducing harms. This is why it is impossible to deploy a strategy of *general* risk aversion or harm avoidance: reducing one's exposure to one kind of risk necessarily involves increasing exposure to others. Secondly, the strategy runs the converse risk from that of building coalitions of the moderate. If most attention goes into combating harms, then there will insufficient attention, commitment and institutional capacity for sustaining the positive relations between the solidarities which are also essential to any viable form of organic solidarity.

Practical policy-making consists firstly in making sense of experience (Peck and 6, 2006). This is something that we can only do through social and political organization, even though the *process* of social and political organization is one of the most difficult things to make sense of (Dunn 2000). Each of the basic forms of social organization has its own style of sense-making, its own peculiar narrative forms and ritual order. The vulnerability of these styles of sense-making is that, in the case of the three active solidarities, they can turn into dogmatic, hubristic and intolerant ways of making meaning. In the case of the passive solidarity of the isolate, the risk is simply of decreasing meaning. In each case, whenever people relentlessly pursue the development of the institutions they understand best and can most readily make sense of, to the point that they extrude all other forms, the tragic irony sets in that they produce such disorganization that their own narratives cease to maintain the very coherence that people in these situations are seeking. In the long run, it has been argued, well-being is practised through settlements between these forms. But settlements are, at least at first blush, less easy to understand than the elements between which they strike accommodations. Both their fragility and their complexity raise risks that sense-making will be undermined by opacity, arbitrariness and banality. The styles of sense-making that are possible in and sustained by organic solidarity – separation, exchange, tolerated spheres and compromise – are indeed complex and fragile narratives reflecting complex and fragile social arrangements of tolerance, multiple faiths or identities and discordant architectures cheek by jowl in crowded, designed civic spaces that are renegotiated rather than designed. The fact that the alternative ways of making sense are, if anything, even more dangerous, even more vulnerable to processes of the corrosion of shared meaning is of central importance. It is a reminder that there are tragic conflicts at the centre of any practice of well-being, and that the task of politics, as the only means we have of sustaining those practices, is to prevent or at any rate contain the worst tragic losses. Crucially, it provides the elements of an account of political responsibility.

In no way do I suggest that policy concern with the material conditions for well-being is not important. Of course the enhancement of employment, health, environmental safety, technological safety, community safety, and all the rest are important. Indeed, for those in the many deprived situations, achievement of these outcomes is necessary to long run improvement in the quality of life and thriving. In destitution, well-being of any kind is hardly possible. The reason for that, however, is not just that of material deprivation: a deeper and sometimes more important reason for well-being (as opposed to passing contentment) is that destitution is both cause and consequence of disorganization that corrodes capacities for sense-making, or else produces sense-making of a vicious and disorganizing kind that undermines the capabilities of other people for viable sense-making.

If the arguments are accepted that all good things do not go together, that tragic conflicts are ineliminable, that even the priority for avoiding harm has only heuristic value since it too is subject to tragic choices between priority harms, then the relationship of public policy to well-being must be understood crucially on two axes: namely, public policy *for* conciliating between rival forms of social organization and their practices of sense-making, and public policy – itself political action and not technical intervention at every stage – *as* sense-making.

What, then, can this approach offer policy-makers interested in well-being? It can offer them no less and no more than any body of intellectual labour can offer policy-makers – namely, a richer way to conceive of framing the problem and of framing the interrelationships between problems (Schön and Rein 1994), different tools, and different forms of social organization. To ask for more than this is, I would argue, for politicians to abdicate their responsibility for the conduct of political process by which settlements are really struck, and for social scientists to engage in a dangerous hubris. On the other hand, what this approach offers is neither trivial nor simply gloomy. To aspire to richer understandings of the dynamics by which problems are related to each other and of the nature of policy tools is surely one of the highest ambitions of the policy sciences. The recognition of the inevitability of tragic conflicts is not, properly understood, disabling. Rather, it is a pointer to a way of thinking more deeply about just how incompatible forms of organization and their values and claims can in practice be related and how settlements can in practice be struck. That is the point of the theory of forms of organic solidarity offered here. Secondly, it is a spur to thinking afresh about how to describe and how to cultivate among policy-makers the nature of the craft skills of iterative design and redesign, at many levels throughout a social and policy system, as accommodation of rival claims, through which we can politically reframe and make new sense of our shared and institutionally shaped lives (Schön 1987).

And that is, I have tried to show, what well-being as a social process is fundamentally about.

Acknowledgements

I am grateful to John Haworth for commissioning this chapter, originally for the seminar on 'Wellbeing: Research and Policy' in the ESRC funded seminar series on 'Wellbeing: Social and Individual Determinants',

King's Fund, Cavendish Square, London, 4 July 2002. Ian Christie, Mary Douglas, John Haworth, Jenny Secker and Mike Thompson gave me invaluable comments on earlier drafts, and John Haworth undertook some drastic editing from what was originally a much longer article. None of these people bears any responsibility for my errors, nor should they be assumed to agree with my arguments.

References

6, P. (2002) 'Governing Friends and Acquaintances: Public Policy and Social Networks', in V. Nash (ed.), *Reclaiming Community*. London: Institute for Public Policy Research.

6, P. (2003a) 'What is There to Feel? A neo-Durkheimian Theory of the Emotions', *European Journal of Psychotherapy, Counselling and Health*. Special issue on theories of the emotions from across the sciences, 5(3): 263–90.

6, P. (2003b) 'Institutional Viability: a neo-Durkheimian Theory', *Innovation: the European Journal of Social Science Research*, 16(4): 395–415.

6, P. (2004a) *E-governance: Styles of Political Judgment in the Information Age Polity*. Basingstoke: Palgrave Macmillan.

6, P. (2004b) 'Can Government Influence our Friendships? The Range and Limits of Tools for Trying to Shape Solidarities', in C. R. Phillipson, G. Allen and D. Morgan (eds), *Social Networks and Social Exclusion: Sociological and Policy Issues*. Aldershot: Ashgate.

6, P. (2006) 'Viable Institutions and Scope for Incoherence', in L. Daston and C. Engel (eds), *Is There Value in Inconsistency?* Baden-Baden: Nomos.

6, P. (2007) 'Rituals Elicit Emotions to Define and Shape Public Life: a neo-Durkheimian Theory', in P. 6, C. Squire, A. Treacher and S. Radstone (eds), *Public Emotion*. Basingstoke: Palgrave Macmillan.

6, P., Goodwin, N., Peck, E. and Freeman T. (2006) *Managing Networks of Twenty-first Century Organisations*. Basingstoke: Palgrave Macmillan.

6, P., Seltzer, K., Leat, D. and Stoker, G. (2002) *Towards Holistic Governance: the New Agenda in Government Reform*. Basingstoke: Palgrave Macmillan.

Adams, J. (1995) *Risk*. London: UCL Press.

Aldridge, S., Halpern, D. and Fitzpatrick, S. (2002) *Social Capital: a Discussion Paper*. London: Performance and Innovation Unit, Cabinet Office.

Allen. J. (2001) 'The Place of Negative Morality in Political Theory', *Political Theory* 29(3): 337–63.

Baron, S., Field, J. and Schuller, T. (eds) (2000) *Social Capital: Critical Perspectives*. Oxford: Oxford University Press.

Carter, N., Klein, R. and Day, P. (1993) *How Organisations Measure Success: the Use of Performance Indicators in Government*. London: Routledge.

Coyle, D. J. and Ellis, R. J. (eds) (1993) *Politics, Policy and Culture*. Boulder: Westview Press.

Crick, B. 1964 [1962] *In Defence of Politics*, 2nd edn. Harmondsworth: Penguin.

Diener, E. and Suh, E. M. (eds) (2000) *Culture and Subjective Wellbeing*. Cambridge, MA: MIT Press.

Douglas, M. (1966) *Purity and Danger: an Analysis of the Concepts of Pollution and Taboo*. London: Routledge.

Douglas, M. (1970) *Natural Symbols: Explorations in Cosmology*. London: Routledge.

Douglas, M. (1977) [1963] *The Lele of the Kasai*. London: International African Institute.

Douglas, M (1982a) [1978] 'Cultural Bias', in M. Douglas, *In the Active Voice*. London: Routledge & Kegan Paul.

Douglas, M. (ed.) (1982b) *Essays in the Sociology of Perception*. London: Routledge & Kegan Paul.

Douglas, M. (1986) *How Institutions Think*. London: Routledge & Kegan Paul.

Douglas, M. (1992a) 'Why Do People Want Goods?', in X. Hargreaves, S. Heap and A. Ross (eds), *Understanding the Enterprise Culture: Themes in the Work of Mary Douglas*. Edinburgh: Edinburgh University Press.

Douglas, M. (1992b) *Risk and Blame: Essays in Cultural Theory*. London: Routledge.

Douglas, M. (1996) *Thought Styles: Critical Essays on Good Taste*. London: Sage.

Douglas, M. and Isherwood, B. (1979) *The World of Goods: Towards an Anthropology of Consumption*. London: Routledge.

Dunn, J. (2000) *The Cunning of Unreason: Making Sense of Politics*. London: Harper-Collins.

Durkheim, E. (1951) [1897] *Suicide: a Study in Sociology*, trans. J. A. Spaulding and G. Simpson. London: Routledge.

Durkheim, E. (1961) [1925; lectures: 1902–3] *Moral Education: a Study in the Theory and Application of the Sociology of Education*, trans. E. K. Wilson and H. Schnurer. New York: Free Press.

Durkheim, E. (1984) [1893] *The Division of Labour in Society*, trans. W. D. Halls. Basingstoke: Macmillan.

Durkheim, E. (1995) [1912] *Elementary Forms of the Religious Life*, trans. K. E. Fields. New York: Free Press.

Evans-Pritchard, E. E. (1940) *The Nuer: a Description of the Modes of Livelihood and Political Institutions of a Nilotic People*. Oxford: Oxford University Press.

Evans-Pritchard, E. E. (1976) [1937] *Witchcraft, Oracles and Magic among the Azande*. Oxford: Oxford University Press.

Fardon, R. (1999) *Mary Douglas: an Intellectual Biography*. London: Routledge.

Fischer, F. and Forester, J. (eds) (1993) *The Argumentative Turn in Policy Analysis and Planning*. London: UCL Press.

Fleck, L. (1979) [1935] *Genesis and Development of a Scientific Fact*, trans. F. Bradley and T. J. Trenn. Chicago: University of Chicago Press.

Frey, B. and Stutzer, A. (2001) *Happiness and Economics: How the Economy and Institutions Affect Human Wellbeing*. Princeton: Princeton University Press.

Fukuyama, F. (1995) *Trust: the Social Virtues and the Creation of Prosperity*. Harmondsworth: Penguin.

Fukuyama, F. (1999) *The Great Disruption: Human Nature and the Reconstitution of Social Order*. London: Profile.

Gamble, A. (2000) *Politics and Fate*. Cambridge: Polity Press.

Goffman, E. (1967) *Interaction Ritual: Essays on Face-to-Face Behaviour*. New York: Pantheon Books.

Griffin, J. (1988) *Wellbeing: Its Meaning, Measurement and Moral Importance*. Oxford: Oxford University Press.

Halpern, D. (2005) *Social Capital*. Cambridge: Polity.

Hood, C. C. (1983) *The Tools of Government*. Basingstoke: Macmillan.

Hood, C. C. (1998) *The Art of the State: Culture, Rhetoric and Public Management*. Oxford: Oxford University Press.

Lin, N. (2001) *Social Capital: a Theory of Social Structure and Action*. Cambridge: Cambridge University Press.

Louis, M. (1980) 'Surprise and Sense-making: What Newcomers Experience in Entering Unfamiliar Organisational Settings', *Administrative Science Quarterly*, 5: 226–51.

Majone, G. (1989) *Evidence, Argument and Persuasion in the Policy Process*. New Haven: Yale University Press.

Mannheim, K. (1936) [1929, 1931] *Ideology and Utopia: an Introduction to the Sociology of Knowledge*, trans. L. Wirth and L. Shils. Orlando, Florida: Harcourt Brace Jovanovich.

Mars, G. (1982) *Cheats at Work: an Anthropology of Workplace Crime*. Aldershot: Ashgate.

Merton, R. K. (1996) [1945] 'Paradigm for the Sociology of Knowledge', in P. Sztompka (ed.), *Robert K. Merton on Social Structure and Science*. Chicago: University of Chicago Press, 205–22, excerpted from R. K. Merton (1945) *Sociology of Knowledge*. Also in G. Gurvitch and W. E. Moore (eds), *Twentieth Century Sociology*. New York: Philosophical Library, 366–405.

Peck, E. and 6, P. (2006) *Beyond Delivery: Policy Implementation as Sense-Making and Settlement*. Basingstoke: Palgrave Macmillan.

Prescott-Allen, R. (2001) *The Wellbeing of Nations*. Washington, DC: Island Press.

Putnam, R. D. (1995) 'Bowling Alone: America's Declining Social Capital', *Journal of Democracy*, 6: 65–78.

Putnam, R. D. (2000) *Bowling Alone: the Collapse and Revival of American Community*. New York: Simon & Schuster.

Putnam, R. D., Leonardi, R. and Nanetti, Y. (1993) *Making Democracy Work: Civic Traditions in Modern Italy*. Princeton: Princeton University Press.

Rayner, S. (1982) 'The Perceptions of Time and Space in Egalitarian Sects: a Millenarian Cosmology,' in M. Douglas (ed.), *Essays in the Sociology of Perception*. London: Routledge & Kegan Paul.

Rayner, S. (1992) 'The Cultural Theory of Risk', in S. Krimsk and D. Golding (eds), *Social Theories of Risk*. Westport: Praeger.

Richards, P. (1996) *Fighting for the Rain Forest: War, Youth and Resources in Sierra Leone*. London: Heinemann; Oxford: James Currey.

Schön, D. (1987) *Educating the Reflective Practitioner*. San Francisco: Jossey-Bass.

Schön, D. A. and Rein, M. (1994) *Frame Reflection: Toward the Resolution of Intractable Policy Controversies*. New York: Basic Books.

Thompson, M. (1979) *Rubbish Theory: the Creation and Destruction of Value*. Oxford: Oxford University Press.

Thompson, M. (1982) 'A Three Dimensional Model', in M. Douglas (ed.), *Essays in the Sociology of Perception*. London: Routledge & Kegan Paul.

Thompson, M. (1992) 'The Dynamics of Cultural Theory', in S. Hargreaves Heap and A. Ross (eds), *Understanding the Enterprise Culture: Themes in the Work of Mary Douglas*. Edinburgh: Edinburgh University Press.

Thompson, M. (1996) *Inherent Relationality: an Anti-Dualist Approach to Institutions*. Bergen: Los Senteret (Norwegian Research Centre in Organization and Management).

Thompson, M., Ell, R. J. and Wildavsky, A. (1990) *Cultural Theory*. Boulder: Westview Press.

Thompson, M., Grendstad, G. and Selle, P. (1999) *Cultural Theory as Political Science*. London: Routledge.

Vickers, Sir G. (1995) [1965] *The Art of Judgment: a Study of Policy Making.* London: Sage.

Weick, K. E. (1995) *Sensemaking in Organisations.* London: Sage.

Weick, K. E. (2001) *Making Sense of the Organisation.* Oxford: Blackwell.

Wildavsky, A. (1998) 'Cultural Pluralism Can Both Strengthen and Weaken Democracy', in S. K. Chai and B. Swedlow (eds), *Culture and Social Theory.* New Brunswick, NJ: Transaction Publishers.

Woolcock, M. (1998) 'Social Capital and Economic Development: Towards a Theoretical Synthesis and Policy Framework', *Theory and Society,* 27: 151–208.

Zerubavel, E. (1997) *Social Mindscapes: an Invitation to Cognitive Sociology.* Cambridge, MA: Harvard University Press.

Part 2

8

Is Well-Being Local or Global?
A Perspective from Ecopsychology

John Pickering

> Human kind
> Cannot bear very much reality.
>
> T. S. Eliot (1942) *Burnt Norton*

Introduction[1]

Well-being has both noun and verb senses. The noun sense will here mean the feeling of having a place, of being at home in the world. The verb sense will here mean living in balance with the trials of life. It is important to note that neither sense implies that all life's problems have been solved. It means being aware of what is going on, both good and bad, without that unease that comes from feeling something's wrong but not knowing what it is or what to do about it.

Here I suggest that well-being is being diminished as media technology brings us conflicting messages. On the one hand we are bombarded by explicit images of a life of plenty and of opportunity – more so perhaps than any previous generation. At the same time we get clear indications, the more powerful for being implicit, that all is not right.

What seems to be going wrong is that our relationship with the environment is increasingly violent and destructive. We are beginning to realize that the effects of our technologized lifestyles are leading to damage on a global scale that we may not be able to repair. The unease that this creates is fundamentally detrimental to well-being. It needs to be studied within an appropriate theoretical framework and with appropriate styles of enquiry. I shall propose that ecopsychology provides both.

The Long War

Ecopsychology (e.g. Roszak et al. 1995) is roughly at the centre of a cluster of related disciplines, such as ecological psychology (e.g. Winter 1996), deep ecology (e.g. Tobias 1988; Deval and Sessions 1985) and environmental psychology (e.g. Cassidy 1997). Lester Brown, founder and until 2000 the director of the Worldwatch Institute in Washington, commended ecopsychology like this: 'Ecopsychologists believe there is an emotional bond between human beings and the environment out of which we evolve... Ecopsychologists are drawing upon the ecological sciences to reexamine the human psyche as an integral part of the web of nature' (Brown 1995: xvi).

Now in recent times this web has had another thrown over it. The internet reminds us that the world is one place. It was a dark irony that the seminar for which this chapter was originally prepared should have been held on 11 September 2001. Unknown to those taking part in it, events elsewhere were providing a violent backdrop to their discussions of well-being. Witnessed around the world in real time, the events of the day were a trauma for some and a triumph for others, signifying both the interconnectivity of the global community and the deep divisions within it.

The response to the attacks over the intervening years has increased hatred of America and its allies, as their perpetrators intended. It has made further attacks more likely. As what was the 'War Against Terrorism' becomes what is now called 'The Long War', we are moving closer to the permanent global warfare depicted in Orwell's *1984*. The war is not so much between states as between the rich and the poor. While this divide has always been with us, it has now reached pathological proportions. The grotesque disparities within the world community that have emerged with globalization are no longer simply a matter of more advanced nations outperforming less advanced ones. They result from an aggressive manipulation of the conditions of international trade to increase the wealth of those already rich and the power of those already powerful. The results are patently unjust, especially for vulnerable people whose cultures and economies are distorted by market manipulation (see, e.g., Chossudovsky 2003). The hegemony of the wealthy nations is so abusive that it has to be maintained by economic and military force. It is, accordingly, resisted by force. The resulting violence, often amplified by ancient cultural enmities, is literally brought home to us via globalized communications.

Globalization and the growth of the internet have dominated cultural change over the past few decades. Indeed, they can be seen as different aspects of the same process. In analysing what he calls the 'Runaway World', Anthony Giddens puts it like this: 'I see globalisation as a fundamental shift in our institutions . . . an underlying shift in the way we live. The main driver of globalisation isn't economic globalisation as such, it is information and communication' (Giddens 1999: 4–5). Communication networks have shrunk the world. Digitally mobilized information circulates and blends within them. The value this creates is the currency of the weightless economy, the recombinant culture of postmodernity (Harvey 1990).

Giddens puts a positive spin on all this, seeing globalization as the means to wealth creation and even to fairer distribution. For him, it means that those in the poor world now have a greater chance to benefit by participating in postmodern capitalism. By contrast, the anti-capitalist movement sees globalization as leading to more disparity, not less. In their eyes it reflects the unsustainable exploitation of people and environments by transnational corporations (Klein 2000). Others see global communications as promoting the evolution of capitalism towards a more ecologically responsive condition (Porritt 2005).

Whether it is for good or ill, and of course it will be for both, globalization is unstoppable. Images of Western lifestyles spread via the internet become the hypermobile shock troops of postmodern capitalism. Dreams of unsustainable wealth sear into vulnerable minds, creating desires that cannot be fulfilled. Well-being diminishes as cultural diversity disappears and economic autonomy shrinks.

The significance of the internet is not only economic but semiotic and double coded at that. It signifies the interconnectivity of our economic and political lives but also demonstrates how that interconnectivity is fragmented as globalization exaggerates disparities of wealth and power. The internet actively creates what it signifies through its power to transform. The turbulent, space-less interconnectivity of the internet is a reminder of the braided lives of all those who live in our world. Unlike films and television, which bring images to where you are, the images got by exploring the internet have an aura of being 'elsewhere'. Although the notions of taking a 'virtual holiday' or of travelling a 'highway' by using the internet are transparent nonsense, discovering strange internet sites can feel like the exploration of exotic places. The medium is indeed the message and the message, appropriately, is that we have been living in McLuhan's global village for decades.

The double coding, though, brings another message: the village is a violent place. This is made clear to us in a new and intimate way as images rather than words demonstrate the direct connection between rich lifestyles and violent resistance to them. More immediately and vividly than even a decade ago, wealthy people are being reminded that their secure and abundant lifestyles do not come for free. The cost is violence done to people, to cultures and to the environment. Some of this violence, as the events of 11 September 2001 and of 7 July 2005 show, is coming home.

The nature of this violence was described by Walter Benjamin, writing amid the dark geopolitics of the 1930s. He realized that when society cannot contain the power of technology, the result is not only violence but also the celebration of violence. The media frenzy that greeted the attacks in New York and London, along with the highly controlled presentation of the warfare in Iraq and Afghanistan, demonstrate how enduring and penetrating his analysis was. For many people in the West, the warfare of recent years has become somewhat like a film. It reaches them through reports from journalists embedded in the military who work for highly partisan media companies like Fox TV. All stages of the process are bought and paid for by political and economic organizations who have an enormous stake in creating the meaning of what is happening. This control of information is as strong as that in any totalitarian state, the more so for being hidden. The view that the violence in Iraq and Afghanistan is fundamentally an aggressive war for oil struggles to be heard. The view that it is the heroic struggle of the forces of freedom and democracy against a worldwide conspiracy of mad terrorists is hard to avoid. This fable, which might have been crafted by Disney Corporation, not only conceals much of what led to the warfare but also satisfies the desire for spectacular on-screen violence.

Now, we cannot disown this violence, since we know much more than Benjamin did about what produces it. The pursuit of unsustainable levels of living by the rich requires there to be cheap energy. The effort to control sources of energy leads directly to violent damage being inflicted on the people of other cultures and on the environment. As people resist there is more violence, some of which appears in the wealthly cultures, aggravated by poverty elsewhere and by the 'clash of cultures' depicted by contemporary commentators such as Fukuyama and Huntington. Events in Manhattan, Washington and London, along with protests in Seattle and Genoa, show that violence does not occur 'elsewhere' in a world shrunk by globalization. There is more trouble ahead and it is likely to be ever closer to home. Violence from which we benefit or which is connected with the way we live belongs to us. Since it is done in our names, we are involved. We feel responsible.

But this violence is out of control. Even those in power are powerless, given the decline of the nation-state as a global political player (Hutton 1996). Transnational corporations exert enormous geopolitical influence and yet are beyond political restraint. People have disengaged with the political processes, disenchanted by spin and misrepresentation. Fewer people vote than ever before and the democratic deficit is growing. We are witnessing a transition from party politics to issue politics, which may be beneficial. However, in the transition, tradtitional politcal structures will be weakened. They will consequently exert even less restraint on those with control of the media, who will have more power than ever before to distort the presentation of events. Distortion, intentional and not, makes it impossible to trust the ever-present media barrage. Real geopolitical events are obscured and misrepresented in what Baudrillard has termed 'hyper reality' (Baudrillard 1983: 166). We feel powerless.

To feel responsible and yet powerless surely diminishes well-being. The effects may not be close to the surface of our conscious lives, but they are important nonetheless. Of course, they are overlaid by a host of distractions. Distant tragedies may evoke sympathy, but unless they directly affect our lives, they are soon forgotten. What's happening elsewhere may be distressing, but it *is* elsewhere, even though elsewhere is closer than it used to be. Things closer to home will still be more significant if they are sources of stress and anxiety. Even in the rich world, someone living in poor conditions has got enough to worry about. Without work or security we are not likely to feel much concern about events in Afghanistan or even in New York. Only when our basic needs are met is there the space to feel concern for others; when they are not, our concerns are for ourselves.

Maslow represented human needs as a pyramid. At the bottom are basic needs to do with the preservation of life, which we share with all other living beings that must have air, water, food, shelter and safety to survive. Next up are social and emotional needs, some of which we share with other social animals. These are our needs to belong and to relate. At the top comes the uniquely human need for self-actualization: to understand ourselves and our place in the world and to strive for the maximum of consciousness. Meeting higher needs is conditional on lower ones having been met. If you can't breathe, you won't notice being hungry; if you're hungry you forget you're lonely, and so on. Once needs at lower levels are met, needs at higher levels may receive attention, if our social environment encourages us to do so.

Now, over the past few centuries those in industrialized societies have found it increasingly easy to meet their basic needs, and since the mid-twentieth century people in the rich world have enjoyed what Franklin Roosevelt called the 'more abundant life'. Of course, our needs have not always been met. The poverty amidst wealth depicted in *Hard Times* and *The Ragged-Trousered Philanthropists* was real enough. And remains real, since the monstrous disparities of Victorian England are now globalized, as many commentators show (Shiva 2000; Chossudovsky 2003).

If well-being primarily depends on needs being met and if people in wealthy societies are becoming more able to meet them, then well-being should be increasing. Surveys show that economic indicators like GDP and unemployment levels do indeed predict reported well-being, at least in the developed countries (di Tella et al. 2001). At the same time, other surveys reveal a steadily increasing incidence of mental and psychosomatic illnesses coupled with consumption of anti-depressants (e.g. Skaer et al. 2000; Blanchflower and Oswald 2004). There are bound to be complex demographic and economic factors at work here, such as the increasing pressure on people with jobs, different patterns of family life and so on. However, an underlying driver for all of these, surely, is the creation of an increasingly unsustainable image of what life should offer. Our basic needs may be met, but all is not well.

But then, it never was. Suffering is the universal condition, as the Buddha realized. Western philosophers from Schopenhauer to Sartre have also detected discontent at the core of human experience. It would be well to bear this in mind as we enquire into well-being. We should not try to eliminate that which cannot be eliminated, especially as it can be a source of growth (Young-Eisendrath 1996; Gilbert 1989).

Nonetheless, there does seem to be something amiss, over and above the normal trials of life. The last century or so has been called 'the age of anxiety', something that McLuhan explained as 'the result of trying to do today's job with yesterday's tools, with yesterday's concepts' (McLuhan and Fiore 1967: 8). In one sense, however, 'today's job' is what it has always been: to seek well-being and to feel whole, secure in a stable identity. But this is made more difficult when identity itself is open to indefinite redefinition. Our job today, as one celebrant of the postmodern condition puts it, is to 'eclect' what to be (Jencks 1996). Our tools, however, are those of yesterday, the notions of personal autonomy, enduring identity and responsibility bequeathed us by Locke, Kant and Mill.

The postmodern turn has provided new tools with which to probe these notions and has prompted a reappraisal of our assumptions of stable personal identity and of individual autonomy. Instead of taking them as absolute, we now regard them as relative to the social system in which they are constructed and maintained. The psychology of post-modern selfhood now 'focuses on the way in which we construct our experience, especially our sense of self, from messages in our quickly changing culture' (Winter 1996: 17). Our culture is indeed changing quickly and we are immersed in a sea of digitally enhanced options. Images, slogans and intellectual fashions are recommendations, both explicit and not, about how to look, speak and think – in short, about what to be. This has always been the case but it is now more powerful, ubiquitous and it appears earlier and earlier in the life cycle.

This choice of identity is exciting while at the same time contributing to the 'stress of modern life'. Clearly 'stress', like 'well-being', is a complex condition with folded layers of components. One of these, at the somewhat neglected global end of the range, may be a growing awareness of the troubled relationship between the self and the world. Selfhood is constructed using what the culture around it provides. What we take ourselves to be is in turn taken from what our cultural context defines a self to be. In the wealthy world selfhood is bound closely to the variety of lifestyles a rich and abundant culture can offer. But these cannot be separated from the relationships with the rest of the world that make them possible. Globalized communications are showing us that rich lifestyles are unsustainable and that they make a major contribution to the causes of violence. Yet even as the personal and geopolitical costs of such lifestyles are becoming clearer, images that create expectations and desires for them are spreading around the world. Those enjoying the lifestyles are unconcerned for the most part. At the Earth Summit held in Rio in 1992, the developing nations drew the attention of the then US president, George Bush senior, to the over-consumption by the US and other rich countries. He dismissed their concerns with the remark: 'The American Way of Life is not up for negotiation'. Despite recent moves explicitly to abandon this way of life, by some US states and by European countries such as Germay and Sweden, the violence in the oil-rich countries is a dark testament to how effectively this policy has been followed.

Now, George Bush junior has declared the 'Long War' in defence of that way of life. Although, like any complex geopolitical campaign, it has many interleaved objectives, there remains a central driver: to maintain control of dwindling energy resources, especially oil. Rich lifestyles need cheap energy and energy is cheap so long as extraction costs can be kept low and the environmental costs are not met, or are met by others.

The wealthy nations are now consuming the global commons at an unsustainable rate and leaving other nations and those yet to be born with the resulting environmental damage. But degrading the environments of those who do not benefit from the resources obtained is not only unjust but also unsafe. The tragedy of the commons is being played out on a global scale. It will be increasingly difficult for the poor and for primary resource producers to maintain their independence and meet their needs in the future. They will do whatever they can to protect themselves and their resources. Sometimes this will be done by peaceful means, as is happening in South America. Sometimes it will be done by armed resistance to transnational companies, as is happening in Africa. Present indications are that this geopolitical situation will worsen over the next century or so.

The base of Maslow's hierarchy of needs is universal. Our needs to breathe, to be nourished or to feel safe are not imposed by culture. As we move further up the hierarchy, universal needs may be transformed by cultural influences into acquired ones. When these include a media-born flood of imperatives about what to wear, about what shape to be and about what it is fashionable to say and think, the middle and upper levels of Maslow's hierarchy become bloated with acquired needs. While children in the poor world look to their parents for food, those in the rich world nag theirs for clothes and electronic toys that will make them feel 'cool', a process inflamed by skilfully targeted media campaigns (Freedland 2006). Their intrinsic need for social identity has been converted by advertising into the need to possess. A brand of trainers, functionally identical to a host of others, can be made so desirable that children are violently robbed for their sake.

Advertising converts natural needs into desires that are hard to recognize and impossible to meet. The meanings attached to products often tap into Maslow's hierarchy at the social level. Clothes can come to mean group membership and hence to satisfy a need to belong. Guided by digitally mobilized sales data, advertising campaigns constantly retune the meanings of products, often choosing targets earlier and earlier in the life cycle. If from the earliest stages of someone's life, needs can be imposed that are hard or even impossible to meet, demand will remain high. Even when we have enough, it must be made to seem unsatisfactory. A sales executive put it this way in the 1950s: 'It's our job to make women unhappy with what they have.' Advertising in 1950 was a cottage industry compared with the corporate enterprise it is today. Its cumulative global impact on well-being is immense. In a recent anthology on ecopsychology, it was put like this:

> Corporate advertising is likely the largest single psychological project ever undertaken by the human race, yet its stunning impact remains curiously ignored by mainstream Western psychology. We suggest that large scale advertising is one of the main factors that creates and maintains a particular form of narcissism ideally suited to consumerism. As such, it creates artificial needs within people that directly conflict with their capacity to form a satisfying and sustainable relationship with the natural world. (Kanner and Gomes 1995: 80)

A satisfying and sustainable relationship with the natural world has been, over the history of human kind, the basis of well-being. That is what 'feeling at home in the world' means. This is not a static condition but depends on a healthy balance between met and unmet needs. Advertising creates artificial needs which are designed to be permanently unmet. They act as an irritant, undermining our sense of balance between what we have, what we need and what we want. Unmet needs are those of which we are generally most conscious, but, being conscious they are subject to scrutiny and, with luck, proper management. Basic needs actually provide the information required to satisfy them. If you're thirsty or hungry, you know what you lack. Artificially imposed needs, by contrast, are often pre-conscious and hence harder to recognize. They are harder to meet because we don't know what we want – only that we want it very badly. When they are specifically designed and constantly modified to stimulate consumption, they are virtually impossible to satisfy.

Gandhi remarked that 'The world has enough for everyone's needs, but not for some people's greed'. Someone who experiences the world from this viewpoint will feel fundamentally secure. Corporate greed, acquired second-hand via the advertising industry, makes people feel insecure. The world cannot seem ever to provide enough. It has been clear for decades that the natural needs of the world's peoples can be met, and met sustainably, given the technological resources we now possess (e.g. Seabrook 1985). Artificial needs created through media stimulation, by contrast, are designed specifically not to be met. Unmet needs create violence. If the needs in question threaten our existence in the short term then the violence is correspondingly immediate. If we are being choked, we will fight for air, if we are being ignored, we will fight for attention. If the needs are longer-term ones then although the response may be more planned and strategic, it will still be a fight for all that.

The technology for imposing artificial needs is violently out of control and is producing violence in the process. Someone who feels incomplete without this or that commodity will struggle to obtain it. There's nothing wrong with the commodity, nor in fact with the struggle to feel complete. The problem arises when one is attached to the other. A child who kills another for their trainers or a nation that subverts the government of another for their own economic ends are two symptoms of a single disorder.

We become more aware of this as global networks bring the evidence to us. Inevitably, this evidence will be distorted and sensationalized in hyper-reality. But despite the smoke and mirrors, it is unmistakable that there is a crisis, and a deep one, of which globalized violence is a symptom.

The ecopsychology perspective on this is that we need to seek an appropriately deep solution and, since the ecological crisis is a psychological crisis, the solution will lie with social changes rather than technological fixes. Much of what threatens well-being arises from the massive over-consumption required to meet pathological needs inflamed by media technology. In *The Fear of Freedom*, written in 1940, Eric Fromm noted that as the 'More Abundant Life' loosened traditional constraints in the name of freedom, the result was a type of emotional vacuity ideal for consumerism to fill. The condition was even more noticeable some thirty years later when he wrote *To Have or To Be?*

Now it is not so much noticeable as starkly definitive of contemporary lifestyles. What some ecopsychologists have called the 'all-consuming self' is a narcissistic condition in which selfhood becomes too strongly defined by possession, having been detached from its more natural supports by a barrage of consumerist images in the media. In this pathological condition, the boundary between the self and the world becomes indefinitely expandable and virtually disappears (Hillman 1995). To be a self is now to possess this or that thing which is not self. If this need to possess is pathologically inflated, the self/world boundary becomes a moving frontier of greed. The answer to the question: 'How much is enough?' is now: 'What's "enough"?' A media-induced trance of unlimited, consequence-free consumption is a global danger. Cultures in which it has taken hold will violently wrest what they want from the environment and from other cultures. This violence can be concealed within hyper-reality to some extent, but pre-consciously the news leaks out. Combined with pre-conscious needs for self-actualization that cannot be met, it makes for a powerful degradation of well-being.

Self-actualization, lying at the top of Maslow's hierarchy, is our most important need and it is crucial to well-being. When the integrity of the self is threatened, well-being is impaired. The technologies of desire that have appeared within post-industrial societies have fundamentally diminished the integrity of the self. Weber described the world as transformed by the industrial revolution as 'disenchanted' (Weber 1958). One of the drivers of colonialism and the westward expansion in America was an effort to re-enchant the world by the appropriation of exotic lands (Berman 1981). To those already living there, the invaders were seen as maddened by the need to consume. The Hopi Indians, as their way of life was being destroyed, recognized the malaise of the white people. It was a mental illness that they called *koyaanisqatsi*, meaning, 'a life out of balance'.

Well-being depends on a life in balance. Our way of life is being driven deeply out of balance by artificial and unsustainable needs, and this has to be addressed if we are to carry out research that is appropriate and useful. Most social sciences, reflecting the ethos of modernity, model their research on the natural sciences. They mainly deal with things that can be counted and with the more immediate, rational, determinants of well-being. The contribution of ecopsychology is to complement this with research that reflects the methodological diversity of the postmodern era (Gergen 2001). It strikes a more even balance between quantitative and qualitative methods. Pre-conscious psychological determinants are treated as seriously as contributing to the rational actions of both groups and individuals. Researchers are no longer neutral external observers but participants.

Following this line suggests that the ESRC, in making well-being one of its thematic priorities, needs to enquire into the deeper qualitative issues raised by the way we live as well as carrying out quantitative studies. Studying social relations can be done on many levels and the wider world community should not be ignored. Healthy outcomes may be sought at both the individual and the collective levels. But the latter is primary: it is harder to promote healthy individuals in sick societies than it is to help sick individuals in healthy ones. The teaching and learning of ecopsychology makes sense since we all inhabit the same environment. Ecopsychology seeks to make people aware of the deep reciprocity between the way we live and the impact this has on other cultures and on the biosphere. In making sense of the world we cannot ignore our impact on it.

If research simply takes growth and abundant consumption for granted and then bolts them onto modernist notions of selfhood, it will not be doing anything radically new. Of course, research carried out in order to inform policy is not meant to address anything radically new. Quite the reverse. Its role is to stabilize and consolidate the power of those who fund it. Hence, it is normative and consensual. It is about finding out what will keep people happy so they will continue to support political institutions. Investigating the effect of the built environment on well-being could be an illustrative case. Most people in the UK live in cities. Helping to make the urban environment good to live in seems worthwhile, as indeed it is, in a limited sense. But if the life support for the world community is threatened by urbanized lifestyles, it is parochial and short-sighted. Quantitative studies of urban well-being do not address the problem deeply enough. What is needed is a complementary qualitative investigation of, for example, why people so often seek alternatives to urban living on retirement.

For ecopsychologists, the object of research needs to be the geopolitical pathology that threatens global well-being. Such research integrates with and complements conventional research very well (Bragg 1997). It is not a luxury to be enjoyed by those with leisure and freedom from more immediate needs. If we are to promote well-being in the longer term and on a global scale, we must recognize the interdependence of self and environment. Then, harm to the environment would be experienced as harm to the self. This is far more effective in helping those in the rich world to change their consumptive lifestyles. Moralizing, scolding and alarmism, what Roszak calls 'guilt trips and scare tactics', certainly don't work (Roszak 1995).

Summary

Well-being depends on a feeling of being in a balanced relationship with our environment. This relationship is obscured by massive propaganda that converts natural needs into the need to consume. Nonetheless, consciously or unconsciously, we know that violence is being done in our name, we fear things are going to get worse and we feel we are powerless.

Ecopsychology is an attempt to recognize and remedy all this. As a psychological analysis of human well-being, it suggests that research has to extend beyond the human sphere. We should not confine our research to quantitative surveys of satisfaction with wealthy lifestyles. Otherwise we will not even be rearranging the deckchairs on the *Titanic*, but merely asking their occupants how comfortable they are.

Note

1. An earlier invited paper on this topic was presented at an ESRC seminar series on 'Wellbeing: Social and Individual Determinants', Seminar 1: 'Well-Being; the Interaction between Person and Environment', 11 September 2001, Queen Mary University London.

References

Baudrillard, J. (1983) *Simulations*, trans. P. Foss, P. Patton and P. Beitchman. New York: Semiotext[e].

Benjamin, W. (1970) 'The Work of Art in the Age of Mechanical Reproduction', in H. Arendt (ed.), *Illuminations*. London: Jonathan Cape.

Berman, M. (1981) *The Re-enchantment of the World*. Ithaca, NY: Cornell University Press.

Blanchflower, D. and Oswald, A. (2004) 'Well-Being Over Time in Britain and the USA', *Journal of Public Economics*, 88: 1359–86.

Bragg, E. (1997) 'Ecopsychology and Academia: Bridging the Paradigms', *Ecopsychology Online*, no. 2 (internet resources below for URL).

Brown, L. (1995) 'Ecopsychology and the Environmental Revolution', in T. Roszak, M. Gomes and A. Kanner (eds), *Ecopsychology: Restoring the Earth, Healing the Mind*. San Francisco: Sierra Club Books.

Cassidy, T. (1997) *Environmental Psychology: Behaviour and Experience in Context*. Hove: Psychology Press.

Chossudovsky, M. (2003) *The Globalization of Poverty and the New World Order*. Ontario: Global Outlook.

Deval, W. and Sessions, G. (1985) *Deep Ecology: Living as if Nature Mattered*. Salt Lake City: Peregrine Smith Books.

di Tella, R. et al. (2001) 'The Macroeconomics of Happiness', *Warwick Economic Research Papers*, No. 615, University of Warwick: Department of Economics.

Freedland, J. (2006) 'Pester Power', *Resurgence*, 235: 40–1.

Fukuyama, F. (2006) *The End of History and the Last Man*. Second edition. New York: Simon & Schuster.

Gergen, K. (2001) 'Psychological Science in a Postmodern Context', *American Psychologist*, 56(10): 803–13.

Giddens, A. (1999) *Runaway World*. London: Profile Books.

Gilbert, P. (1989) *Human Nature and Human Suffering*. Hove: Erlbaum.

Harvey, D. (1990) *The Condition of Postmodernity*. Oxford: Blackwell.

Hillman, J. (1995) 'A Psyche the Size of the Earth', in T. Roszak, M. Gomes and A. Kanner (eds), *Ecopsychology: Restoring the Earth, Healing the Mind*. San Francisco: Sierra Club Books.

Hutton, W. (1996) *The State We're In*. London: Vintage.

Jencks, C. (1996) *What is Postmodernism?* London: Academy Editions.

Kanner, A. and Gomes, M. (1995) 'The All Consuming Self', in T. Roszak, M. Gomes and A Kanner (eds), *Ecopsychology: Restoring the Earth, Healing the Mind*. San Francisco: Sierra Club Books.

Klein, N. (2000) *No Logo: Taking Aim at the Brand Bullies.* London: Flamingo.

McLuhan, M. and Fiore, Q. (1967) *The Medium is the Message.* New York: Random House.

Porritt, J. (2005) *Capitalism as if the World Matters.* London: Earthscan.

Roszak, T. (1995) 'Where Psyche Meets Gaia', in T. Roszak, M. Gomes and A. Kanner (eds), *Ecopsychology: Restoring the Earth, Healing the Mind.* San Francisco: Sierra Club Books.

Roszak, T., Gomes, M. and Kanner, T. (eds) (1995) *Ecopsychology: Restoring the Earth, Healing the Mind.* San Francisco: Sierra Club Books.

Seabrook, J. (1985) *Landscapes of Poverty.* Oxford: Blackwell.

Shiva, V. (2000) 'Globalisation and Poverty', *Resurgence,* 202, September/October.

Skaer, T., Sclar, D., Robison, L. and Galin, R. (2000) 'Trends in the Rate of Depressive Illness and Use of Antidepressant Pharmacotherapy by Ethnicity/Race: an Assessment of Office-Based Visits in the United States, 1991–1997', *Clinical Therapeutics: the International Journal of Drug Therapy,* 22(12): 1575–89.

Tobias, M. (ed.) (1988) *Deep Ecology.* San Marcos, CA: Avant Books.

Weber, M. (1958) *The Protestant Ethic and the Spirit of Capitalism,* trans. Talcott Parsons. New York: Scribners.

Winter, D. (1996) *Ecological Psychology: Healing the Split Between Planet and Self.* New York: HarperCollins.

Young-Eisendrath, P. (1996) *The Gifts of Suffering.* New York: Longman.

Internet sources:

Bragg on ecopsychology: http://isis.csuhayward.edu/ALSS/ECO/0197/newresch.htm

Ecopsychology in general: http://isis.csuhayward.edu/ALSS/ECO/Final/index.htm#intro

The World Watch Institute: http://www.worldwatch.org/

Koyaanisqatsi,'A Life Out of Balance': http://www.koyaanisqatsi.org/index.php

Anthony Giddens on globalization: http://www.polity.co.uk/giddens/pdfs/Globalisation.pdf

9
Societal Inequality, Health and Well-Being

Dimitris Ballas, Danny Dorling and Mary Shaw

Introduction

A house may be large or small; as long as the neighboring [*sic*] houses are likewise small, it satisfies all social requirement for a residence. But let there arise next to the little house a palace, and the little house shrinks to a hut. The little house now makes it clear that its inmate has no social position at all to maintain, or but a very insignificant one; and however high it may shoot up in the course of civilization, if the neighboring [*sic*] palace rises in equal or even in greater measure, the occupant of the relatively little house will always find himself more uncomfortable, more dissatisfied, more cramped within his four walls. (Marx 1847)

In three dozen neighbourhoods of London and three in Glasgow most children aged under five are living in housing, provided by the state, with too few rooms for their family according to the 2001 census. The same source suggests that most under fives in Britain are growing up in homes, small palaces, with a surfeit of rooms. (Thomas and Dorling 2007)

This chapter considers well-being at the ecological level and investigates the relationship between happiness and inequality across Britain. The chapter briefly reviews the theoretical background of happiness research and also considers its relevance to public policy. It can be argued that societies that are extremely polarized and divided are less desirable, and less 'well' than those which have elements of equity and communitarianism as their core values and principles.

The first section presents evidence for the recent widening of the gap between the rich and the poor leading to unprecedented post-World

War Two socio-economic polarization and income inequalities in Britain and reviews the literature that investigates the relationship between inequalities, health and happiness. The second section explores the spatial dimensions of socio-economic polarization by investigating the geographies of income and wealth in Britain. The third section explores the geographical distribution of happiness in Britain using data from the British Household Panel Survey. Finally, the fourth section offers some concluding comments.

Inequalities, health and happiness: a review of evidence so far

> Within each of the developed countries, including the United States, average life expectancy is five, ten, or even fifteen years shorter for people living in the poorest areas compared to those in the richest. (Wilkinson 2005: 1)

There has been extensive research on the relationship between income, wealth, happiness and health. Most relevant studies suggest that there is a positive relationship (e.g. see Hagerty and Veenhoven 2001; Oswald 1997) such that more income and wealth is associated with greater happiness and better health. However, as Clark and Oswald (2002) point out, while higher income is apparently associated with higher happiness for poor countries, the evidence is less strong among richer countries. In addition, it has long been argued that it is *inequality* that affects happiness rather than levels of income (Jencks 2002). Further, a number of studies have shown a connection with health such that health is better in less unequal societies. This finding was recently disputed by, among others, Lynch et al. (2004) and their criticism has in turn been disputed with new evidence by Ram (2006). Thus, as the quote from Marx at the start of this chapter suggests, the relationship between inequalities and happiness has long been identified, but also long disputed. This debate has raged in the context of a huge growth in wealth and 'mini-palaces' amongst the rich in Britain: people tend to compare themselves to their colleagues, friends, neighbours or so-called 'reference groups' and this in turn has an impact on happiness and health.

> When we are at home, most of us like to live in roughly the same style as our friends or neighbours, or better. If our friends start giving more elaborate parties, we feel we should do the same. Likewise if they have bigger houses or bigger cars. (Layard 2005: 43)

People compare themselves most with their 'near equals' (Runciman 1966). In particular, as Clark and Oswald (2002) point out, the group of people to whom we compare our income is thought to be our 'peer group', defined as 'people like me' (of the same sex, age and education). It could also be 'others in the same household', 'myself in the past', 'friends and neighbours', etc. As Layard (2005) points out, income is much more than a means to buy things. It is also an indicator of how we are valued and for some a measure of how they value themselves.

Research by Wilkinson (1992) suggested that a more equal distribution of income was related to improved life expectancy in rich countries. Subsequent work showed that mortality was also lower in American states and metropolitan areas where incomes were more equally distributed. There are a growing and large number of studies supporting the view that inequality has a negative relationship with population health and happiness (Wilkinson and Pickett 2006). As Jencks (2002) points out:

> while economic goods and services are obviously important, many people believe that inequality also affects human welfare in ways that are independent of any given household's purchasing power. Even if my family income remains constant, the distribution of income in my neighbourhood or my nation may influence my children's educational opportunities, my life expectancy, my chance of being robbed, the probability I will vote and perhaps even my overall happiness. (Jencks 2002: 57)

Nevertheless, it is unclear at which geographical level inequality is most damaging. As noted above, inequality matters because people compare themselves with their 'peer groups'. But do they compare themselves to 'peer groups' in their neighbourhood, city, region, country or possibly to diaspora groups in other countries or with peoples of whom they know little? There are many other kinds of non-geographical groups as well as diaspora to which we may compare ourselves and with whom we consider ourselves to be of a similar social standing. It is far from clear how reference groups are constituted. Given this confusion, some have elected to simply focus on inequality at the small area level, aiming to capture social comparisons within that level, without reference to the wider social structure (Wilkinson and Pickett 2006). Wilkinson (1997) has argued that income inequality in small areas (such as streets, wards, or even towns) is affected by the degree of residential segregation of rich and poor and that the health of people in deprived neighbourhoods is poorer not because of the inequality within their neighbourhoods but because they are deprived in relation to the wider society:

> the broad impression is that social class stratification establishes itself primarily as a national social structure, though there are perhaps also some more local civic hierarchies – for instance within cities and US states. But it should go without saying that classes are defined in relation to each other: one is higher because the other is lower, and vice versa. *The lower class identity of people in a poor neighbourhood is inevitably defined in relation to a hierarchy which includes a knowledge of the existence of superior classes who may live in other areas some distance away.* (Wilkinson and Pickett 2006: 1774, our emphasis)

Endeavouring to investigate this issue Wilkinson and Pickett (2006) compiled a list of 155 published peer reviewed reports of research on the relation between income distribution and measures of population health. They classified these studies as 'wholly supportive' or 'unsupportive' according to whether they were international studies, using data for whole countries, whether their data were for large sub-national areas such as states, regions and metropolitan areas or whether they were for smaller units such as counties, census tracts or parishes. The proportion of analyses classified as wholly supportive falls from 83 per cent (of all wholly supportive or unsupportive) in the international studies to 73 per cent in the large subnational areas, to 45 per cent among the smallest spatial units. The implication of this is that the spatial scale at which people make their social comparisons is more likely to be the nation-state (arguably reflecting socio-economic position) than it is to be locality (reflecting position within neighbourhood).

On the basis of the above, it can be argued that the degree of societal inequality expressed through the income and wealth distribution may have a huge impact on levels of happiness and well-being (Wolfson 2003). It can be argued that if money is transferred from a richer person to a poorer person, the poor person gains proportionately more income, and thereby happiness, than the rich person loses. But the overall effects of redistribution may be greater still (the whole benefit being greater than the sum of the individual benefits). Along similar lines, as Jencks (2002) points out, when social scientists measure income inequality they assume that inequality has not changed if everyone's income rises by the same percentage. Therefore, it can be argued that a 1 per cent increase in income is equally valuable to the rich and the poor, even though a

1 per cent increase represents a much larger absolute increase for the rich. Jencks describes this assumption as the 'One Percent is Always the Same' (OPIATS) rule:

> This rule implies that if my income is $100,000 and I give $20,000 of it to the poor, my well-being falls by a fifth. If I divide my $20,000 equally between ten people with incomes of $10,000 ten people's well-being will rise by a fifth. The gains from this gift will thus exceed the losses by a factor of ten. The utilitarian case for governmental redistribution almost always reflects this logic: taxing the rich won't do them much harm, and helping the poor will do them a lot of good. If you look at the actual relationship between income and outcomes like health and happiness the OPIATS rule seldom describes the relationship perfectly but it comes far closer than the 'One Dollar is Always the Same' rule, which is the only rule under which income inequality does not affect health or happiness. (Jencks 2002: 57)

Nevertheless, what Jencks's economic example omits is the sociological argument that in losing $20,000 the individual earning $100,000 actually gains a better life through helping to create and feel part of a better society. This actual benefit is not included in the OPIATS rule – let alone any projected theological benefits involving rich men fitting through the 'eye of the needle' for future lives! (All world religions are pro-redistribution!) The unhappiest man in the universe of hypothetical worlds would presumably be the one with an income of $1 trillion a day, in a world where everyone else lived on $1 a day. We rarely think clearly about income and wealth distributions as so much of our own identity is subsumed within them (if you are reading this you know you are relatively well-off – or are most probably a student and expect to be richer soon!)

The above brief review of literature on the impact of inequality on well-being and happiness suggests that public policies should aim to reduce income and wealth inequalities if their aim is to maximize population health and well-being. In this context, it is interesting to explore what has been happening in Britain over the last century in terms of the distribution of income, health and well-being. Social equity grew most clearly from the start of the century to the middle of the century. The absolute and relative gaps between rich and poor fell in what was most important: in the chances of children dying as infants, in the wealth of their parents, in their opportunities for education, and in the importance that where they lived – their geography – had on their lives. Analysing the results of a survey in the early 1950s, comparing it to one he had commissioned over half a century earlier, Seebohm Rowntree declared that poverty had all but been eliminated by social reform (Rowntree 2000). It had not (see Hatton and Bailey 1999), but it is easy to forget just what had been achieved in those years and how hard it was fought for (Bevan 1990). Social equality was further abated in the late 1950s. The income shares of the 'richest of the rich' as analysed by others show that clearly. This is seen in Figure 9.1, which describes the proportion of income that the richest segments of the UK and Dutch societies hold (Atkinson and Salverda 2005). As Atkinson and Salverda (2005) point out, in the UK the share of the top 1 per cent increased from 4.2 per cent in 1977 to 7.1 per cent in 1989, and rose a further 2 percentage points from 1990 to 1999. In addition, the share of the top 0.1 per cent rose from 0.66 per cent in 1977 to 1.81 per cent in 1989, and a further 1.2 percentage points from 1990 to 1999. The same pattern is exhibited by the 'shares within shares' shown in Figure 9.1 (where 1 per cent is a tenth of the richest 10 per cent): convergence up to 1977 and then the UK trend-line rises steadily, while the Netherlands' lines are near-horizontal.

Interestingly, analysis of mortality trends over time reaches almost identical conclusions as those for income (Dorling 1997); wealth too shows the same pattern. The 1960s Labour governments presided over a period of slight increases in equality again, as did the late 1970s government, but their efforts when viewed over the course of the whole of the last century appear now to simply have been to have held back a revival in inequality. The economic 'restructuring' and monetarist neo-liberal

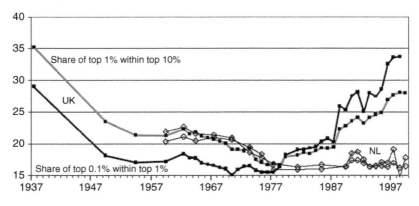

Figure 9.1: What proportion of income do the richest of the rich hold?
Source: Atkinson and Salverda 2005: 906

policies of the 1980s and early 1990s have significantly increased income and wealth inequalities. There is little doubt that the distribution of income in Britain has become even more unequal since 1979 (Atkinson 1996; Hills 1996, Hills and Stewart 2005). Although average real incomes have grown significantly, at the bottom of the scale there has been little or no rise in real income, while top incomes have risen a great deal faster than the average (Atkinson 1996; Green 1996, 1998; Pearce and Paxton 2005). This revival of inequality brought us – by the start of this century – to levels of inequality we last experienced at the height of the 1930s depression. In terms of absolute wealth, especially in comparison to most of the rest of the world, we are much richer. In terms of relative chances between social groups we are as unequal now as we were then (Dorling et al. 2005).

More recent research suggests that the situation in the last decade has been deteriorating. In particular:

1. Housing wealth per child rose 20 times more in the best-off tenth as compared to the worst-off tenth of areas in Britain 1993–2003 (Shelter 2005).
2. The majority of 'extra' higher education places have gone to children from already advantaged areas and so the participation gap between social groups has been increasing (1997–2003 graduating cohorts, HEFCE Widening Participation report, January 2005 – note however that for cohorts graduating in 2004 and 2005 this trend may be changing).
3. 'Work rich' and 'work poor' geographical divisions are growing by area and by income to at least mid-2005 (for more details see Dorling 2006).

From a geographical perspective, a decade ago Green (1996) pointed out that the social and economic processes, which determined the distribution of income, were spatially uneven. The regions which suffered the least in the recession of the early 1980s tended to gain most in the subsequent recovery. In contrast, the most depressed regions had not recovered the ground lost in the early 1980s (Green 1996). A decade later and using census material from 2001, compared to 1991, the same process was seen to be continuing if not accelerating (Dorling and Thomas 2004a). The social polarization that Figure 9.1 above illustrates as having grown most rapidly in the 1980s, and even more so in the 1990s, was matched by spatial polarization of the growth between regions, cities and neighbourhoods. The south-east of England and especially its more affluent neighbourhoods (such as Kensington and Chelsea in London and the county of Surrey) saw wealth, opportunity and incomes concentrate within their populations. Few of the top 1 per cent or 0.1 per cent of income earners lived outside of the most affluent parts of the country and so when their wealth rose dramatically geographical inequalities rose too. Furthermore, those rises were reflected in smaller but still significant rises further down the income distribution – stretching it at every point and exacerbating difference and inequality between both people and places (Hills and Stewart 2005).

Geographical inequalities of income and wealth: what people want and need

> By necessities, I understand not only the commodities which are indispensably necessary for the support of life, but whatever the customs of the country renders it indecent for creditable people, even of the lower order, to be without. A creditable day labourer would be ashamed to appear in public without a linen shirt. (Smith 1952: 383)

This section presents the most recent socio-geographical data currently available on polarization and discusses the changing geographical distribution of inequality through income and poverty in England and Wales, highlighting how the trends identified through the 1970s, 1980s and 1990s are continuing unabated as social inequalities rise. We have had to exclude Scotland and Northern Ireland from this analysis because of lack of comparable data on income. Figures 9.2 and 9.3 show the regions and cities we are considering. In all cases cities are defined as the built-up area of each city approximated by aggregations of parliamentary constituencies.

Incomes matter: even the smallest amounts can have vital implications. Money is a ticket to social interaction, to dignity and respect. This is easy to overlook when you have enough to get by:

> Interviewing single mothers on council estates a few years ago it was striking that most spoke about their depressing social isolation. They couldn't afford to keep up with former friends, because they hadn't the money to make even the most minimal gestures required of a friendship – sending birthday cards or buying rounds of drinks. As one said at the time, 'My friends will offer to buy me a round – but I have to say no, because I can't buy the next'. As a consequence, these women's social circles had shrunk to their mothers and their lovers, because these were the only relationships which could be maintained without the expectation of financial reciprocity. (Russell 2006: 93)

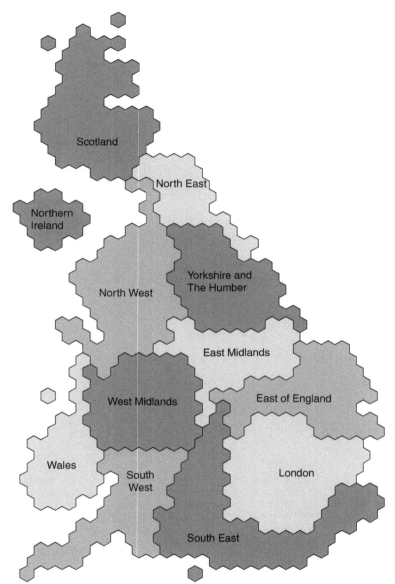

This is a population cartogram map of the regions of the UK. To map the two key indicators of what people want and need we first divide people by region. Each hexagon in the map above is a parliamentary constituency.

Figure 9.2: UK regions by population

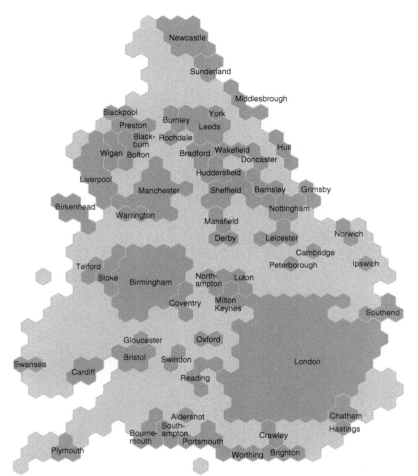

We have identified the main cities of England and Wales and approximated their extent through the parliamentary constituencies that cover their built-up area. All the statistics below are shown for these cities and the more rural remainder of each region. You'll need to refer to this map to see where is where.

Figure 9.3: English and Welsh cities

As Layard (2005) points out, friendship is one of the biggest sources of happiness and well-being. However, the ability to make and maintain friends, as suggested by the above quote, is significantly affected by income. Looking at income distributions can therefore be seen as the equivalent of looking at a proxy of the 'ability to make and keep friends and friendship' in your 'peer group' and hence well-being and happiness distributions. We are not saying that income is necessary to create and maintain friendship. For instance, homeless people report friends as being very important, and rich folk can have very shallow friendship networks. However, the ability to make friends is facilitated by income. Poor homeless people cannot choose to be friends with the rich man or woman (although the contrary is not true). Figures 9.4 and 9.5 show the degree to which average incomes vary across these areas and how that inequality has risen in just the most recent two years (in addition to rises recorded between 1991–2001, 1981–1991 and 1971–1981 in proxies for income by area).

As can be seen in Figure 9.4, there is a very clear North–South divide. According to the December 2005 data released by one of the largest high street banks on its customers' incomes the 'rural remainder of the south-east' (excluding London and other cities) had the highest average income (per person) in England and Wales (£26,539) followed by Crawley (£25,746), London (£25,153), Reading (£24,388) and Oxford (£23,239). In addition, there are relatively high average incomes in the 'remainder of the east of England' (£22,778), Bournemouth (£22,733), the 'remainder of the south-west' (£22,512), Milton Keynes (£22,334) and West Midlands (£22,116).

In contrast, Hull has the lowest average income (£15,916). Just above Hull are the cities of Bradford (£15,950), Stoke (£16,448), Leicester (£16,841), Birmingham (£16,909), Blackpool (£17,005), Rochdale (£17,070), Sunderland (£17,268) and Liverpool (£17,406). Money in and of itself cannot be eaten, provides no warmth and makes poor company. Above subsistence level money buys the right to leisure time and activities – Rowntree's postage stamp, Adam Smith's linen shirt, to escape Marx and Engels' hovels, to have a drink with friends, to have friends, to pay for a phone call. Although crude summaries, the differences between the average incomes flowing through bank accounts in different British cities are a marker for a collective measure of respect. In 2005 incomes were lowest, at £12,875, across all of England and Wales in the Birmingham, Sparkbrook and Small Heath constituency (where riots took place on the Lozells road in 2005). They were highest in Kensington and Chelsea at £50,438 (which has not experienced rioting since 1958 in Notting Hill).

Figure 9.5 shows the degree to which some cities and regions are catching up with the rest of the country. As can be seen, there is a general trend of ever-increasing social and economic polarization: most of the

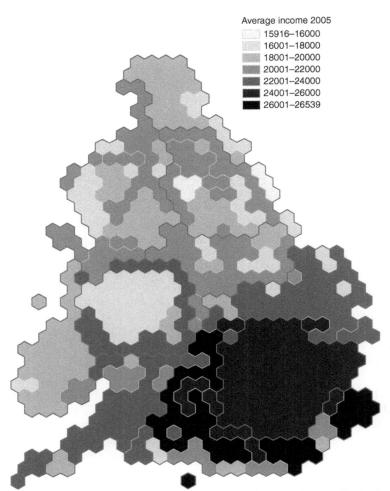

In December 2005 a major bank released estimates of average income flowing into its customers' bank accounts by parliamentary constituency for England and Wales. Here we show that by city these average incomes range from less than £16,000 per income bearing account in Hull and Bradford, to over £26,000 per account in the more rural parts of the south-east region of England (combined).

Figure 9.4: Income inequality 2005

areas experiencing the highest increases in average income are located in the south. In particular, the city of Bournemouth experienced the highest income increase, followed by the remainders of the south-west

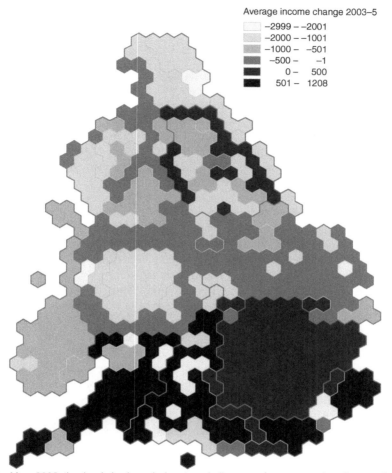

In May 2003 the bank had carried out a similar exercise – scanning the regular incomes entering the current accounts of its customers to estimate annual average income. This map shows the changes over this time period. Where average incomes have fallen it is possible that more young (and/or poorer) people have opened bank accounts – but the patterns shown here are the best reflection of recent social change that we have – on the key indicator of income.

Figure 9.5: Rising inequality 2003–2005

and south-east, Brighton and London. In contrast, most of the cities which are at the bottom of the 2005 average income distribution, seem to have experienced a decline between 2003 and 2005. For instance, Hull and Stoke are amongst the cities that experienced significant declines in average income between 2003 and 2005. Other towns and cities and regions that experienced considerable decline include Middlesbrough, Luton, Newcastle, Wigan, Coventry, Doncaster, Milton Keynes, Birmingham, Mansfield and Bradford.

There is a similar geographical pattern when we look at the distribution of poverty. Figure 9.6 shows the geographical distribution of poverty around 1999/2001, on the basis of preliminary estimates made using the Poverty and Social Exclusion (PSE) survey sponsored by the Joseph Rowntree Foundation and the 2001 census of population in collaboration with David Gordon at the University of Bristol. The survey was based on the 'Breadline Britain method' (Gordon et al. 2000), which measures relative poverty based on a lack of the perceived necessities of life. This has been widely accepted as a relative poverty measure whereby poverty is defined as a lack of having the items people need to play a normal part in society. Therefore Figure 9.6 shows the percentages of households living in poverty in each place when poverty is defined by people themselves. There are immediate material consequences to – for instance – not having a warm coat for your child to wear (one of the items used to calculate the measure). Thus the poverty map is a map of what people *need* (at a basic level of need) but can also be read as a map of the basic things in life that people need to maintain dignity.

Hull, which, according to Figures 9.4 and 9.5 had the lowest average income, has also the highest poverty rate in the country in 2001 (39.7 per cent). Hull is followed closely by Liverpool (38.5 per cent), Sunderland (36.8 per cent), Bradford (36.2 per cent), Newcastle (36 per cent), Birmingham (35.6 per cent), Blackburn (35.4 per cent), Rochdale (35.2 per cent), Nottingham (35 per cent) and Leeds (33.8 per cent). In contrast, the lowest poverty rates are observed in Aldershot (18.8 per cent), Reading (19.3 per cent) and the rural remainder of the south-east (19.6 per cent).

Figure 9.7 shows the change in these rates between 2001 and 1991. As can be seen, poverty rates using this relative measure have increased everywhere since 1991. In addition, the proportion rises to almost 2 out of 5 households in the worst off places. In particular, the highest rise in the poverty rate has been experienced in Bradford (11 per cent change) followed by Birmingham (10.7 per cent), Hull (10.5 per cent), Huddersfield (10.3 per cent), Liverpool (10 per cent), Blackburn (10 per cent), Leeds (9.3 per cent) and Nottingham (9.3 per cent). It is noteworthy that London is also amongst the cities experiencing a high rise in poverty rates. Poverty rates have increased everywhere, but

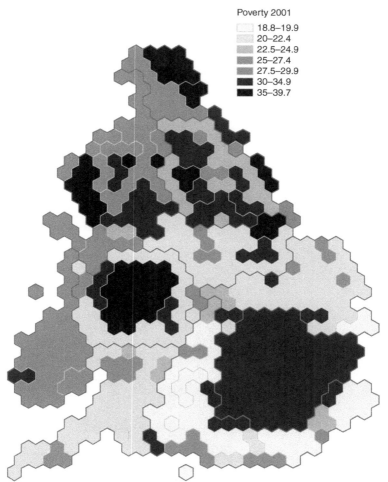

Poverty 2001

	18.8–19.9
	20–22.4
	22.5–24.9
	25–27.4
	27.5–29.9
	30–34.9
	35–39.7

Roughly a quarter of households lived in poverty around 1999/2001. These prelim-inary estimates were made using the Poverty and Social Exclusion (PSE) survey sponsored by the Joseph Rowntree Foundation and the 2001 census of population in collaboration with David Gordon at the University of Bristol. The figures above are the percentages of households living in poverty in each place when poverty is defined by the people.

Figure 9.6: Poverty 2001

amongst the cities and regions that experience the lowest increases are Aldershot (3.8 per cent increase), Reading (4.3 per cent), the 'rest of the south-east' (4.4 per cent) and Bournemouth (4.5 per cent).

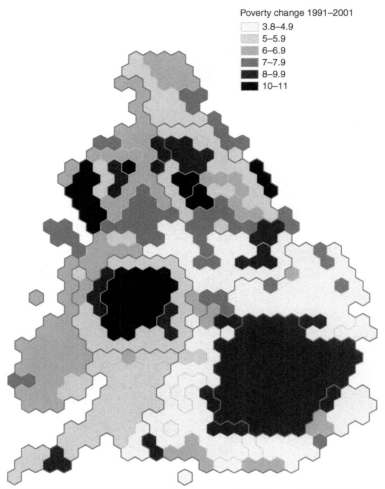

The 1999 survey and 2001 census can be compared with the equivalent 1990 survey and 1991 census which were used to produce the Breadline Britain index of household poverty – most comparable with the PSE survey. Everywhere poverty rose between 1990/1991 and 1999/2001 and most quickly where it was most prevalent to begin with. The figures above are the percentage point rise in poverty over this decade by household.

Figure 9.7: Rising povery rates 1991–2001

Regional distributions of 'unhappiness' in Britain

So far we have discussed the relationship between inequalities, health and happiness suggesting that there is a strong relationship between them. We have reviewed recent evidence suggesting that socio-economic polarization and income inequalities in Britain have been rising considerably. Admittedly, given the available evidence all we can do to date is to suggest that there is a relationship, but it is difficult to believe that greater inequality improves health and increases aggregate happiness. We now turn to look at empirical evidence on the geographies of happiness and well-being. In particular, we attempt to investigate the geographical distribution of happiness in Britain based on data from the British Household Panel Survey (BHPS). This survey was also recently used by Clark and Oswald (2002) who attempted to measure the importance of material goods in relation to happiness. The BHPS is one of the most comprehensive surveys in Britain drawn from a representative sample of over 5000 households. The aim of the survey is to deepen the understanding of social and economic change at the individual and household level in Britain, as well as to identify, model and forecast such changes, their causes and consequences in relation to a range of socio-economic variables (Taylor et al. 2001). In the context of this chapter we use BHPS data to explore the geographical distribution of responses to the following question: *Have you recently been feeling reasonably happy, all things considered?*

Table 9.1 shows the percentage of individuals (by social class) who answered that they were *less happy* or *much less so* (sorted in ascending order by the column for all social classes). Note that there are many subtle differences between the social classes, but that people tend to be happier in rural and southern areas. Figure 9.8 shows a cartogram depicting the spatial distribution of unhappiness for all social classes combined (column 4 in Table 9.1).

As can be seen, the North–South divide, which was evident earlier, is to an extent replicated in this simple map of unhappiness in Britain (excluding the affluent 'Remainder of Yorkshire and the Humber' and somewhat less affluent Tyne and Wear region). Note that by class the best off are most unhappy in the 'Rest of the North', class 2 (skilled) in outer London suburbia and class 3 (unskilled) in South Yorkshire. Different places suit different groups worse or better: skilled appear least unhappy in Inner London, unskilled in Tyne and Wear and the professional and managerial occupations seem to be most at ease in rural Yorkshire and Humberside. Figure 9.8 enhances further the argument that income and wealth level as well as income and wealth inequalities appear to be related to happiness, but it also suggests other possible factors at play. The latter may include quality of life indicators such as life expectancy, educational attainment, low work-related benefit

Table 9.1: Distribution of 'unhappiness' in Britain (*Class 1* comprises 'professional and managerial & technical' occupations, *Class 2* comprises 'skilled non-manual and manual' occupations and *Class 3* comprises 'partly-skilled' and 'unskilled' occupations)

Region by social class	Class 1	Class 2	Class 3	Classes 1–3	N
Rest of Yorks & Humberside	3.3	7.1	7.0	5.9	328
Tyne & Wear	10.0	7.1	3.4	7.2	264
East Midlands	5.3	8.1	11.2	7.9	782
Inner London	10.3	5.2	8.8	7.9	418
Rest of North-west	4.9	9.2	12.3	8.5	454
South-west	11.7	6.7	8.9	8.7	930
Scotland	11.29	7.95	7.81	9.0	957
Greater Manchester	14.5	8.2	4.8	9.3	416
West Midlands conurbation	10.5	8.9	8.8	9.3	453
East Anglia	10.7	6.5	13.3	9.5	390
Merseyside	17.6	9.2	0.0	9.5	233
West Yorkshire	14.5	7.7	9.6	10.2	364
Rest of South-east	10.5	10.8	8.7	10.3	1,875
Outer London	8.9	13.3	6.9	10.7	668
Rest of West Midlands	8.9	11.6	14.9	11.5	506
Rest of North	19.7	10.4	8.5	12.4	400
Wales	11.1	12.9	15.3	13.0	533
South Yorkshire	17.6	11.6	24.2	15.4	293
Great Britain	*10.5*	*9.3*	*9.7*	*9.8*	*10,264*

claims, low rates of poverty and high house prices. It is interesting at this stage to examine relevant recent research findings pertaining to the state of English cities. Table 9.2 shows a number of the key indicators mentioned above, that are combined to create a very simple overall index of the quality of life in English cities.

The units constructed for the score are analogous to life expectancy and can be thought of as a crude indicator of quality of life. They are simply the sum of the five measures in the other columns, each standardized to have the mean and standard deviation of life expectancy. Change over time in this score can also be calculated and is given in Table 9.2, but note that the indicators start from a variety of dates and are only indicative of changing position from the early to mid-1990s. The largest increases of an additional 6.7 points are found in Oxford, Brighton and London. The next three largest increases are in Cambridge, Reading and York. The smallest three increases have been in Hull (least improvement), Burnley and Bradford, followed by Stoke, Huddersfield and Blackburn.

Table 9.2: Key state of the city indicators, sorted by an overall score and change measure given (after Pritchard et al. 2005)

City	Life expectancy 2001–2003	% of adults with a degree 2001	% working age claiming JSA/IS 2003	% of poverty by PSE 1999–2001	Average housing price 2003 (£)	Average score 2003	Change in score over time
Cambridge	79.5	41	5.1	29	244862	82.3	5.6
Aldershot	79.0	22	3.7	17	238991	81.9	4.6
Reading	79.6	26	4.7	20	211794	81.5	5.3
Oxford	79.2	37	6.1	30	255181	80.9	6.7
Crawley	79.6	19	4.8	22	205506	79.8	4.7
Bournemouth	79.7	17	7.1	21	214296	79.1	5.0
York	79.4	23	5.4	25	147513	78.2	5.4
Worthing	78.8	16	6.4	20	186992	78.0	4.1
Southend	79.0	13	7.5	19	186481	77.6	4.2
Brighton	78.4	29	9.3	27	212361	77.6	6.8
London	78.6	30	10.3	33	283387	77.5	6.7
Bristol	78.9	23	7.7	25	160708	77.1	4.6
Southampton	78.8	19	6.9	25	172585	76.9	4.9
Norwich	79.8	18	7.5	27	138187	76.3	3.9
Portsmouth	78.8	16	6.6	25	157145	76.2	4.0
Swindon	78.2	15	6.6	22	150689	76.0	4.1
Milton Keynes	78.2	18	6.6	25	161625	76.0	4.2
Gloucester	78.4	16	8.5	22	141690	75.5	3.4
Northampton	78.2	17	7.8	24	135871	75.1	4.1
Warrington	77.9	17	6.8	23	119668	75.1	4.6
Ipswich	79.0	16	10.1	25	134514	74.7	3.5
Chatham	77.7	12	7.7	23	142374	74.2	2.8
Preston	77.7	17	7.2	26	97038	73.6	3.6
Derby	78.1	18	10.5	27	114280	73.1	4.2
Leeds	78.2	19	8.9	32	119262	72.8	3.1
Nottingham	77.5	18	9.8	28	123663	72.7	3.4
Telford	77.9	13	9.0	27	115722	72.6	2.9
Leicester	78.0	17	11	28	124812	72.6	2.3
Blackpool	77.2	13	8.9	24	103656	72.5	2.2
Plymouth	78.1	13	9.8	28	118978	72.4	3.5
Hastings	77.4	15	13.4	25	163128	72.3	3.7
Luton	77.2	14	9.7	28	143698	72.2	2.0
Peterborough	77.5	14	9.5	28	123089	72.1	2.1
Wakefield	77.5	14	9.0	28	110407	72.1	3.5
Coventry	77.8	16	10.9	28	111165	72.0	3.8
Huddersfield	77.2	15	8.7	29	97815	71.6	1.8
Manchester	76.7	19	11.6	30	119569	70.9	3.6
Sheffield	77.9	16	10.4	33	96328	70.8	3.6
Wigan	76.5	12	8.6	27	88946	70.7	2.6
Birkenhead	77.9	13	12.2	29	95632	70.6	3.3
Mansfield	77.1	9	9.4	28	94749	70.4	2.0
Bolton	76.8	15	10.4	29	89281	70.4	2.3

Table 9.2: (Continued)

City	Life expectancy 2001–2003	% of adults with a degree 2001	% working age claiming JSA/IS 2003	% of poverty by PSE 1999–2001	Average housing price 2003 (£)	Average score 2003	Change in score over time
Grimsby	77.6	10	11.5	28	77898	70.0	2.6
Doncaster	77.3	11	10.6	30	82267	69.8	3.0
Birmingham	77.4	14	12.8	33	122794	69.7	2.2
Stoke	76.9	11	10.3	29	78834	69.7	1.7
Newcastle	77.1	16	12.8	34	111220	69.2	4.1
Barnsley	77.2	10	10.8	32	79492	68.9	3.0
Rochdale	76.4	14	12.2	31	92523	68.8	2.5
Burnley	76.8	12	10.7	31	55879	68.7	1.5
Bradford	76.9	13	11.5	33	75919	68.6	1.4
Middlesbrough	77.1	12	13.1	32	81760	68.4	3.1
Sunderland	76.6	12	12.4	34	91322	67.8	3.2
Blackburn	75.8	14	12.7	30	70969	67.8	1.9
Hull	76.6	12	17.1	33	72374	66.0	1.4
Liverpool	75.7	14	18	36	87607	64.7	2.8

The indicators are sorted by change in overall score. This overall index confirms the North–South division, which was also described in the previous section. In particular, Table 9.2 suggests that in general, English

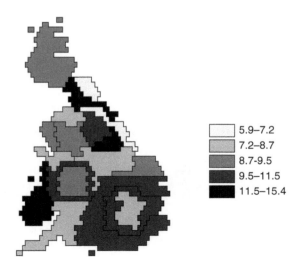

	5.9–7.2
	7.2–8.7
	8.7-9.5
	9.5–11.5
	11.5–15.4

Figure 9.8: Distribution (%) of 'unhappiness' in Britain in 1991

cities are clearly divided between those in the south-east of the country and those situated towards the north-west.

It is interesting to view data such as those presented in Table 9.2 in parallel with geographical distributions of happiness or unhappiness as depicted in Figure 9.8. It can reasonably be expected that the indicators listed in Table 9.2 influence to an extent the distribution of happiness and well-being and there is a need to analyse these and other similar data sets in tandem in order to explore the arguments made in the context of this chapter in more detail.

Concluding comments

This chapter adds a little more evidence to the mounting case being made that there is a relationship between inequalities and well-being that needs to be examined in more detail. In particular, it has been suggested that the relationship between inequalities, happiness and well-being has long been identified, even though there has been considerable debate about the strength of this relationship. This chapter briefly reviews clear evidence that there is an increasing socio-economic polarization and widening of inequalities in Britain. It also argues that this polarization has a geographical dimension at various geographical levels. In particular, there is a clear and growing 'North–South' divide in Britain, but there is also local socio-economic polarization within regions and cities. Given the evidence and recent research on the determinants of happiness and well-being, it has been argued that it is reasonable to assume that widening income and wealth inequalities and the resulting polarization have a detrimental effect on the overall happiness and well-being of the population. Clearly, there is a need to have a closer examination of the data that include measurements of happiness and well-being. The fourth section of this chapter provided a brief discussion of such data and illustrated how it is possible to look at the geographical as well as the socio-economic distribution of happiness, using data from the British Household Panel Survey and some simple measures of well-being. More sophisticated analysis of this data in combination with the data and evidence presented in the third section of this chapter is needed to provide a better understanding of the relationship between happiness and income and wealth inequalities, and by extension a wide range of social justice issues. However, it can be argued that on the basis of the evidence presented here it becomes clearer that public policy that is aimed at income and wealth redistribution and societal equality would probably lead to higher overall levels of happiness and well-being.

Acknowledgements

Funding from the Economic and Social Research Council (research fellowship grant number RES-163-27-1013) and the British Academy (British Academy Research Leave Fellowship) is gratefully acknowledged. Mary Shaw is funded by the South-West Public Health Observatory. The authors would like to thank John Pritchard at the University of Sheffield for all his help with the illustrations. The British Household Panel Survey data used in this chapter were made available through the UK Data Archive. The data were originally collected by the ESRC Research Centre on Micro-social Change at the University of Essex, now incorporated within the Institute for Social and Economic Research. All responsibility for the analysis and interpretation of the data presented in this chapter lies with the authors.

References

Atkinson, A. B. (1996) 'Seeking to Explain the Distribution of Income', in J. Hills (ed.), *New Inequalities: the Changing Distribution of Income and Wealth in the United Kingdom*. Cambridge: Cambridge University Press.

Atkinson, A. B. and Salverda, W. (2005) 'Top Incomes in the Netherlands and the United Kingdom over the 20th Century', *Journal of the European Economic Association*, 3, 4: 883–913.

Bevan, A (1990) [1952] *In Place of Fear*. London: Quartet.

Clark, A. and Oswald, A. (2002) 'A Simple Statistical Method for Measuring How Life Events Affect Happiness', *International Journal of Epidemiology*, 31(6): 1139–44.

Dorling, D. (1997) *Death in Britain: How Local Mortality Rates Have Changed: 1950s–1990s*. Report published by the Joseph Rowntree Foundation.

Dorling, D. (2006) 'Class Alignment', *Renewal*, 14: 8–19.

Dorling, D., Ballas, D., Thomas, B. and Pritchard, J. (2004) *Pilot Mapping of Local Social Polarisation in Three Areas of England, 1971–2001*. New Horizons project report to the Office of the Deputy Prime Minister, available online from: http://www.sasi.group.shef.ac.uk/research/pilot_mapping.htm.

Dorling, D., Mitchell, R., Orford, S., Shaw, M. and Davey Smith, G. (2005) 'Inequalities and Christmas Yet to Come', *British Medical Journal*, 331: 1409.

Dorling, D. and Thomas, B. (2004a) *People and Places: a Census Atlas of the UK*. Bristol: The Policy Press.

Dorling, D. and Thomas, B. (2004b) *Know Your Place: Housing Wealth and Inequality in Great Britain 1980–2003 and Beyond*. Shelter Policy Library (electronic copies available online from: http://www.sheffield.ac.uk/sasi/publications/reports/knowyourplace.htm).

Gordon, D., Adelman, A., Ashworth, K., Bradshaw, J., Levitas, R., Middleton, S., Pantazis, C., Patsios, D., Payne, S., Townsend, P. and Williams, J. (2000) *Poverty and Social Exclusion in Britain*. York: Joseph Rowntree Foundation.

Gordon, D. and Pantazis, C. (eds) (1997) *Breadline Britain in the 1990s*. Aldershot: Ashgate.

Green, A. (1996) 'Aspects of the Changing Geography of Poverty and Wealth', in J. Hills (ed.), *New Inequalities: the Changing Distribution of Income and Wealth in the United Kingdom*. Cambridge: Cambridge University Press.

Green, A. (1998) 'The Geography of Earnings and Incomes in the 1990s', *Environment and Planning C: Government and Policy*, 16: 633–48.

Hagerty, M. and Veenhoven, R. (2001) *Wealth and Happiness Revisited: Growing Wealth of Nations Does Go with Greater Happiness*. University of California-Davis, mimeo 2001 (available online: http://faculty.gsm.ucdavis.edu/~mrhagert/Papers/easterlinreply.pdf).

Hatton, T. J. and Bailey, R. E. (1999) *Seebohm Rowntree and the Post-War Poverty Puzzle*. London: Centre for Economic Policy Research discussion paper 2147.

Hills, J. (1996) 'Introduction: After the Turning Point', in J. Hills (ed.) *New Inequalities: the Changing Distribution of Income and Wealth in the United Kingdom*. Cambridge: Cambridge University Press.

Hills, J. and Stewart, K. (eds) (2005) *A More Equal Society?: New Labour, Poverty, Inequality and Exclusion*. Bristol: The Policy Press.

Jencks, C. (2002) 'Does Inequality Matter?', *Daedalus*, Winter: 49–65.

Layard, R. (2005) *Happiness: Lessons from a New Science*. London: Allen Lane.

Low, A. and Low, A. (2004) Measuring the Gap: Quantifying and Comparing Local Health Inequalities', *Journal of Public Health*, 26(4): 388–95.

Lynch, J., Davey Smith, G., Harper, S., Hillemeier, M., Ross, N., Kaplan, G. A. and Wolfson, M. (2004) 'Is Income Inequality a Determinant of Population Health? Part 1. A Systematic Review', *Millbank Quarterly*, 82: 5–99.

Mackenbach, J. P. and Kunst, A. E. (1997) 'Measuring the Magnitude of Socioeconomic Inequalities in Health: an Overview of Available Measures Illustrated with Two Examples from Europe', *Social Science and Medicine*, 44: 757–71.

Manor, O., Matthews, S. and Power, C. (1997) 'Comparing Measures of Health Inequality', *Social Science and Medicine*, 45: 761–71.

Marx, K. (1847) [online version] *Wage, Labour and Capital*. Marx/Engels Internet Archive (www.marxists.org) 1993, 1999. Available from: http://www.marxists.org/archive/marx/works/1847/wage-labour/index.htm, accessed 15 September 2006.

Mitchell, R., Dorling, D. and Shaw, M. (2000) *Inequalities in Life and Death: What if Britain Were More Equal?* Bristol: The Policy Press.

Oswald, A. J. (1997) 'Happiness and Economic Performance', *Economic Journal*, 107: 1815–31.

Pearce, N. and Paxton, W. (2005) *Social Justice: Building a Fairer Britain*. London: Institute for Public Policy Research/Politico.

Pritchard, J., Thomas, B., Ballas, D. and Dorling, D. (2005) *The State of the Cities Database*, project report submitted to the Office of the Deputy Prime Minister, 30 June.

Ram, R. (2006) 'Further Examination of the Cross-Country Association between Income Inequality and Population Health', *Social Science and Medicine*, 62: 779–91.

Rowntree, B. S. (2000) *Poverty: a Study of Town Life*. Bristol: The Policy Press, centenary edition.

Runciman, W. (1966) *Relative Deprivation and Social Justice*. London: Routledge & Kegan Paul.

Russell, J. (2006) 'Friendship: Needs, Hopes, and Hidden Assumptions', in A. Buonfino and G. Mulgan (eds), *Porcupines in Winter: the Pleasures and Pains of Living Together in Modern Britain*. London: The Young Foundation.

Shaw, M., Dorling, D., Gordon, D. and Davey Smith, G. (1999) *The Widening Gap: Health Inequalities and Policy in Britain*. Bristol: The Policy Press.

Shelter (2005) *The Great Divide: an Analysis of Housing Inequality*. London: Shelter.

Smith, A. (1952) [1759] *The Theory of the Moral Sentiments*, reprint. Indianapolis: Liberty Classics.

Taylor, M. F., Brice, J., Buck, N. and Prentice-Lane, E. (2001) *British Household Panel Survey User Manual Volume A: Introduction, Technical Report and Appendices*. Colchester: University of Essex.

Thomas, B. and Dorling, D. (2007) *People, Places and Identity*. Bristol: The Policy Press.

Veenhoven, R. (1989) 'National Wealth and Individual Happiness', in K. Grunert and M. Olander (eds), *Understanding Economic Behavior*. Dordrecht: Kluwer Academic.

Wagstaff, A., Paci, P. and van Doorslaer, E. (1991) 'On the Measurement of Inequalities in Health', *Social Science and Medicine*, 33(5): 545–57.

Wilkinson, R. (1992) 'Income Distribution and Life Expectancy', *British Medical Journal*, 304: 165–8.

Wilkinson, R. (1997) 'Socioeconomic Determinants of Health: Health Inequalities: Relative or Absolute Material Standards?' *British Medical Journal*, 314: 591.

Wilkinson, R. (2005) *The Impact of Inequality: How to Make Sick Societies Healthier*. New York: New Press.

Wilkinson, R. G. and Pickett, K. E. (2006) 'Income Inequality and Population Health: a Review and Explanation of the Evidence', *Social Science and Medicine* 62(7): 1768–84.

Wolff, J. (2003) *The Message of Redistribution: Disadvantage, Public Policy and the Human Good*. London: Catalyst working paper, Catalyst: (http://www.catalystforum.org.uk/pdf/wolff.pdf), accessed 5 December 2005.

10
A Life Course Approach to Well-Being

Stephani Hatch, Felicia A. Huppert, Rosemary Abbott,
Tim Croudace, George Ploubidis, Michael Wadsworth,
Marcus Richards and Diana Kuh

Introduction

Well-being is characterized by the capacity to actively participate in work and recreation, create meaningful relationships with others, develop a sense of autonomy and purpose in life, and to experience positive emotions. Well-being varies with age, and with personality and age-related attributes such as educational attainment and health status that are known to be shaped by early life experience. Thus we argue for a life course approach that investigates how experiences from the beginning of life promote (or threaten) the development and maintenance of overall well-being, and its physiological, cognitive and psychosocial components. A life course perspective has been actively promoted by many disciplines within the behavioural, biomedical and social sciences (Cairns et al. 1996; Magnusson 1996; Panter-Brick and Worthman 1999; Giele and Elder 1998; Kuh and Ben-Shlomo 2004). Investigating the independent, cumulative and interactive effects of risk and protective factors at each life stage on later health or well-being is methodologically challenging (De Stavola et al. 2006). Up until now more attention has been paid to chains of risk leading to chronic disease or functional loss in later life rather than to protective chains that promote long-term well-being. The life course approach can, and should, accommodate both types of outcome.

An active pursuit of well-being over the life course implies a considerable amount of individual agency, for example in terms of health literacy and preventive behaviours that optimize individual development, function and psychological experience. Individual agency operates within the context of social structure that regulates access to the fundamental resources (e.g. healthy physical environment, power, prestige, money, knowledge, or social connections) through ascribed and achieved socio-economic positions (Link and Phelan 1995).

A life course approach is particularly interested in how access to resources and individual agency in early life have long-term effects, via development and behaviour, on adult physiological, cognitive or psychosocial well-being, and the extent to which these effects can be modified or reversed by later experience. A long-term developmental perspective, focused on early life factors, may promote understanding of how individuals build a foundation for well-being, as well as the far-reaching contribution of positive early life experiences.

In this chapter, we first draw on a conceptual framework for investigating physiological and cognitive well-being across the life course and its early life determinants. We then apply a similar framework to the study of subjective and psychological well-being, explore the life course processes that promote and protect such well-being, and identify areas for further research. We draw particularly on research programmes in the oldest of the three British birth cohorts, the MRC National Survey of Health and Development, commonly known as the 1946 British birth cohort study. This is a prospective study of 5362 individuals (2815 men and 2547 women), followed up repeatedly since their birth in March 1946, until age 60 years.

Physiological and cognitive well-being across the life course

A life course approach to physiological and cognitive well-being begins with some understanding of the natural history and physiological trajectory of biological systems. Many biological functions (such as lung, cognitive or muscle function) display rapid growth and development in the first stages of life followed by a period of stability and then a gradual decline with age (Ben-Shlomo and Kuh 2002). Early life factors may influence the development of this potential or 'capital' and, alongside adult factors, the timing and rate of decline. Physiological and cognitive capital includes the accumulation of biological resources, inherited or acquired during earlier stages of life. Individuals use this capital to adapt to later life challenges, helping to delay physical and cognitive degenerative ageing processes, or their consequences, for well-being.

Tests of physical and cognitive performance to assess developmental potential in children have a long history; they are becoming an increasingly popular approach for assessing ageing processes in older people. Older people with better scores on tests of grip strength, standing balance, and chair rises (i.e. ability to stand from sitting), for example, have higher chances of survival and are less likely to become frail and disabled than those with lower scores (Onder et al. 2005; Guralnik et al. 1995; Rantanen et al. 2003). There is growing evidence that developmental characteristics, such as prenatal and postnatal growth, and childhood motor and cognitive abilities, are associated with better physical performance in later life (Aihie Sayer et al. 2004; Kuh et al. 2006b). In terms of later cognitive performance, childhood cognitive ability protects against cognitive decline in later life (Richards et al. 2004). Early cognitive ability is also associated with longevity (Whalley and Deary 2001; Kuh et al. 2004) and better adult physical health, for example better lung function (Richards et al. 2005) or later age at menopause timing (Kuh et al. 2005). As yet it is still to be clarified whether these associations reflect primarily neurodevelopmental pathways or social pathways, given that early cognitive ability is also associated with safer adult environments and healthy adult behaviours (Whalley and Deary 2001; Power and Kuh 2006).

The early social environment influences adult physiological and cognitive well-being, independently of adult risk factors (Richards and Sacker 2003; Guralnik et al. 2006). In the 1946 British birth cohort study, for example, those raised by well-educated mothers were more likely than others to be in the top 10 per cent on an aggregate physical performance score at age 53 (Guralnik et al. 2006). Those from non-manual rather than manual social class origins were more likely at age 36 to be in the healthiest top 10 per cent (defined by the absence of health problems or poor biological function) (Kuh and Wadsworth 1993). These effects persisted even after taking account of own adult socio-economic circumstances and health behaviours.

This growing evidence of the early developmental and social origins of adult physiological and cognitive well-being needs to be replicated in other cohorts and the underlying long-term biological and social processes elucidated. This approach, based on objective indicators, is complementary to the health and functioning models of quality of life (Brown et al. 2004) that generally rely on scales based on reports of ability to undertake activities of daily living.

Subjective aspects of well-being across the life course

Different perspectives have been utilized in developing operational definitions of subjective aspects of well-being and measurement scales. These measures of well-being form part of a wider, diffuse set of measures of quality of life and successful ageing, that reflect the lack of an agreed definitive theoretical framework in this research area (Brown et al. 2004).

A parsimonious and public health perspective views well-being as the positive end of a single continuum of mental health, from disorder to well-being. However, many mental health measures are derived from screening questionnaires for mental disorders and psychological distress (e.g. the General Health Questionnaire) that include symptoms of illness, not signs of positive well-being, and usually discriminate less well at the positive end of the spectrum (Croudace et al., provisionally accepted).

Other perspectives view subjective aspects of well-being as a multi-dimensional rather than unidimensional construct; they distinguish hedonic or subjective well-being that captures experiences of happiness and life satisfaction (Bradburn 1969; Diener 1984; Kahneman et al. 1999) from eudaimonic or psychological well-being that captures the realization of personal potential, the pursuit of goals, and personal development (Ryff 1989; Ryff et al. 2004; Ryan and Deci 2001). For example, Diener (1984) and colleagues (Diener et al. 1999) argue that hedonic well-being comprises three independent constructs: pleasant affect, lack of unpleasant affect and life satisfaction. Bradburn's (1969) Affect Balance Scale is one of the most well-known instruments measuring the affective dimension of well-being by determining an individual's level of positive and negative affect. Emerging from ageing studies on adaptation, life satisfaction measures refer to a cognitive evaluation of one's general life situation and of various domains (e.g. work, social life, family, marriage) (Pinquart and Sorenson 2000). Neugarten et al.'s (1961) Life Satisfaction Index and Diener et al.'s (1985) Satisfaction with Life Scale are two of the most widely used measures of the cognitive dimensions of well-being.

Ryff and her colleagues (Ryff 1989; Ryff and Keyes 1995) have developed a theoretical-based, multidimensional measure of eudamonic well-Being. Ryff's (1989) Scales of Psychological Well-Being (PWB) purport to identify six separate dimensions of psychological well-being: autonomy, environmental mastery, personal growth, positive relations with others, purpose in life, and self-acceptance. Empirical data have shown that these dimensions are interrelated (Abbott et al. 2006; Cheng and Chan 2005; Kafka and Kozma 2002; Springer and Hauser 2006) and are not independent, as suggested by Ryff's theory.

A number of questions are raised when investigating these measures of the subjective aspects of well-being from a life course perspective. First, should definitions of well-being be tailored to the age or life phase of the population being assessed? For example, Bergman and Scott (2001) argue that measures of adolescent well-being should be based on multidimensional constructs that consider the cognitive and behavioural processes related to identity transitions of a particular life phase. Satisfaction with body image and family are two domains that they postulate to have a qualitatively different meaning for adolescents in comparison to adults, especially in terms of self-esteem and mastery.

Second, what do we know about the life course trajectory of subjective aspects of well-being? Cross-sectional studies using Ryff's PWB items have suggested that the different dimensions of psychological well-being exhibit varying age profiles. Purpose in life and personal growth scores are lower in older age groups, whilst environmental mastery scores are higher. In contrast, self-acceptance shows little age variation (Ryff 1989; Ryff and Keyes 1995). Eudaimonic well-being may change as individuals negotiate various life transitions (Kwan et al. 2003). Longitudinal research shows that life satisfaction generally increases with age, but the results for positive and negative affect are less consistent. Studies demonstrate both improvement and decline in positive affect and both stability and reduction in negative affect (Diener and Suh 1998; Ryff et al. 2004). Clearly then, the trajectory of well-being, whether eudaimonic or hedonic, takes a different form, at least over adult life, than trajectories of physiological and cognitive well-being. This is supported by recent research on quality of life in older people, using an outcome (CASP-19) based on a theory of needs satisfaction that captures the concepts of control, autonomy, self realization and pleasure (Netuveli et al. 2006). In the English Longitudinal Study of Ageing of 11 000 persons aged 50 years and older, quality of life, as measured by CASP-19, increased from age 50 years to peak at 68 years and then gradually declined reaching the same level as at 50 years by 86 years.

Third, to what extent is the foundation for subjective aspects of well-being laid in early life? Huppert (2005) suggests that the origins of positive emotions lie in development, drawing on pioneering human studies of mother–infant attachment styles and animal studies of the effects of maternal care on offspring's stress response. However, evidence that well-being in childhood and adolescence shapes aspects of adult subjective well-being is limited. Personality traits most relevant in assessing happiness, such as extroversion and neuroticism have been linked to well-being (Vitterso and Nilsen 2002), and to the extent that these are stable across the life course, links between childhood and adulthood might be expected. Preliminary analysis on the 1946 British birth cohort showed that early personality measures were associated with psychological well-being in midlife. Measures of extroversion and neuroticism obtained in adolescence and early adult life explained between 12 per cent (autonomy) and 19 per cent (self-acceptance and positive relations) of the variance in the Ryff PWB dimensions of women in their early fifties. Extroversion had a significant positive relationship with all six PWB dimensions explaining from 7.6 per cent (purpose in life) to 15 per cent (positive relationships) of PWB variance. Conversely, neuroticism was negatively related to PWB, particularly environmental mastery, purpose in life and self-acceptance (Abbott et al. under preparation). As expected, an inverse relationship was observed between a traditional mental health outcome (GHQ-28) in mid-life and personality measured in adolescence/early adulthood. Neuroticism was a very strong predictor of mental health outcomes, whereas extroversion had a negligible effect (Ploubidis et al., submitted).

Fourth, to what extent are subjective aspects of well-being dependent upon the development and maintenance of physiological and cognitive well-being (and vice versa)? A better understanding of their dynamic interplay would promote understanding of how people use their 'capital' in these areas to maintain overall well-being over the life course. There is growing evidence from ageing studies that maintenance of good health is a critical influence on aspects of subjective well-being (Brown et al. 2004; Baltes and Mayer 1999), and that the quality of socially productive activities is a critical influence in maintaining physiological and cognitive well-being (Siegrist 2005).

There is little evidence on the effects of early socio-economic circumstances on adult psychological well-being because few long-term cohort studies have measured well-being. Studies generally focus on poor emotional well-being and show, for example, strong relationships between parents' low socio-economic position and higher risks of hopelessness and cynical hostility in adult life (Berkman and Gurland 1998; Lynch et al. 1997) or poor self-rated health and psychological distress (Power et al. 2002). Most of the evidence relates to associations between adult socio-economic circumstances and adult psychological well-being where findings are inconsistent (Diener and Biswas-Diener 2002; Myers 2000). Some US longitudinal evidence showed that increases in income are related to lower subjective well-being (Diener et al. 1993). In contrast, most studies of psychological and subjective well-being show a social gradient whereby the higher the socio-economic position, the higher the well-being and that income is a strong positive predictor of happiness (Helliwell and Putnam 2004; Ryff and Singer 1998a; Ryff et al. 1999; Subramanian et al. 2005). These inconsistent results may be explained if income does little to improve happiness and well-being once individuals have enough money to satisfy basic needs, such as food and shelter (Diener and Biswas-Diener 2002).

In the 1946 birth cohort study we found inconsistent effects of different measures of socio-economic position on PWB in 52-year-old women. Greater levels of household income and higher adult social class were positively associated with higher reported levels of PWB, but women with the lowest levels of education had the highest levels of PWB, significantly so on the dimensions of environmental mastery, positive relations with others and self-acceptance.

Psychosocial capital

The concept of 'psychosocial capital' refers to the accumulation of psychosocial resources such as personal and social skills (e.g. competence), capacity for positive emotions (e.g. hope and optimism), attitudes and values that develop over time, particularly during childhood and adolescence. The development of psychosocial capital is influenced by opportunities for socialization and social integration (through social networks and social support) that are shaped by the social structure and access to material resources (see below). Psychosocial capital can be mobilized proactively or as adversities arise to develop coping strategies (see below) to maintain subjective aspects of well-being. Positive behavioural and emotional responses of individuals to environmental challenges are likely to reinforce psychosocial capital (see below).

We suggest that a number of components of psychosocial capital should be studied from a life course perspective to explore how they develop and are maintained across the life course. These are self-competence, mastery, self-esteem, and 'mattering', by which we mean the degree that individuals feel they matter to significant others.

Various definitions of *self-competence* have been explored (Baltes et al. 1993). Psychological conceptualizations of self-competence consider the process to involve basic cognitions and domain-specific knowledge needed to address and solve issues related to daily living (Pinquart and Sorenson 2000). Baltes et al. (1993) argue that considerations of self-competence must distinguish between competence as a range of skills, as belief about one's abilities (the mastery or self-efficacy perspective) versus competence arising from a match between abilities and environmental demands (the adaptive fit perspective).

The general concept of *mastery* (also referred to as self-efficacy) is defined as an individual's understanding and perceptions of their ability to control the forces that affect their lives (Pearlin and Schooler 1978). Mastery is not a fixed element of personality, but is a dynamic aspect of the self-concept that has the potential to change as individuals' lives change (Skaff et al. 1996). Mastery is a potential moderator in the stress process (i.e. exposure to adversity, acute stressors, chronic strain) for two reasons: people with a high level of mastery are less threatened by stressors in comparison to those with more limited mastery, and people who believe they can exert some control over adverse conditions are more likely to act in a manner consistent with their beliefs. As Rosenberg suggests with self-esteem, Pearlin (1999) contends mastery may be captured globally, as well as role and situation specific.

Self-esteem refers to both global and specific cognitive evaluations of the self (Rosenberg 1979). Rosenberg (1965) defines self-esteem as positive attitudes one takes towards oneself. In order to fully understand self-esteem, the selection of reference groups and significant others referred to in making social comparisons and evaluations must be known. Some evidence suggests that self-esteem and life satisfaction reflect long-term, stable judgements of well-being in contrast to happiness which reflects more short-term assessments of subjective well-being that vary by situation (Pinquart and Sorenson 2000).

Mattering, the degree to which we feel we matter to significant others, is a motive that propels us towards actions that benefit our well-being. Mattering to another person makes one feel the object of attention, important to others, and that others depend on us. Rosenberg believed that mattering binds us to society through social obligations and operates as a source of social integration. Rosenberg and McCullough (1981) provide empirical evidence suggesting the importance of mattering on an individual level in relation to self-esteem and mental health, specifically depression and anxiety, and on a societal level, as a significant source of social cohesion. A sense of mattering is hypothesized to change across the life course. Rosenberg hypothesizes young children ('the world revolves around me') and adults ('I run the world') possess a higher sense of mattering than adolescents and the aged, whose roles are less socially defined, in part, because family units are less dependent on their contribution.

Resilience

Resilience is the capacity for positive adaptation in the face of ever-changing environmental challenges (Cicchetti and Cohen 1995). Since large numbers of people do not show negative outcomes in the presence of acute or chronic stressors, we need to understand what protects them from adversity, facilitates effective coping and confers resilience.

Resilience depends on extrinsic and intrinsic protective factors. Extrinsic factors operate indirectly to modify exposure to, or the impact of, adverse events. Intrinsic protective factors are the accumulated physiological, cognitive and psychosocial capital that individuals can mobilize. The result of previous experiences can also reinforce or mitigate the impact of negative life events (Rutter 1985). Positive outcomes are characterized by successful adaptation where a sense of mastery is reinforced; negative outcomes are characterized by poor adaptation that reinforces a sense of failure.

Existing research has focused on the intrinsic and extrinsic factors associated with educational, emotional and behavioural resilience of children (Luthar et al. 2000). In the 1946 cohort, we have explored early life factors associated with maintaining adolescent well-being in the face of adversity. Initial findings show that protective parental characteristics, such as low maternal neuroticism, were associated with high well-being in adolescence in the presence of high levels of material disadvantage from early childhood. Generally, there has been less focus on physiological resilience, adult resilience, whether childhood resilience is associated with later adult resilience, or whether resilience in one domain increases the chance of resilience in another. Ryff et al. (1998) have explored pathways to psychological resilience in middle-aged women using person-centred techniques to construct individual narratives. They found that the life course trajectories of a small group of women with high levels of psychological well-being despite a history of depression involved one or more of the following: good starting resources, quality social relationships, realization of desired trajectories, and positive social comparisons (Ryff et al. 1989).

Life course processes that develop psychosocial capital and promote subjective aspects of well-being

Socialization and social integration are two primary processes unfolding over the life course that develop psychosocial capital and promote subjective aspects of well-being. These processes are strongly influenced by the social structure and the resources that are differentially mobilized depending on social position. They also require an active and growing involvement by the individual in social interactions as they develop and mature.

Socialization

The early development of psychosocial capital is influenced by socialization and social integration efforts by parents, teachers and caregivers (Schooling and Kuh 2002). Socialization is defined as the manner in which individuals selectively acquire skills, knowledge, values, motives and roles that are associated with certain status position in society or groups (Bush and Simmons 1992; Sewell 1963). There are four contexts present during the life course with the explicit purpose to socialize and integrate individuals at both the community and societal level (Gecas 1992).

First, family life can be a vital source of meaning and purpose, and variation in the structure and functioning of the family influences patterns of power and authority in familial socialization. The family socialization process potentially benefits both the child and the parents. Ryff and colleagues developed an extensive research programme to investigate the relationship between parenting and well-being. One study found that parents in middle age with adult children had higher well-being if they perceived their children to be doing as well, or better, than themselves and if they believed they had raised children who were more self-confident and happy (Ryff et al. 1994).

Second, school has a more narrowly defined socialization goal that primarily involves formal instruction and cognitive development (the acquisition of knowledge, development of analytic and verbal skills). The structural features of the classroom encourage students to make social comparisons and develop their response to a system of costs and rewards.

Third, peer groups are an avenue for socialization that are uniquely characterized by being voluntary associations where boundaries are more fluid and independence can be exercised. Friendships are, more often than other relationships, associations between status equals. They help to develop competence and validation of the self and provide an opportunity to acquire knowledge not introduced in family and school contexts.

Finally, the work (occupational) context is often the most dominant setting for socialization outside of the family. It is organized around a bureaucratic structure and the socialization of adults in this context varies by the levels of autonomy, conformity, supervision, routinization, and complexity experienced (Kohn 1980). Certain jobs give access to status, prestige, knowledge and other resources that enhance well-being, especially when accompanied by a sense of mastery.

Social integration

Social integration refers to individuals' embeddedness in social structures that results from involvement with and attachment to individuals and networks through participation in social organizations (Lin et al. 1999). A feeling of belonging, which comes from a high level of social integration, is a fundamental human motive, and is likely to contribute to enduring well-being over the life course (Ryff and Singer 1998b).

The process of social integration extends from entry into the earliest social milieux (e.g. playgroups and nursery) in childhood and continues throughout life to old age. Social organizations provide anchorage for people integrated into them and serve as stabilizing forces that furnish a potential protective function. Social integration gives people access to the interpersonal relationships where values, norms and beliefs are set and collective sentiments shared by its members. Greater social integration often results in more opportunities to gather social support through increasing social network size and strengthening social ties (Hong and Seltzer 1995).

There is growing evidence of the beneficial effect on well-being of reciprocity in social exchange, which is having opportunities to give as well as receive social support. Evidence suggests that receiving help (social support) buffers against negative well-being, whereas giving help (social contribution) is more influential for positive well-being (Huppert and Whittington 2003). The study of lifetime influences on social participation, and on the quality and quantity of social relationships is gaining momentum (Marks and Ashleman 2002; Hatch and Wadsworth, under review) and should continue to be pursued, particularly the implications for well-being.

Protecting aspects of subjective well-being

Coping

Coping refers to behaviours that individuals employ in an effort to prevent or avoid adversity and its consequences (Lazarus and Folkman 1984; Pearlin 1999; Pearlin and Schooler 1978). These behaviours function to shape the meaning of adversity, to reduce threat, and to hinder stress proliferation. Successful coping efforts ultimately change the situations from which stressors arise. More research has focused on identifying coping responses than assessing whether or not coping is efficacious in preserving well-being.

The stressors that people have to cope with are not evenly distributed in the population and are not the result of rare situations, such as exposure to a traumatic event. Stressors are, in fact, persistent and relatively common adverse situations and events that are often socially patterned, and can affect well-being over the life course. For example, caregiving burden and community relocation are associated with significant changes in well-being over time (Kling et al. 1997).

People have distinct responses (i.e. behaviours, cognitions and perceptions) that are used in coping repertoires when confronted with deleterious circumstances. Pearlin and Schooler (1978) differentiate psychological resources (or what we call capital) from coping responses. The former refers to a matter of being or who people are, while the latter refers to actions or concrete efforts to confront adversity.

Aspinwall and Taylor (1997) differentiate *coping with stressful events* (actions to reduce or minimize perceived harm or losses), *anticipatory coping* (preparation for the stressful event that is likely to result in potential harm or losses), and *proactive coping*. Proactive coping is action that is temporally prior to other types of coping and involves the accumulation of resources and the acquisition of skills for general preparation for encountering stressors. Aspinwall and Taylor argue that proactive coping requires a different set of skills related to the ability to identify potential sources of stress before it occurs. These sets of skills and activities are related to processing information and making positive reappraisals (see below) and may be particularly important to develop early in life.

In Fredrickson's (2001) 'broaden-and-build' theory, positive emotions, such as joy, contentment and pride, are seen as beneficial in broadening thought–action repertoires and building psychosocial capital to be utilized in coping. Research on small groups by Fredrickson and colleagues reveals that positive emotions contribute to finding positive meaning and enhancing coping resources in the face of negative events and circumstances (Tugade et al. 2004; Tugade and Fredrickson 2004).

Two competing theoretical views about coping efficacy are of interest from a life course perspective and will be tested in the 1946 British birth cohort study. Do positive experiences or a particular temperament in early life underpin the ability of adults to cope with adversity, or determine their likelihood of exposure to adversity? Or are coping resources for adult life developed only when children have been challenged by adversity?

Cognitive appraisal

Cognitive functioning has a primary role in relation to subjective well-being and the capacity for resilience in the face of adversity (Masten et al. 1999). Cognitive processes generally involve some type of appraisal, both positive and negative, of a major event or situation. Primary appraisals involve judgements about whether the individual is in jeopardy and secondary appraisals involve judgements about the options and resources available to the individual in response to the event (Lazarus and Folkman 1984). Hence cognitive appraisal underlies the choice of coping strategies. Tertiary appraisals (Janoff-Bulman 1992) are ongoing evaluations, potentially over many years, of the impact of the experience after it has occurred. From a life course perspective, tertiary appraisals may be of particular interest because they involve time and potential change in the meaning of events and circumstances. In contrast to appraisals of situations, reflective appraisals refer to how individuals perceive others view them (Cooley 1902). There are reciprocal influences of well-being on reflective appraisals in times of negotiating a major life transition (Kwan et al. 2003).

Motivation and reinforcements

A less developed area related to the protection of well-being concerns the processes that turn experiences of positive affect into sustained well-being. Prolonged regulation of behaviours over the life course largely depends on both intrinsic motivation (i.e. the tendency to explore, exercise one's capacities, to assimilate, and seek out challenges for the inherent satisfaction of the activity) and extrinsic motivation (i.e. performing an activity in order to obtain a discrete outcome) (Ryan and Deci 2000).

Often individuals are extrinsically motivated to engage in behaviours because they are modelled on or valued by significant others to whom they feel they matter. Internalizing and integrating behaviours potentially beneficial to sustaining well-being begin in childhood socialization. Prolonging extrinsically motivated behaviours, to a large extent, depends on perceived self-competence and mastery. To this end, external reinforcements may provide a concrete marker of successful socialization and integration in that they represent a 'life of productive activity' (Becker 1992). The accumulation of reinforcements, such as public acknowledgements and accolades received from educational sources, involvement in social organizations, and advancement in work settings, serve to further internalize and integrate behaviours, improve a sense of self-competence, and preserve well-being (Ryan and Deci 2000).

Conclusions

There is growing recognition that the well-being of individuals or populations cannot be understood simply in terms of the absence of risk factors for negative outcomes. A life course framework offers a dynamic model of the interplay over time between the individual, his or her accumulated capital, and the environment that can be used to understand the factors that develop and maintain well-being and successful adaptation over the life course. The physiological, cognitive and psychosocial components of capital, well-being and resilience are intertwined over the life course and should be studied together. There is growing evidence from the 1946 British birth cohort study and other longitudinal studies that developmental factors, the early social environment, early behaviour and temperament have long-term effects on adult physiological, cognitive and psychosocial well-being through the capacity to accumulate capital and promote resilience. Further longitudinal research is needed to identify common psychosocial and biological life course pathways that underlie these associations so that early interventions to promote individual and societal well-being and resilience can be identified. We have identified some theoretical constructs and processes that could be operationalized in longitudinal studies that may help to elucidate these pathways.

References

Abbott, R. A., Ploubidis, G. B., Huppert, F. A., Kuh, D., Wadsworth, M. E. and Croudace, T. J. (2006) 'Psychometric Evaluation and Predictive Validity of Ryff's Psychological Well-Being Items in a UK Birth Cohort Sample of Women', *Health and Quality of Life Outcomes*, 4: 76.

Aihie Sayer, A., Syddall, H. E., Gilbody, H. J., Dennison, E. M. and Cooper, C. (2004) 'Does Sarcopenia Originate in Early Life? Findings from the Hertfordshire Cohort Study', *Journal of Gerontology: Biological Sciences and Medical Sciences*, 59: 930–4.

Aspinwall, L. G. and Taylor, S. E. (1997) 'A Stitch in Time: Self-Regulation and Proactive Coping', *Psychological Bulletin*, 121: 417–36.

Baltes P. B. and Mayer, K. U. (eds) (1999) *The Berlin Ageing Study: Ageing from 70 to 100*. New York: Cambridge University Press.

Baltes, M. M., Mayr, U., Borchelt, M., Maas, I. and Wilms, H. (1993) 'Everyday Competence in Old and Very Old Age: the Inter-disciplinary Perspective', *Ageing and Society*, 13: 657–80.

Barker, D. J. P. (1998) *Mothers, Babies and Health in Later Life*. Edinburgh: Churchill Livingstone.

Becker, L. C. (1992) 'Good Lives: Prolegomena', *Social Philosophy and Policy*, 9: 15–37.

Ben-Shlomo, Y. and Kuh, D. (2002) 'A Life Course Approach to Chronic Disease Epidemiology: Conceptual Models, Empirical Challenges, and Interdisciplinary Perspectives', *International Journal of Epidemiology*, 31: 285–93.

Bergman, M. M. and Scott, J. (2001) 'Young Adolescents' Well-Being and Health-Risk Behaviours: Gender and Socio-economic Differences', *Journal of Adolescence*, 24: 183–97.

Berkman, C. S. and Gurland, B. J. (1998) 'The Relationship Among Income, Other Socioeconomic Indicators, and Functional Level in Older Persons', *Journal of Ageing and Health*, 10: 81–98.

Bradburn, N. M. (1969) *The Structure of Psychological Well-Being*. Chicago: Aldine.

Brown, J., Bowling, A. and Flynn, T. N (2004) 'Models of Quality of Life: a Taxonomy and Systematic Review of the Literature'. European Forum on Population Ageing Research (http:///www.shef.ac.uk/ageingresearch/pdf/).

Bush, D. M. and Simmons, R. G. (1992) 'Socialization Processes Over the Life Course', in M. Rosenberg and R. Turner (eds), *Social Psychology: Sociological Perspectives*. New Brunswick, NJ: Transaction Publishers.

Cairns, R. B., Elder, G. H. and Costello, E. J. (eds) (1996) *Developmental Science*. Cambridge: Cambridge University Press.

Cheng, S. T. and Chan, A. C. (2005) 'Measuring Psychological Well-Being in the Chinese', *Personality and Individual Differences*, 38: 1307–16.

Cicchetti, D. and Cohen, D. (1995) 'Perspectives on Developmental Psychopathology', in D. Cicchetti and D. Cohen (eds), *Developmental Psychopathology. Vol. I: Theory and Methods*. New York: Wiley and Sons, pp. 3–22.

Cooley, C. H. (1902) *Human Nature and the Social Order*. New York: Scribner.

Croudace, T. J., Abbott, R., Ploubidis, G. B., Colman, I., Jones, P. B., Huppert, F. A., Kuh, D. and Wadsworth, M. E. 'Psychometric Modelling of Goldberg's General Health Questionnaire (GHQ-28): Modified Likert Scoring [0-0-1-2] is Preferred for Measuring a Continua of Psychological Distress in the Population', *Journal of Clinical Epidemiology* (provisionally accepted).

De Stavola, B. L., Nitsch, D., dos Santos Silva, I., McCormack, V., Hardy, R., Mann, V., Cole, T. J., Morton, S. and Leon, D. A. (2006) 'Statistical Issues in Life Course Epidemiology', *American Journal of Epidemiology*, 163: 84–96.

Diener, E. (1984) 'Subjective Well-Being', *Psychological Bulletin*, 95: 542–75.

Diener, E. and Biswas-Diener, R (2002) 'Will Money Increase Subjective Well-Being: a Literature Review and Guide to Needed Research', *Social Indicators Research*, 57: 119–69.

Diener, E., Horwitz, J. and Emmons, R. A. (1985) 'Happiness of the Very Wealthy', *Social Indicators Research*, 16: 263–74.

Diener, E., Sandvik, E., Seidlitz, L. and Diener, M. (1993) 'The Relationship between Income and Subjective Well-Being: Relative or Absolute?', *Social Indicators Research*, 28: 195–223.

Diener, E. and Suh, E. (1998) 'Age and Subjective Well-Being: an International Analysis', *Annual Review of Gerontology and Geriatrics*, 17: 304–24.

Diener, E., Suh, E., Lucas, R. and Smith, H. (1999) 'Subjective Well-Being: Three Decades of Progress', *Psychological Bulletin*, 125: 276–302.

Dubos, R. (1965) *Man Adapting*. New Haven and London: Yale University Press.

Fredrickson, B. L. (2001) 'The Role of Positive Emotions in Positive Psychology: the Broaden-and-Build Theory of Positive Emotions', *American Psychologist*, 56: 218–26.

Gecas, V. (1992) 'Contexts of Socialization', in M. Rosenberg and R. Turner (eds), *Social Psychology: Sociological Perspectives*. New Brunswick, NJ: Transaction Publishers.

Giele, J. Z. and Elder, G. H. Jr. (1998) 'Life Course Research: Development of a Field', in J. Z. Giele and G. H. Elder Jr. (eds), *Methods of Life Course Research: Qualitiative and Quantitative Approaches*. Thousand Oaks, CA: Sage Publications Inc.

Guralnik, J., Butterworth, S., Wadsworth, M. E. J. and Kuh, D. L. (2006) 'Childhood Socioeconomic Status Predicts Physical Functioning a Half Century Later', *Journal of Gerontology: Biological Sciences and Medical Sciences*, 61A: 694–701.

Guralnik, J. M., Ferucci, L., Simonsick, E. M. and Wallace, R. B. (1995) 'Lower Extremity Function in Persons Over the Age of 70 Years as a Predictor of Subsequent Disability', *New England Journal of Medicine*, 332: 556–61.

Hatch, S. L. and Wadsworth, M. E. J. 'Does Adolescent Affect Impact Adult Social Integration? Evidence from the British 1946 Birth Cohort', *Sociolgy* (in press).

Helliwell, J. and Putnam, R. D. (2004) 'The Social Context of Well-Being', *Philosophical Transactions of the Royal Society*, series B, 359: 1435–46.

Hong, J. and Seltzer, M. M. (1995) 'The Psychological Consequences of Multiple Roles: the Non-normative Case', *Journal of Health and Social Behavior*, 36: 386–98.

Huppert, F. A. (2006) 'Developmental, Neuroscience and Health Perspectives', in J. P. Forgas (ed.), *Affect in Social Thinking and Behaviour*. New York: Psychology Press, 235–52.

Huppert, F. A. and Whittington, J. (2003) 'Evidence for the Independence of Positive and Negative Well-Being: Implications for Quality of Life Assessment', *British Journal of Health Psychology*, 8: 107–22.

Janoff-Bulman, R. (1992) *Shattered Assumptions: Toward a New Psychology of Trauma*. New York: Free Press.

Kafka, G. and Kozma, A. (2002) 'The Construct Validity of Ryff's Scales of Psychological Well-Being (SPWB) and their Relationship to Measures of Subjective Well-Being', *Social Indicators Research*, 57: 171–90.

Kahneman, D., Diener, E. and Schwarz, N. (eds) (1999) *Well-Being: the Foundations of Hedonic Psychology*. New York: Russell Sage Foundation.

Kling, K. C., Seltzer, M. and Ryff, C. D. (1997) 'Distinctive Later Life Challenges: Implications for Coping and Well-Being', *Psychology and Ageing*, 12: 288–95.

Kohn, M. (1980) 'Job Complexity and Adult Personality', in N. Smelser and E. Erikson (eds), *Themes of Love and Work in Adulthood*. Cambridge, MA: Harvard University Press.

Kuh, D. L. and Ben-Shlomo, Y. (eds) (2004) *A Life Course Approach to Chronic Disease Epidemiology: Tracing the Origins of Ill-health from Early to Adult Life*. 2nd edn. Oxford: Oxford University Press.

Kuh, D. L., Butterworth, S., Kok, H., Richards, M., Hardy, R., Wadsworth, M. E. J. and Leon, D. A. (2005) 'Childhood Cognitive Ability and Age at Menopause: Evidence from Two Cohort Studies', *Menopause*, 12: 475–82.

Kuh, D., Hardy, R., Butterworth, S., Okell, L., Wadsworth, M. E. J., Cooper, C. and Aihie Sayer, A. (2006a) 'Developmental Origins of Adult Grip Strength: Findings from a British Birth Cohort Study', *Journal of Gerontology: Biological Sciences and Medical Sciences*, 61, 7: 702–6.

Kuh, D., Hardy, R., Butterworth, S., Okell, L., Wadsworth, M. E. J., Cooper, C. and Aihie Sayer, A. (2006b) 'Developmental Origins of Midlife Performance: Evidence from a British Birth Cohort Study', *American Journal of Epidemiology*, 164: 110–21.

Kuh, D., Richards, M., Hardy, R., Butterworth, S. and Wadsworth, M. E. J. (2004) 'Childhood Cognitive Ability and Deaths Up Until Middle Age: a Postwar Birth Cohort Study', *International Journal of Epidemiology*, 33: 408–13.

Kuh, D. L. and Wadsworth, M. E. J. (1993) 'Physical Health Status at 36 Years in a British National Birth Cohort', *Social Science and Medicine*, 37: 905–16.

Kwan, C. M. L., Love, G., Ryff, C. and Essex, M. (2003) 'The Role of Self-enhancing Evaluations in a Successful Life Transition', *Psychology and Ageing*, 18: 3–12.

Lazarus, R. S. and Folkman, S. (1984) *Stress, Appraisal, and Coping*. New York: Springer.

Lin, N., Xiaolan, Y. and Ensel. W. (1999) 'Social Support and Depressed Mood: a Structural Analysis', *Journal of Health and Social Behavior*, 40: 344–59.

Link, B. G. and Phelan, J. C. (1995) 'Social Conditions as Fundamental Causes of Disease', *Journal of Health and Social Behavior* (Extra Issue): 80–94.

Lucas, R., Diener, E., Grob, A., Suh, E. and Shao, L. (2000) 'Cross-cultural Evidence for the Fundamental Features of Extraversion', *Journal of Personality and Social Psychology*, 79: 452–68.

Luthar, S. S., Cicchetti, D. and Becker, B. (2000) 'The Construct of Resilience: a Critical Evaluation and Guidelines for Future Work', *Child Development*, 71: 543–62.

Lynch, J. W., Kaplan, G. A. and Salonen, J. T. (1997) 'Why Do Poor People Behave Poorly? Variation in Adult Health Behaviours and Psychosocial Characteristics by Stages of the Socioeconomic Lifecourse', *Social Science and Medicine*, 44: 809–19.

Magnusson, D. (ed.) (1996) *The Lifespan Development of Individuals: Behavioral, Neurobiological and Psychosocial Perspectives*. Cambridge: Cambridge University Press.

Marks, N. F. and Ashleman, K. (2002) 'Life Course Influences on Women's Social Relationships at Midlife', in D. Kuh and R. Hardy (eds), *A Life Course Approach to Women's Health*. Oxford: Oxford University Press.

Masten, A. S., Hubbard, J. J., Gest, S. D., Tellegen, A., Garmezy, N. and Ramirez, N. (1999) 'Competence in the Context of Adversity: Pathways to Resilience and Maladaptation from Childhood to Late Adolescence', *Development and Psychopathology*, 11: 143–69.

Myers, D. (2000) 'The Funds, Friends, and Faith of Happy People', *American Psychologist*, 55: 56–67.

Netuveli, G., Wiggins, R. D., Hildon, Z., Montgomery, S. M. and Blane, D. (2006) 'Quality of Life at Older Ages: Evidence from the English Longitudinal Study of Ageing (wave 1)', *Journal of Epidemiology and Public Health*, 60: 357–63.

Neugarten, B. L., Havighurst, R. and Tobin, S. (1961) 'The Measurement of Life Satisfaction', *Journal of Gerontology*, 16: 134–43.

Onder, G., Penninx, B. W., Ferucci, L., Fried, L. P., Guralnik, J. M. and Pahor, M. (2005) 'Measures of Physical Performance and Risk for Progressive and Catastrophic Disability: Results from the Women's Health and Ageing Study', *Journal of Gerontology: Biological Sciences and Medical Sciences*, 60: 74–9.

Panter-Brick. C. and Worthman , C. M. (eds) (1999) *Hormones, Health and Behaviour*. Cambridge: Cambridge University Press.

Pearlin, L. I. (1999) 'The Stress Concept Revisited', in C. S. Aneshensel and J. Phelan (eds), *Handbook of the Sociology of Mental Health*. New York: Kluwer Academic/Plenum.

Pearlin, L. I. and Schooler, C. (1978) 'The Structure of Coping', *Journal of Health and Social Behavior*, 19: 2–21.

Pinquart, M. and Sorensen, S. (2000) 'Influences of Socio-economic Status, Social Networks, and Competence on Subjective Well-Being in Later Life: a Meta-analysis', *Psychology and Ageing*, 15: 187–24.

Ploubidis, G. B., Abbott, R. A., Kuh, D., Wadsworth, M. E. J., Huppert, F. A. and Croudace, T. J. 'Life-course Associations Between Personality Traits in Early Adulthood and Multiple Measures of Mental Health through Mid-life: a Prospective Birth Cohort Study', *British Journal of Psychiatry* (submitted).

Power, C. and Kuh, D. (2006) 'Life Course Development of Unequal Health', in J. Siegrist and M. Marmot (eds), *Socioeconomic Position and Health: New Explanations and Their Policy Implications*. Oxford: Oxford University Press.

Power, C., Stansfeld, S. A., Matthers, S., Manor, O. and Hope, S. (2002) 'Childhood and Adult Risk Factors for Socio-economic Differentials in Psychological Distress: Evidence from the 1958 British Birth Cohort', *Social Science and Medicine*, 55: 1989–2004.

Rantanen, T., Volpato, S., Ferrucci, L., Heikkinen, E., Fried, L. P. and Guralnik, J. M. (2003) 'Handgrip Strength and Cause-specific and Total Mortality in Older Disabled Women: Exploring the Mechanism', *Journal of the American Geriatrics Society*, 51: 636–41.

Richards, M. and Sacker, A. (2003) 'A. Lifetime Antecedents of Cognitive Reserve', *Journal of Clinical and Experimental Neuropsychology*, 25: 614–24.

Richards, M., Shipley, B., Fuhrer, R. and Wadsworth, M. E. J. (2004) 'Cognitive Ability in Childhood and Cognitive Decline in Mid-life: Longitudinal Birth Cohort Study', *British Medical Journal*, 328: 552–4.

Richards, M., Strachan, D., Hardy, R., Kuh, D. L. and Wadsworth, M. E. J. (2005) 'Lung Function and Cognitive Ability in a Longitudinal Birth Cohort Study', *Psychosomatic Medicine*, 67: 602–8.

Rosenberg, M. (1965) *Society and the Adolescent Self-Image*. Princeton: Princeton University Press.

Rosenberg, M. (1979) *Conceiving the Self*. New York: Basic Books.

Rosenberg, M. and McCullough, C. (1981) 'Mattering: Inferred Significance and Mental Health Among Adolescents', in R. G. Simmons (ed.), *Research in Community and Mental Health*. Greenwich, CT: JAI Press, pp. 163-80.

Rutter, M. (1985) 'Resilience in the Face of Adversity: Protective Factors and Resistance to Psychiatric Disorder', *British Journal of Psychiatry*, 147: 598–611.

Ryan, R. M. and Deci, E. L. (2000) 'Self-determination Theory and the Facilitation of Intrinsic Motivation, Social Development, and Well-Being', *American Psychologist*, 55: 68–78.

Ryan, R. and Deci, E. L. (2001) 'On Happiness and Human Potentials: a Review of Research on Hedonic and Eudaimonic Well-Being', *Annual Review of Psychology*, 52: 141–66.

Ryff, C. D. (1989) 'Happiness is Everything, Or Is It? Explorations on the Meaning of Psychological Well-Being', *Journal of Personality and Social Psychology*, 57: 1069–81.

Ryff, C. D. and Keyes, C. L. (1995) 'The Structure of Psychological Well-Being Revisited', *Journal of Personality and Social Psychology*, 69: 719–27.

Ryff, C. D., Lee, Y. H., Essex, M. J. and Schmutte, P. S. (1994) 'My Children and Me: Midlife Evaluations of Grown Children and of Self', *Psychology and Ageing*, 9: 195–205.

Ryff, C. D., Magee, W. J., Kling, K. C. and Wing, E. H. (1999) 'Forging Macro-Micro Linkages in the Study of Psychological Well-Being', in C. D. Ryff and V. W. Marshall (eds), *The Self and Society in Ageing Processes*. New York: Springer, pp. 247-78.

Ryff, C. D. and Singer, B. (1998a) 'Middle Age and Well-Being', *Encyclopedia of Mental Health*, 2: 707–19.

Ryff, C. D. and Singer, B. (1998b) 'The Contours of Positive Human Health', *Psychological Inquiry*, 9: 1–28.

Ryff, C. D., Singer, B. and Love, G. (2004) 'Positive Health: Connecting Well-Being with Biology', *Philosophical Transactions of the Royal Society*, series B, 359: 1383–94.

Ryff, C. D., Singer, B., Love, G. D. and Essex, M. J. (1998) 'Resilience in Adulthood and Later Life: Defining Features and Dynamic Processes', in J. Lomranz (ed.), *Handbook of Ageing and Mental Health: an Integrative Approach*. New York: Plenum Press, pp. 69-96.

Schooling, M. and Kuh, D. (2002) 'A Life Course Perspective on Women's Health Behaviours', in D. Kuh and R. Hardy (eds), *A Life Course Approach to Women's Health*. Oxford: Oxford University Press.

Sewell, W. H. (1963) 'Some Recent Developments in Socialization Theory and Research', *The Annals of the American Academy of Political and Social Science*, 349: 163–81.

Siegrist, J. (2005) 'Social Reciprocity and Health: New Scientific Evidence and Policy Implications', *Psychoneuroendocrinology*, 30: 1033–8.

Skaff, M. M., Pearlin, L. I. and Mullan, J. T. (1996) 'Transitions in the Caregiving Career: Effects on Sense of Mastery', *Psychology and Ageing*, 11: 247–57.

Springer, K. W. and Hauser, R. M. (2006) 'An Assessment of the Construct Validity of Ryff's Scales of Psychological Well-Being: Method, Mode and Measurement Effects', *Social Science Research*, 35: 1080-1102.

Subramanian, S. V., Kim, D. and Kawachi, I. (2005) 'Covariation in the Socioeconomic Determinants of Self Rated Health and Happiness: a Multivariate Multilevel Analysis of Individuals and Communities in the USA', *Journal of Epidemiological Community Health*, 59: 664–9.

Tugade, M. M. and Fredrickson, B. L. (2004) 'Resilient Individuals Use Positive Emotions to Bounce Back from Negative Emotional Experiences', *Journal of Personality and Social Psychology*, 86: 320–33.

Tugade, M. M., Fredrickson, B. L. and Barrett, L. F. (2004) 'Psychological Resilience and Positive Emotional Granularity: Examining the Benefits of Positive Emotions on Coping and Health', *Journal of Personality*, 72: 1161–90.

Vitterso, J. and Nilsen, F. (2002) 'The Conceptual and Relational Structure of Subjective Well-Being, Neuroticism, and Extraversion: Once Again, Neuroticism is the Important Predictor of Happiness', *Social Indicators Research*, 57: 89–118.

Whalley, L. J. and Deary, I. J. (2001) 'Longitudinal Cohort Study of Childhood IQ and Survival Up to Age 76', *British Medical Journal*, 322: 1–5.

11
Organizational Commitment: a Managerial Illusion?

Michael White

This chapter examines one of the main ways in which working life can become more fulfilling: through a sense of involvement with and commitment to an organization. This type of commitment, and the committed experience it can offer, is in principle available to most working age people, and there is a widespread belief that it can be effectively fostered by certain kinds of management practice that are becoming increasingly prevalent. The main purpose of the chapter is to provide new evidence about the nature of organizational commitment, and especially to test the claims for the positive influence of management practices on commitment. In the first three sections of the chapter the concepts and background are sketched, while subsequent sections provide the evidence and draw conclusions.

The OC concept

Organizational commitment (OC) vies with job satisfaction as the leading current indicator of well-being at work.[1] Commitment in working life shares and draws upon current society's wider approval of committed behaviour. Applied to personal relationships, committed implies long-term, deep and true, while uncommitted means half-hearted, uncertain or insincere. Beyond personal relationships, commitment is deemed to be a condition for active and fulfilled life. One needs (so it is assumed) commitment to a cause, to a community, to a lifestyle, to an organization, or better still to all these. By being committed, we demand more of ourselves and express more of our potential. Through our commitments taken as a whole, we also express the values that we wish to shape our lives (Anderson 1993). Our commitments define our selves, and so commitment is closely linked to two other foci of contemporary desire: personal choice and identity.

Management, and its theorists, have vigorously promoted commitment as a workplace goal and an ideal. They responded to changing attitudes in society and saw how these could be linked to the needs of corporate success or survival. Employees were manifestly becoming more frustrated and soured by the dull and futile experience of life at work, while the economic dominance of the West faltered in the face of the challenge from Japan. OC became an element in the project of improving – or more boldly, 'transforming' – the nature of employment relations and the performance of organizations. For example, Richard Walton (1985, 1987), who was much impressed by the innovative successes of Japanese companies, argued that organizations needed to move from an employment relationship based on control (the traditional managerial mode) towards one based on commitment, where the employee would engage fully and without coercion in innovation and change. This change project has come to be known as human resource management (HRM). HRM, as a coherent set of practices, was by the early 2000s becoming widespread in British workplaces (White et al. 2004: Chapter 9).

It is easy to see why OC has an important role in management thought. A workforce that is highly committed to the organization and its goals is likely to be motivated and responsible, loyal and flexible. Management can rapidly translate this picture into one of high performance and lowered labour costs. This is not to say, however, that the well-being of employees has been of no interest in HRM. Much of the early thinking about workplace transformation grew out of the belief that conditions in many US manufacturing plants had to be changed because they were generating conflict and alienation (Blauner 1964; Walton 1972). Additionally, there is ample evidence that the attitudes expressing OC are positively correlated with those expressing job satisfaction, and with indicators of psychological well-being such as the General Health Questionnaire.

An important attraction of the idea of OC, for employees as much as for management, is its inclusiveness. Even someone in the most routine job can feel attachment to the organization, for example because of what it stands for or how it treats people, and gain an identity through becoming a committed member. In contrast, commitment to an occupation or a career is perhaps more available to those in professions or in 'career jobs', and so has something elitist about it. From this viewpoint, the goal of building OC fits well with ideas of harmonizing the treatment of employees and removing class distinctions in the workplace.

Linking HRM to performance

Despite the links to employee welfare, over the past decade or so the dominant model for HRM has come to focus chiefly on business performance. OC has been subsumed within that model, as the link between management's HRM practices and improved organizational performance. As David Guest (2002) has remarked, this model has become so widely *assumed* that little attention has been paid to verifying links between HRM practices and OC. Instead, the prevalent form of research in this field is to look directly at practices and performance, with the (often tacit) presumption that if a positive link exists, then employees must be getting well motivated (committed) along the way.[2]

A still stronger version of this assumed model is that there exists 'best practice' HRM that achieves good outcomes for both employees and employers – referred to in the USA as 'win-win' HRM – across most types of organization.[3] The cluster of policies and practices which are believed to have these desirable properties has come to be known variously as 'high commitment strategy' (Walton 1985, 1987), 'high performance management' (Kochan and Osterman 1994), 'high commitment management' (Wood and Albanese 1995; Wood 1999), 'high performance work organisation' (Osterman 2000), and 'high performance work systems' (Appelbaum et al. 2000). The practices include involvement and consultation, team-based organization, continuous development of individuals' skills and capabilities, and recognizing and rewarding performance. In this chapter, with its focus on OC, the label 'high commitment management' (HCM) will be used. But it should be emphasized that, although there are differences in detail between one version and another (some, for instance, include job security policies while others do not), the underlying model differs little across brand-labels.

Two further points should be noted. First, HCM practices are applied systematically across whole swathes of employees, through 'schemes' and 'programmes' rather than through one-on-one supervisory motivation of employees. This in principle permits HCM to impact on large numbers of employees: a critical requirement for the goal of workplace transformation. Secondly, most of the authorities in this field maintain that HCM practices are more effectual when 'bundled' (meaning, applied in sets) than when applied singly, because they tend to support one another. This claim is commonly made when referring to the effects of HCM on organizational performance, but if the path to performance lies through commitment, then presumably as HCM practices become denser on the ground, OC should rise more than proportionally.

Critiquing the HCM model

There has been a great deal of critical comment, especially in Britain, directed at the notion of HCM, and indeed more generally at the whole HRM movement (Guest's 2002 review signposts some of this material). Much of this criticism accuses HCM/HRM of bad faith: of professing to offer something for employees while in reality seeking the advantage of the employer. Indeed, as private sector employers have overriding aims of profitability and asset preservation, it would be inexplicable if they devoted considerable resources to HCM/HRM unless it was to improve business performance. This also applies to public sector employers, now that they are dominated by financial and efficiency criteria. Yet this does not mean that employees cannot benefit from altered practices, nor does it mean that they are gullible: they too can play their own game to get more of what they want.

Delusions about HCM and OC are perhaps more likely on the management than on the employee side. The connection between the practices (HCM) and the desired outcome (OC) is mediated by individual choice. Accordingly any hope of controlling the outcome is likely to be deceptive; indeed, as the earlier management thinkers like Walton appreciated, fostering commitment involves some letting go of control. Management, with its ethos of control and 'can-do', may be prone to overestimate the extent to which OC can be *produced* by its own intervention.

Apart from that basic point, there are other limitations that bound OC, at least from a managerial perspective. One is that the impact of HCM on OC may depend in part on a sense of breaking down the restraints of the conventional employment relationship. Employees are more likely to see something worth committing to when management dares to be open to transformed relations. But this spirit of the early years is hard to sustain when innovation becomes replaced by mere good practice. The leaders and innovators continually strive to reinvent themselves and stay fresh, but this can only apply to a small fraction of organizations: most aspire to no more than the industry standard. As HCM becomes ordinary, it may lose its capacity to enthuse and involve employees.

One early writer on commitment with a clear view of the value constraints was Amitai Etzioni (1975). Etzioni argued that 'utilitarian' (i.e. economic) organizations chiefly had to rely upon their 'remunerative power' in order to produce 'calculative commitment', a commitment of an intrinsically low order. He went on to say that calculative commitment produces an individual response of low intensity – as much effort as is paid for, but no more. In contrast, organizations such as in the arts, religions or the higher professions such as medicine, can evoke a 'moral commitment' with more intense and far-reaching effects on behaviour. It is this moral commitment that is more like the idea of commitment in everyday usage. The question that Etzioni's discussion raises, then, is whether workaday organizations are seeking to foster something akin to moral commitment, something which stands above the calculative nature of the employment relationship. If they are not, then is any genuine commitment involved? But if they are, do they really have the means at their disposal?

This questioning leads to some of the more general critiques of employer policies which have been mounted in recent years. It has been argued, for instance by Richard Breen (1997), that the increasingly competitive and deregulated nature of advanced market economies makes it impossible for the employment relationship to be based on long-term commitment. These competitive conditions reinforce employers' need to extract the maximum of performance from employees and, at the same time, to hedge commitments towards them. As a result, employers tend to become more exploitative and more willing to 'dump' employees when it is financially advantageous. According to this critique, then, contemporary conditions lead to an undermining of job security and a corrosion of trust (Sennett 1998).

HCM and OC in practice

These critiques suggest that the promise of widespread improvement in well-being at work through OC may be limited by various features of the employment relationship and of the economic environment. But what has been happening in reality? Have employers been pressing ahead with the currently accepted ideas for making the workplace more engaging and fulfilling, and has this then been translated into active commitment by employees? Or has the growth of OC been stunted by one or other of the constraining forces?

These and similar questions can be answered by means of two sample surveys of employed people, the Employment in Britain survey (EIB) of 1992, and the Working in Britain survey (WIB) of 2000/1. A detailed description of the surveys will not be given here, since this can be found elsewhere (Gallie et al. 1998; White et al. 2003). The main points are as follows: the surveys were nationally representative of people in paid work aged 20–60; the information was collected by means of personal interviews in the employed people's homes; and WIB was to a large extent designed as a *replication* of EIB, so as to get a high degree of comparability over time. This included the use of the identical attitudinal measure of OC in both surveys. It consists of six statements about possible feelings towards the organization: loyalty, pride, similarity of values, willingness to give effort, willingness to do any job, and unwillingness to move elsewhere even for more pay. Responses are on an agreement scale and the OC measure sums the six responses.[4]

To interpret the surveys, one must appreciate their differing context. In the early 1990s, Britain was in the midst of an acute recession with high unemployment and a brooding sense of insecurity and anxiety. On the other hand, the skill-level of jobs had been rising rapidly in an emergent economy of services. By the start of the next decade, a long period of economic growth and prosperity had made recession a distant memory, despite a scary new vocabulary of globalization. The intervening years also witnessed a step-change in information and communications technology (ICT), as e-mails and the internet created a novel business and services infrastructure. These years of prosperity and change were, surely, a propitious time for the promised transformation of employment relations.

What then do employees tell us about their experiences and attitudes, at these two rather contrasting points in time? Two findings emerge starkly from the surveys:

- Over the decade, the diffusion of HCM practices continued steadily, with an *increased* prevalence in employees' experience of around 14 per cent.[5]
- Over the same period, the average level of OC expressed by employees *decreased*. Reasonable figures, which depend on how OC is scored, lie in the range from 4 to 10 per cent.[6]

Over the period, then, HCM and OC moved in opposite directions. Managements on average did pursue the HCM agenda, and there were appreciable increases in the prevalence of management–employee meetings with two-way exchanges, in participation in problem-solving groups or quality circles, in group working and group-based financial incentives, in personal appraisal systems that help plan personal training and development, and in both individual incentives and workplace-wide bonus or profit shares. Out of thirteen practices that form generally accepted facets of HCM, *none* registered an appreciable fall. Yet, despite this steady advance in implementing HCM, there was no evidence of increased OC among employees – if anything, the reverse.

These findings seem at first sight to support the critics of HCM who see such practices as essentially manipulative, and so unlikely to enthuse any but the most gullible employees. But before drawing any such conclusion, one needs to look more closely at the relationships between the practices and the committed (or uncommitted) attitudes expressed by employees (for an outline of the method involved, see the Appendix to this chapter).

One finds that, on the whole, employees who experienced HCM practices in their own workplaces *tended to express above-average levels of OC, and this was true of both 1992 and 2000*. It is true that the majority of the positive relations between HCM practices and OC were, viewed on their own, statistically non-significant, but as the claims made for HCM practices refer to their *cumulative* effect, it is appropriate to take account of the general direction of the relationship. Practices linked in a significant way to higher commitment included two-way meetings with management, taking part in problem-solving groups or quality circles, having pay increases based on performance ('merit pay'), and appraisals to plan training and development. In each year there was only one practice that pulled OC down to a significant degree: appraisal systems determining pay (in 1992), and group financial incentives (in 2000/1).

There is therefore substance in the claims of those who have argued (or assumed) that HCM generates higher OC. But how can this be reconciled with the evidence that, over a decade in many ways highly favourable for HCM, the practices grew but commitment did not?

Why more HCM did not 'produce' more OC

If insecurity makes employees cynical and untrusting, that could perhaps pull down commitment levels, so offsetting employers' efforts to engage and involve them through new HCM practices. There is a substantial amount of information in the EIB and WIB surveys to assess this potential explanation, with questions about temporary contracts, the expectation of being made redundant, actual experiences of unemployment, and recent contraction of the workplace. Certainly, all these circumstances are associated with lower levels of OC. Nonetheless, insecurity did *not* pull down OC over this particular period. There was a simple reason for this: with improved economic conditions over the decade, considerably *fewer* employees were in a precarious situation at the second survey than at the first.[7]

There is a more direct explanation of why increasing HCM practices did not produce increasing OC, one that lies within the HCM–OC relationship. It was because HCM's influence was (though positive) less powerful and also *less stable* than often supposed. To see how this conclusion is reached requires a closer look at the details.

First, how much difference did HCM practices make to OC at the start of the period being reviewed? One way of visualizing this is to imagine all employees positioned along a scale of OC. As the scale is not absolute, we cannot define the 'distance' between any two employees, but we can estimate what proportion of all the employees separates their respective positions. On this basis, let us compare an individual with the average level of OC, and in a workplace with *none* of the HCM practices, and another individual, with identical characteristics but in a workplace with every one of the thirteen HCM practices. According to the 1992 statistics, 15 per cent of the population of employees would separate these two individuals.[8]

This does not seem a huge impact for such a large set of changes in workplace practices. Most workplaces are still at a low level of HCM practice, and each new practice involves a great deal of effort to install. The realistic picture for the average employer is not to raise HCM practices from none to thirteen, but to go from (say) four to five: this would be twice the average rate of advance actually observed between 1992 and 2000! Accordingly, the gains in OC that are realizable through feasible HCM expansion are rather modest, even without any other complications.

There are, however, further complications. One is that the links between particular HCM practices and OC vary in strength, so the overall effect on OC depends on *which* HCM practices are implemented. Two growing areas of HCM practice – problem-solving groups and appraisal systems to shape training and development – were particularly good choices over this period, as employees' OC was very responsive to these practices. There was also some expansion of two-way communication meetings, another practice to which OC appears responsive. But many employers expanded the use of team-working and of group financial incentives: these choices were counter-productive at this time, with employee OC tending to *fall* in response. Overall, the choices to expand HCM in particular ways were 'right' for OC in about only half the cases.

Most problematically, the overall effectiveness of HCM, in terms of OC responsiveness, itself changed over time. If OC is to rise predictably as a result of HCM practices, then not only do employers need to install more practices, but these practices have to be responded to by employees *in a reliable way.*[9] On balance, this did not happen. While (as noted earlier) the prevalence of HCM practices rose by 14 per cent, the responsiveness of OC to HCM – that is, how much OC rose, on average, for each additional HCM practice experienced by the employee – shrunk by 20 per cent. According to taste, one can attribute this to initially gullible employees becoming less gullible, or to enthusiasm declining as novel practices become standards. Whatever the interpretation, the changing employee response was, in this period, offsetting the growth of HCM in its impact on OC.

These findings suggest that the managerial model of OC, whereby the employer can 'produce' or 'generate' OC by taking certain actions, is misconceived. A model that better fits the findings is one where employees actively look for what they can engage with and commit to because it matches their preferences. What attracts them towards a commitment at one time may attract them less at a later time, or vice versa.

Committing to learn

To illustrate this interpretation further, we can turn from HCM practices – which are *systems* for involving substantial groups of employees – to features of the individual employee's job. A voluminous literature (for review, see Gallie et al. 1998) has grown up around the idea that a central issue for the individual employee is a job that permits her or him to express an existing range of skills, and to acquire new skills. These aspects of jobs should then be of considerable importance, also, for OC.[10] Again, though, an underlying assumption is that the relation between OC and skill use or skill acquisition is a stable one over time. Skill has certainly been presented as having an enduring centrality in working life by influential voices both in psychology and in sociology. For example, full development and exercise of one's skills is an important element in self-actualization, the summit of Maslow's hierarchy of needs, a theory that purports to describe the permanent structure of human well-being. Loss of skills through technological change was characterized as the dehumanization or degradation of work by writers in the 'labour process' tradition, again signalling the fundamental role of skills for social status and self-esteem. Such ideas have had large practical effects, influencing attempts to improve the quality of working life over several decades. Surely, then, employees are more likely to commit to an organization that provides them with the opportunities to express themselves through their skills?

In fact, the 1990s witnessed a marked change in the responsiveness of employees, in terms of OC, to skill opportunities in their jobs. In 1992, the use of existing skills had a rather strong positive link with OC, appearing to justify the high importance traditionally attributed to this job dimension. Yet by 2000/1, a job that used existing skills had virtually ceased to matter, from the viewpoint of its effect on employees' OC. This was despite the fact that skill use, as reported by employees, was increasing over the period.

What came to the forefront of employees' commitment, instead, was the opportunity to go on learning in the job. In 1992 this was already important for OC, but between 1992 and 2000/1 the link between learning in the job and OC became very much stronger, so as to emerge as a remarkably powerful influence on commitment.[11] Figure 11.1

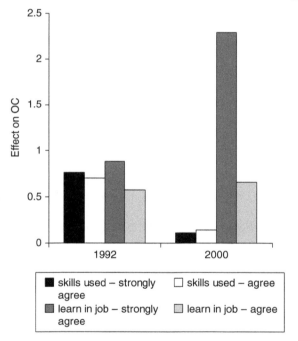

Figure 11.1: Changing effects of skills-use and learning in job on OC, 1992–2000
Sources: EIB and WIB surveys.
Note: The estimated effects on OC are coefficients from regression analyses for the two years, with organizational commitment (OC) as the dependent variable. The questions are whether existing skills are used in the current job, and whether the job requires learning new things.

summarizes these changes. Implicitly, employees appear to be accepting a world where formerly acquired skills decay rapidly and are less valuable to them than the opportunity to go on learning things that will be required in the future.

Someone seeing only the results for 2000/1 might suppose that the 'learning organization' (see Boyett and Boyett 1998: Chapter 3) offers the true pathway to higher commitment, with employees being drawn into a culture where they are encouraged and required to pursue in-the-job learning opportunities. Putting the results for the two surveys together, however, one sees how uncertain are any predictions about commitment. If learning in the job is one decade's magic bullet, by the next decade something else may have taken over and learning may have lost much of its charm, as happened with skill use in the previous decade.

How does OC make a difference?

So far the assessment has focused on what circumstances employees respond to in their commitment. An equally relevant question is what other (behavioural) outcomes OC is involved with. Is OC merely a willingness to speak loyal words about the organization, or does it involve living the work in a different way? There is simple evidence to show that OC does 'make a difference', yet this too must be qualified by change over time.

Among the ways that OC might be expected to connect with behaviour are through good attendance at work, through wanting to stay with the organization, and through taking on a job that requires a high level of effort. In each of the two surveys, there was indeed a marked inverse relationship between the level of OC and the frequency of sickness absence that individuals reported of themselves. (This of course is also consistent with the interpretation that OC is a form of well-being.) After allowing for the fact that the overall level of OC had declined across surveys, the relationship was highly consistent. The findings were similar for intentions of leaving the employer over the coming year. Those who intended to stay had on average significantly higher levels of OC than those thinking of leaving, and this applied equally to both years.

These findings confirm that OC is interwoven with employees' conduct, in ways that make it valuable to employers. When, however, we look at OC in relation to jobs that require a high level of effort,[12] we see signs of the relationship growing weaker over time. In both years, those who felt their jobs required them to work hard had higher than average levels of OC, but the strength of this association was roughly twice as great in 1992 as in 2000/1.[13] Shifts were also appearing in the link between OC and working hours. Those who worked long hours in the job in 1992 tended to have somewhat higher than average OC; by 2000/1, this connection had disappeared – indeed if anything it was those in the lower third of the hours distribution[14] who had the higher OC.

One possible explanation lies in changing attitudes towards 'work-life balance' and growing sensitivity to the conflicts between time spent at work and time spent with one's family (see also Chapter 12 by Lewis and Purcell, this volume). These issues were continually being aired in news media and in popular drama in Britain during the late 1990s and early 2000s.[15] This growing rift between work and family is reflected in comparisons between the two surveys. In 1992, there was no correlation between OC and individuals' feelings of conflict between work and family, suggesting they were seen as entirely separate issues. In 2000/1, however, the two measures had become associated to a moderate but significant degree: employees experiencing a high degree of work–family conflict tended to have somewhat lower OC, and vice versa.[16] Work–family conflict was biting back on OC.

Management's increasing use of HCM practices probably forms part of the explanation for this development. Other research (using the same two surveys as in this chapter) has shown that some HCM practices have led to negative feelings about work–family conflict (White et al. 2003). As certain HCM practices such as intensive team-working (Barker 1993) are extended to create a more committed and performance-orientated workforce, they begin to push employees into a conflict with their commitments to the family. Individuals then attempt to reconcile family and work by scaling back their own emphasis on effort. This can be seen in sharp focus in the case of those male employees who are entrusted with choosing and controlling their own working times. In 1992, these on average had particularly *high* work–family conflict, whereas in 2000/1 they had *below average* work–family conflict. It appears that over the decade, they began to use their self-determination to escape pressurized working, rather than to volunteer for more of it (White et al. 2003).

Discussion

The idea underlying this chapter is that in important respects people construct their own well-being, and one of the ways in which they do so is by choosing commitments which make them more fully or more actively the people they want to be (Anderson 1993). Organizational commitment may seem somewhat lowly by comparison with commitments to loved ones, to a religion, or to a political cause, yet *if it is genuinely a commitment* then it should have the same nature as other commitments. Appreciation of this similarity is perhaps reflected in phrases such as 'married to the job'.

One alternative view, that of Etzioni (1975), is that in most (economic) organizations commitment is of a lower-level type. As this commitment is calculative (it is offered in return for inducements), employers can develop it in a dependable way by implementing practices that please and benefit employees. Something like this seems to be assumed (tacitly) in recent mainstream discussions of 'high commitment management', since they visualize higher performance resulting via committed employees once the proper set of practices is introduced.

The evidence presented in this chapter suggests that OC is *not* of this simple, reliable, manipulable type. True, HCM practices in each of the two years studied were (on average) positively related to OC. But an increase in HCM practices was *not* accompanied by increased OC. In part, this was because the response in terms of OC to many of the HCM practices was rather modest, and in part because this response changed – either up or down – across years. Overall, the response was declining, but it is the variability in response, rather than the decline as such, that needs emphasis. For it is this variability that gainsays the assertion that OC can reliably be produced by having the right managerial practices.

A likely objection, from those who advocate HCM, is that more positive results would be obtained by focusing on more powerful examples of practice. For instance, 'group working' is now so commonplace that it doubtless includes many rather feeble specimens, whereas examples involving high levels of team autonomy and responsibility are rarer, and perhaps more able to inspire high and lasting commitment. Certainly, the evidence in this chapter is compatible with the existence of high and sustained levels of OC in particular, exceptional workplaces. Yet if HCM is put forward as 'best practice' or as a management standard, then it is the average effect on employees of implementing these practices across all kinds of organization that one needs to consider, not the effect in the smartest companies. Moreover, if employee well-being is part of the agenda, it is unsatisfactory to focus on outcomes in a small and special minority of workplaces.

In any case, the variability and lack of predictability in OC across time was by no means limited to HCM schemes and programmes. It also extended to some aspects of individual employees' jobs that have usually been regarded as central to well-being. Skill use in the job, long regarded as of fundamental importance to employees, had a strong relation to OC in 1992, which justified the conventional wisdom, yet by 2000/1 it no longer had any significance for commitment. Learning in the job rose correspondingly to being a central factor in OC, with a strength of relationship that greatly exceeded that of 1992. This evidence, even more than the evidence concerning HCM practices, illustrates how different features of working life can provide the key to employees' commitment at different times. People are capable of jettisoning their attachment to features of their jobs they once valued highly.

Similarly, there are indications that commitment to the organization is changing its behavioural implications. Committed employees refrain from sick-days and do not intend to quit, but they are no longer quite so apt to define themselves in terms of hard work. The reason for this shift has to be inferred from a variety of hints, which suggest growing tensions between commitment to the organization and commitment to the family. In a period when work-life balance came to the forefront of public debate, employees had to face the adverse family consequences of work-centred commitment. This was an issue notable by its absence from the key texts of the 1980s on managerial innovations. It was, however, clearly seen by scholars who approached the issue from the family side: for example, a landmark paper by Bielby and Bielby (1989) argued that roles and relations within families were affected by both work identification and family identification. Commitments and identifications with family life impose constraints on OC, and changes in these external constraints are another source of uncertainty about the effects of management practices.

The findings have obvious implications for corporate policy. There is little to be gained by trying to predict or control OC through elaborate sets of HCM practices. Nobody can know what next year's successful recipe is going to be. People search out for themselves what they can value as a reason for commitment, but values themselves are shifting. Organizations accordingly can do less about commitment than their managements tend to suppose.

None of this, of course, should lead to the conclusion that HCM practices are not worth developing. They do have some positive effect on OC, and so on well-being, even if it is modest and uncertain. As Edwards and Wright (2001) have argued more generally, the direct effects of such practices are weak but cumulatively they still make some positive contribution to wider goals of performance and to the foundations of improved employment relationships.

What *positive* recommendation could be made to employers and managements about OC? Simply to assume that commitment is an individual matter, and then consider what the implications are. This line of thought could lead to seeing a connection between OC and 'diversity policy', another area of great current interest for employers (see Kandola and Fullerton 1998; Liff 2003). As management practice pays increasing respect to the diversity of personal circumstances and values among employees (including those that relate to life outside of work), this will not only help to unify HCM with diversity policy, but may possibly provide a more nurturing environment for employees' spontaneous commitments.

From the viewpoint of individual well-being, the overall findings indicate that it is probably rather hard for employees to find rich sustenance for their commitment in most organizations, even those that have benign human resource policies. Over a period that was in many ways very favourable – both in terms of general economic conditions and in terms of active development of employer practices – OC on average failed to rise, and even declined a little. With changing social values influencing many employees to seek an improved work-life balance and a more equitable family life, it is hard to see OC rising much in the coming years. However, our ability to predict is probably no better than our ability to control what people will choose.

Appendix: an outline of measures and methods

Full technical details of the analyses used in this chapter are available on the author's website (http://www.psi.org.uk/people/person. asp?person_id=24). This Appendix provides a brief overview.

The measure of OC consists of six items selected from Mowday's Organizational Commitment Questionnaire or OCQ (Mowday et al. 1982). Meyer and Allen (1984, 1997) showed that the OCQ is multidimensional; the selection used here is the same as in Gallie et al. (1998) and Appelbaum et al. (2000), and is unidimensional. A summative score of the six items is used as the measure; it correlates 0.988 with the factor score of these items. It is approximately normally distributed and has a reliability of 0.79 in each year. The items are also similar to those in the organizational commitment scale of Cook and Wall (1980).

In selecting the thirteen HCM practices, the conceptual scheme of Appelbaum et al. (2000) was followed: the practices relate to participation/communication, group organization, skills/development, and incentives. As an illustration, work improvement groups (quality circles) relate to both participation and to group organization. The practices were of a systematic type that could only apply across groups of employees, or across the whole workplace, rather than selectively to individual employees.

The surveys had response rates of 72 per cent in 1992 and 65 per cent in 2000/1. They provided analysis samples of 3339 and 2099 employees respectively. Further details of the surveys can be found in the cited references.

The relations of HCM practices to OC were assessed through regression analysis, with OC as the dependent variable. Each HCM practice was represented by a dummy variable. Additional variables in the analyses were as follows: job security variables (temporary contract, expects to be made redundant, experience of long-term unemployment, perception of employment change at workplace); own job characteristics (skill use in job, learning in job, supervisor who coaches, influence on decisions regarding own work); other characteristics (sex, age, occupational class, whether use IT in own job). In making statistical inferences, account was taken of the complex survey design by means of robust variance estimation.

Acknowledgements

The survey 'Working in Britain in the Year 2000' was funded by the Economic and Social Research Council as part of its Future of Work Research Programme under grant number L212252037. Additional support was provided from the Work Foundation. Acknowledgements for the comparator survey, Employment in Britain 1992, are given in Gallie et al. (1998). The usual disclaimers apply.

Notes

1. A literature search on a bibliographic database revealed nearly 1200 academic articles relating to organizational commitment in the period 2001–5. Over the same period, job satisfaction featured in a little less than 1800.
2. A study cited in support of this presumption is that of Appelbaum and colleagues (2000), where 'high performance work systems' (HPWS) were assessed in terms of employees' OC, job satisfaction, and trust towards the employer, as well as in terms of business performance. However, this study, despite its generally positive findings, provides a weak platform for generalization: it was based on purposive samples drawn from three manufacturing

industries in certain areas of the USA. Other studies using more representative samples have found weaker or more patchy relationships between HRM practices and employee attitudes and commitment (see, for Britain, Ramsey et al. 2000; for Canada, Godard 2001; for Australia, Harley 2002).

3. There are other models that assert a contingent relationship between subsets of HR practices and the circumstances of an organization. See Wood (1999) and Guest (2002) for review.

4. For the sources of the questions, see the Appendix. For the full wording of the questions, and for a detailed account of the findings from the 1992 survey, see Gallie et al. 1998.

5. HCM is measured through a set of 13 practices, see the Appendix.

6. The lower figure is obtained by scoring the OC questions (Figure 11.1) from 0 to 3, summing the responses, and expressing the change as a proportion of the average in 1992. The higher figure is calculated by giving a score of 2 to responses that 'strongly agree' with each of the six committed statements and a score of 1 to those that 'agree', while the other responses are scored 0.

7. The supposed adverse effects of precarious employment may in any case have been overstated in the past. Guest (2004) reviews evidence and finds that for many people, 'flexible' contracts have positive psychological outcomes.

8. This figure is derived by taking the estimated difference in OC between the two situations, in standard deviation units, and assuming a normal distribution of OC. With a normal distribution, changes on the percentile scale depend on where the two points being compared are located in the distribution.

9. The employee response is assessed through the average statistical relationship (regression coefficient) of each HCM practice with respect to the OC score: see the Appendix.

10. While the analysis assumes that job characteristics such as skill use influence OC, it is also possible that OC influences skill use or other job characteristics. A committed individual may feel an obligation to put all her skills into the job, to go on learning in the job, etc. If this is so, then the assumed influence of job characteristics on OC may be overestimated. This, however, does not reduce the interest of the changes over time in the relationships between job characteristics and OC.

11. The analysis also considered employee perceptions of whether their supervisor helped employees to learn in their jobs. Here also there was a positive relationship with OC, which increased considerably over the two surveys.

12. The OC scale itself includes a question about *willingness* to work exceptionally hard. The question considered here is a different one, focusing on whether the current job *actually involves* working very hard.

13. To assess this, the OC scores were divided into terciles (equal thirds) of the distribution, for each survey separately, and then cross-tabulated with the question about how hard employees' jobs required them to work (very hard, hard or not hard). The relative odds-ratio for high OC versus low OC employees being respectively in 'very hard' and 'not hard' jobs fell from 2.65 in 1992 to 1.49 in 2000/1.

14. This is based on dividing up the hours distribution separately for women and for men.

15. A major debate arose in the USA somewhat earlier, with the publication of Schor's best-selling book *The Overworked American* in 1991.
16. In 2000/1 the correlation was −0.123, p<0.001. In 1992 it was −0.018, p=0.48.

References

Anderson, E. (1993) *Value in Ethics and Economics*. London: Harvard University Press.

Appelbaum, E., Bailey, T., Berg, P. and Kalleberg, A. L. (2000) *Manufacturing Advantage: Why High-Performance Work Systems Pay Off*. Ithaca, NY: Cornell University Press.

Barker, J. R. (1993) 'Tightening the Iron Cage: Concertive Control in Self-Managing Teams', *Administrative Science Quarterly*, 38: 408–37.

Bielby, W.T. and Bielby, D. D. (1989) 'Family Ties: Balancing Commitments to Work and Family in Dual Earner Households', *American Sociological Review*, 54: 776–89.

Blauner, R. (1964) *Alienation and Freedom: the Factory Worker and His Industry*. Chicago: University of Chicago Press.

Boyett, J. H. and Boyett, J. T. (1998) *The Guru Guide: the Best Ideas of the Management Thinkers*. New York: Wiley.

Breen, R. (1997) 'Risk, Recommodification and Stratification', *Sociology*, 31: 473–89.

Cook, J. and Wall, T. (1980) 'New Work Attitude Measures of Trust, Organisational Commitment and Personal Need Non-fulfilment', *Journal of Occupational Psychology*, 53: 39–52.

Edwards, P. and Wright, M. (2001) 'High-involvement Work Systems and Performance Outcomes: the Strength of Variable, Contingent and Context-bound Relationships', *International Journal of Human Resource Management*, 12: 568–85.

Etzioni, A. (1975) [1961] *A Comparative Analysis of Complex Organisations*, revised and enlarged edition. New York: Free Press.

Gallie, D., White, M., Cheng, Y., and Tomlinson, M. (1998) *Restructuring the Employment Relationship*. Oxford: Oxford University Press.

Godard, J. (2001) 'High Performance and the Transformation of Work? The Implications of Alternative Work Practices for the Experience and Outcomes of Work', *Industrial and Labour Relations Review*, 54: 776–805.

Guest, D. (2002) 'Human Resource Management, Corporate Performance, and Employee Wellbeing: Building the Worker into HRM', *Journal of Industrial Relations* 44(3): 335–58.

Guest, D. (2004) 'Flexible Employment Contracts, the Psychological Contract and Employee Outcomes: an Analysis and Review of the Evidence', *International Journal of Management Reviews*, 5/6: 1–19.

Harley, B. (2002) 'Employee Responses to High Performance Work System Practices: an Analysis of the AWIRS95 Data', *Journal of Industrial Relations*, 44(3): 418–34.

Kandola, R. and Fullerton, J. (1998) *Managing the Mosaic: Diversity in Action*, 2nd edn. London: Institute of Personnel and Development.

Kochan, T. A. and Osterman, P. (1994) *The Mutual Gains Enterprise*. Cambridge, MA: Harvard Business School Press.

Liff, S. (2003) 'The Industrial Relations of a Diverse Workforce', in P. Edwards (ed.), *Industrial Relations: Theory and Practice*, 2nd edn. Oxford: Blackwell.

Meyer, J. P. and Allen, N. J. (1984) 'Testing the "Side-Bet" Theory of Organisational Commitment: Influences on Work Positions and Family Roles', *Journal of Applied Psychology*, 69: 372–8.

Meyer, J. P. and Allen, N. J. (1997) *Commitment in the Workplace: Theory, Research and Application*. Thousand Oaks, CA: Sage Publications.

Mowday, R., Porter, L. W. and Steers, R. H. (1982) *Employee–Organisation Linkages: the Psychology of Commitment, Absenteeism and Turnover*. New York: Academic Press.

Osterman, P. (2000) 'Work Reorganisation in an Era of Restructuring: Trends in Diffusion and Effects on Employee Welfare', *Industrial and Labour Relations Review*, 53: 179–96.

Ramsey, H., Scholarios, D. and Harley, B. (2000) 'Employees and High-Performance Work Systems: Testing Inside the Black Box', *British Journal of Industrial Relations*, 38: 501–32.

Schor, J. (1991) *The Overworked American: the Unexpected Decline of Leisure*. New York: Basic Books.

Sennett, R. (1998) *The Corrosion of Character: the Personal Consequences of Work in the New Capitalism*. New York: W.W. Norton & Company.

Walton, R. (1972) 'How to Counter Alienation in the Plant', *Harvard Business Review*, 72(6): 70–81.

Walton, R. (1985) 'From Control to Commitment in the Workplace', *Harvard Business Review*, 85(2): 77–84.

Walton, R. (1987) *Innovating to Compete*. London: Jossey-Bass.

White, M., Hill, S., McGovern, P., Mills, C. and Smeaton, D. (2003) ' "High Performance" Management Practices, Working Hours and Work–Life Balance', *British Journal of Industrial Relations*, 41(2): 175–96.

White, M., Hill, S., Mills, C. and Smeaton, D. (2004) *Managing to Change? British Workplaces and the Future of Work*. Basingstoke: Palgrave Macmillan.

Wood, S. (1999) 'Human Resource Management and Performance', *International Journal of Management Reviews*, 1: 367–413.

Wood, S. and Albanese, M. T. (1995) 'Can We Speak of High Commitment Management on the Shop Floor?', *Journal of Management Studies*, 32: 215–47.

12
Well-Being, Paid Work and Personal Life

Suzan Lewis and Christina Purcell

Positive well-being and 'work-life balance'

Positive well-being is increasingly conceptualized in terms of the satisfactory integration or harmonization of work and family – often referred to as 'work-life balance' in popular discourse. This has become more salient as technological developments and new ways of working increasingly blur the boundaries between paid work and the rest of life, and more people struggle to find time for family, leisure and other activities beyond paid work (Taylor 2002; Lewis 2003). In this chapter we explore some links between well-being and the integration of work and family. We first consider traditional, largely survey-based research linking work-life integration with well-being or lack of it, and discuss the limitations of this approach. In particular we argue that survey approaches underestimate the complexity of well-being and neglect the impact of social and temporal context on the meanings people attach to their experiences of well-being in paid work and beyond. We then illustrate a more contextualized, qualitative approach to well-being in relation to work and family by drawing on a study of well-being in the transition to parenthood.

Research linking work-life experiences with well-being or lack of it

The integration of work and family has long been examined in relation to well-being (e.g. life satisfaction, job satisfaction, family satisfaction) or lack of it (particularly work-family conflict and stress), in survey-based research (Lewis and Cooper 1987, 1988; Swanson 1999). This approach has tended to test two competing models, either explicitly or implicitly: the role conflict model which assumes that multiple roles in paid work and family (or other domains) create the potential for stress and conflict, and the role expansion model, which constructs multiple commitments as providing multiple sources of potential well-being and satisfaction (Noor 2004). More recent research in this tradition examines the conditions under which multiple roles can be more satisfying than stressful, for example, examining relationships between organizational policies or practices and well-being (for example, job satisfaction) with rather mixed findings (Kossek and Oseki 1999).

Survey-based research on work-life experiences and well-being, although useful for indicating certain trends, is often decontextualized, neglecting the impact of time and place on affective experiences and neglecting the complexity of experiences of well-being. More recently interpretist approaches have used qualitative methods to examine the dynamic meanings attached to experiences in employment and in private life, in order to generate more in-depth understandings of the relationships between work and non-work roles and experiences of well-being (Thompson and Bunderson 2001) often going beyond the individual focus to acknowledge the role of social contexts and processes (e.g. 6, 2002; Sointu 2005). For example, Sointu (2005), drawing on changing social representations of well-being in newspapers across time, suggests that in contemporary consumer society, well-being emerges as a normative obligation chosen and sought after by individual agents. Well-being is produced within social contexts at particular points in time, and is dynamically shifting across time and space (Sointu 2005; Gambles et al. 2006).

Transitions: a study of well-being in the transition to working parenthood, in specific contexts

To illustrate the value of a more qualitative and contextualized approach to work-life experiences and well-being that takes account of time and place, we draw on data from an EU Framework Five study. Transitions (full name Gender, Parenthood and the Changing European Workplace). is a cross-national study which examined qualitatively how young European women and men negotiate motherhood and fatherhood and work–family boundaries and how this impacts on their well-being, in the context of different national welfare state regimes, substantial ongoing organizational change, and different family and employer support. The countries represented were Bulgaria, France, Norway, Portugal, Slovenia, Sweden, the Netherlands and the UK.

Eleven organizational case studies were conducted in private (mostly finance) and public (social services) sector workplaces, each involving document analysis, interviews with managers, focus groups with employees who were parents of young children or expecting their first child, well-being questionnaires and home-based biographical interviews with selected parents from the focus groups and, where possible, their partners. In this chapter we draw on one case study, Peak[1] a finance sector organization in the UK, although our discussion of this case is contextualized within the wider study. We first discuss relevant aspects of the national context (and some comparison with other national contexts) and then aspects of the organizational context. Well-being among the new parents in the Peak case study is then examined in relation to multiple layers of context.

Context

Societal (national)

The first stage of the Transitions project involved a context mapping exercise to highlight the major aspects of national contexts seen to be relevant to the study of work, family and well-being, as well as broader societal well-being, in the eight countries represented in the wider study.[2] These included levels of affluence and social equality, fertility rates (sustainability of future generations), working conditions, opportunities for developing a range of work–family strategies, national work–family social policies and the gender contract that this represents, and general government initiatives and pubic debates and concerns relating to the integration of work and family.

It is interesting to look at how the UK fares in relation to the other national contexts in the Transitions study in these respects. Using an overall index of labour market well-being for OECD countries developed by Osberg and Sharpe (2003), Britain ranked fifth out of the eight countries (Fagnani et al. 2004: 140). Better labour market well-being is defined in this index in relation to (low) level of social inequalities, (high) GDP per capita and (generous) national family friendly policies. However, insofar as fertility rates may also be related to well-being as an indicator of the possibilities for reconciling paid work and family, it is worth noting that the fertility rate in the UK is relatively stable and higher than the other countries, except Norway (Fagnani et al. 2004:8), despite the UK having minimal childcare support and limited parental leave rights. One explanation may be the possibilities of part-time work in Britain (the double edged nature of part-time work is illustrated later in the chapter).

British social policy has historically reflected the notion of individual rather than public responsibility for families. However, recent shifts in government approaches, influenced by both EU directives and economic concerns, have included the introduction of paid paternity and extended maternity leave, unpaid parental and sick children leave, and the right to request flexible working. A government campaign on 'work-life balance', encourages employers to implement work-life policies by promoting the idea of 'win-win' arrangements. There is much general concern about long working hours and pressure of work (Bunting 2004; Lapido and Wilkinson 2002) and in this context the work-life balance debate, for men and women, is frequently discussed in the media and everyday life (Smithson et al. 2005).

Organizational context

The UK private sector case study organization, Peak, is a large insurance company undergoing massive organizational changes: mergers, downsizing, reorganization and introduction of new regulations, structures and technology. Insurance companies face competition with supermarkets and other bodies selling insurance as well as the negative effects of pension miss-selling scandals. In this context, organizational change was regarded as a fact of life and was widely accepted by managers and other employees as inevitable in the face of business imperatives and changes or anticipated shifts in regulation. However, downsizing and reorganization were associated with increasing job insecurity and intensification of work.

> I do think there's an awful lot more expected of people. Nowadays. I mean if you look at like the basic, the lowest job, which is like the lowest ranked job now, to what it was when I started here which was only 9 years ago, what's expected of them now is so much more than what we expected then. I think they're expected to do a lot more work for the money. (Mother of 1-year-old child, in focus group at Peak)

The experience of intensification of work was not limited to Peak but was reported in all eleven case studies in the Transitions project, in both public and private sectors, thus appearing to be a widespread characteristic of contemporary workplaces.

At Peak, mergers were seen by managers as an opportunity to develop a distinctive culture for the merged company. The mergers were cited in the manager interviews as the catalyst for many other changes, notably a drive to develop policy, practice and culture change to increase flexibility and trust. Managers presented this as a strategic initiative to enhance performance through a focus on people and their needs and well-being, in the context of changing workplace demands. This reflected the national rhetoric of the business case for 'win-win' forms of flexibility (DTI 2003) and was implemented at Peak by the introduction of an informal 'trust-based' flexitime system which replaced the formal flexitime system. Subsequently, support for part-time and other forms of flexible working became more dependent on management discretion. Employees' experiences of change thus varied across departments as new formal and informal policies were inconsistently applied, depending on how supportive line managers were. In addition, despite the apparent drive for flexibility, trust and support, there was a prevailing assumption that supervisory or management roles could only be fulfilled on a full-time basis – usually with long hours, beyond contracted time. Managers who requested reduced hours work on return from maternity leave were permitted to work less than full-time but, in most cases, were demoted to non-managerial jobs. Ideal worker assumptions that overvalue those who can work full-time and continuously (Lewis 1997; Rapoport et al. 2002) prevailed.

Family contexts

All participants in the study were at some point within the transition to parenthood and were working and caring for young children. They included both two-parent and single-parent families and had various levels of intergenerational support for working and caring, for example, support from grandparents. Within two-parent families, the division of labour also varied, from one couple in which the mother was the main earner and the father undertook much childcare to more traditional arrangements. Most lone parents in the study were mothers but there was one lone father at Peak. Despite changes in national policies to encourage mothers to work, and shifts in the behaviours of some fathers, mothers remained largely regarded as the main carers at Peak and in the other case studies (Smithson et al. 2005).

Economic context

Although the parents participating in the study came from a range of occupations, from call centre workers to actuaries, salaries at Peak were low for the sector. Peak was located in an area with high housing costs and high childcare costs. Many parents therefore lived in less expensive areas and faced long commutes to work.

The nature of well-being and the processes that influence it in relation to work and family integration within multiple levels of context

Well-being is complex and multidimensional

A biographical interview guide was developed for exploring well-being in relation to various dimensions of parents' lives, taking a temporal aspect of narrative, as well as national and workplace context into account. The interviews demonstrated that well-being is not a static state, but a multifaceted process situated in time, both life course and everyday time, and dependent upon the different layers of context in which a person's life is embedded (Nilsen and Brannen 2005). Context influences perceptions, which influence expectations, which in turn influence judgement/appraisal and feelings of well-being that can fluctuate even over a typical day, as parents feel stressed at some points of the day and happy at other times. It is also clear from the interviews that positive and negative well-being are not mutually exclusive. This can be illustrated by the case of Charlotte, a 24-year-old, partnered mother of two children aged 18 months and 6 months. At the time of the focus group she was a customer service 'consultant' at Peak, and pregnant with her second child, commuting to Peak from an area with cheaper housing while her child was cared for by her mother-in-law. By the time of the home-based interview, she had left Peak after difficulties with her inflexible boss who objected to her arriving slightly late on occasions due to traffic problems, and she now worked in a local school. Charlotte talked a great deal about how much she 'enjoyed' motherhood and how 'happy' she was as a mother, but also talked of being unhappy and stressed:

> I'm just really happy being a Mum ... It's just very, very tiring. There's some days when you just can't keep your eyes open past 7 o'clock and you've still got baths to do, and get everybody to bed ... it can just get sometimes a bit, a bit much.

In the focus group Charlotte talked about enjoying motherhood and also many aspects of the job at Peak, especially the socializing, and the training in new skills. At the same time she found aspects of her job stressful. At the time of the home-based interview she was happier in her new job, which affirmed her sense of identity and mattering as an individual. Yet she still felt ambivalent about being a working mother:

> Because it sounds funny, but I matter at the school because it's such a small office and everybody knows one another. I'm known by my name rather than a number, and being at like Peak or in any call centre, it's like being a battery hen, and you don't really matter but being within a team and having to work in such a small team then I matter to the school so...And I think I'm at the minute, I'm quite happy...but...it comes down to the fact that I'm Mum, and somebody else is dealing with my child and I just...I feel as if it's been taken off me.

Charlotte's vivid experience of life, with many emotional peaks and troughs, as reported in her focus group and her interview, were not reflected at all in her questionnaire responses. The individual interview permitted investigation of the emotional aspects of parenting at this life course phase – the guilt, the pleasures, the anxiety – often experienced silmultaneously, thereby demonstrating the complexity of well-being.

The life course: the child as central to well-being at this phase

Clearly Charlotte's role as a mother and her feelings about her children were central to her sense of well-being, but not in a simple way. Analysis of the well-being questionnaires indicated that being a mother or a father contributed most to the positive experiences of well-being for those with young children in all the national case studies, although the influence of social desirability factors cannot be ruled out. A greater sense of well-being emerged in the home-based interviews than in focus groups at the workplace, which suggests that for new parents, and perhaps especially for new mothers, the new baby is the central aspect of their life at this time. Paid work tends to be less important at this transitional point in the life course than before or afterwards. Job pressures were not always to the fore, especially once the parents were back at home.

The role of social comparison and sense of entitlement in determining expectations and subsequent well-being

Feelings of well-being are strongly influenced by parents' expectations and by sense of entitlement to support for work-life balance (Lewis and Smithson 2001), which in turn are based in processes of social comparison. For example, processes of social comparison are central to participants' feelings about their workplace. Even when dissatisfaction was expressed with some aspect of the organization, many parents used social comparison to construct Peak as a better place to work than other organizations on the basis of the flexibility they experienced and/or the pleasant working environment, and hence felt satisfied. So notions of a good place for parents to work may emanate from limited aspirations or sense of entitlement to support, with little expectation of 'caring' as part of the employment deal (Lewis and Smithson 2001).

> I worked for another company and, and you get paid, a higher salary...but you're expected to earn that higher salary whereas here is slightly less well paid than...market rates. But to me it's justified in so much as I can go home and I don't have to think about work...the hours are fairly flexible. (Mother of two aged 3 and 2)

> It's not as bad as other places, 'cos I left for eight weeks and came back, so, when you work here sometimes you think oh God this company and then when you go somewhere else you realize it's really not that bad. (Father, one baby)

Sense of entitlement to support for work and family tends to be generally low in Britain, where managing paid work and family care is typically viewed as a private matter (Lewis 1997; Lewis and Smithson 2001). This remained largely true at Peak:

> To be honest they should just be more understanding. And a bit more flexible. I don't think we should be given everything on a plate just 'cos we've got children, I don't think it should be like oh well you can have all the flexible time off, because it's not fair on the people who haven't...Just to understand, and to, to let them sort of work with you, to find a solution. (Mother, one baby, Peak focus group)

> I think, I'd feel really guilty asking for some unpaid leave with all my colleagues and my manager haven't got children and they're very understanding but, to turn around and say 'Oh by the way, I want the summer off...for 4 weeks', you know. (Father, two children, Peak focus group)

Nevertheless, the management discourses of culture change and flexibility at Peak, and parents' perceptions of support in the wider context, including the government work-life balance campaign and new national regulations, appeared to raise expectations for support amongst mothers and some fathers, and led to feelings of frustration and dissatisfaction when these supports were not forthcoming. Employees with less supportive managers compared themselves with others across the organization. If raised expectations for flexibility and support were not met, parents, particularly but not exclusively mothers, experienced this as a violation of their entitlements. The perceived discrepancy between what 'ought to be' and what 'is' (Reichle 1996) was constructed as one which is socially unjust:

> There's managers that go part-time ... so if they can have the time off why can't the supervisors, so you've got managers can have the time off why can't we? (Expectant mother, focus group, Peak)

Thus, while sense of entitlement to support for reconciling work and parenting was generally quite limited at Peak, there were signs that it was growing, reflecting specific national and organizational contexts. The most immediate social referents for parents at Peak were colleagues, including managers, across the company, with whom they compared themselves as a basis for whether they felt justly treated and hence relatively satisfied or dissatisfied.

Nevertheless, sense of entitlement to modify work for family remained gendered. Although many fathers took advantages of opportunities to work more flexibly, none asked to reduce working hours and part-time work continued to be regarded as a policy for women. Sense of entitlement was also gendered within households. Mothers at Peak were more likely than fathers to talk about feeling guilty – about both their children and their work. Fathers, on the other hand, were more likely than mothers to feel entitled to time for leisure. One mother from Peak who was working long hours at the workplace and also managing childcare with minimal support from her partner reported high levels of satisfaction and well-being, illustrating the subjective nature of sense of entitlement to support and its impact on well-being. The mothers in Peak tended to compare their male partners' contributions to childcare with that of their own fathers, and to husbands or partners of other women, and subsequently defined their partners as involved fathers. These perceptions of partner support, however, appeared to be real in their consequences for aspects of positive well-being such as happiness.

In contrast, other parents at Peak and particularly in case studies elsewhere (e.g. Norway) who had higher expectations of egalitarian couple relationships, were stressed or dissatisfied if this was not realized. Higher expectations and sense of entitlement, whether to workplace support or support within the family can thus be associated with transitional stress or poorer well-being, if raised expectations are not fully met.

Well-being for new parents as a gendered experience

Well-being is a gendered experience, both in relation to levels of workplace support and in relation to expectations. The transition to parenthood appears to be a critical tipping point which reinforces gendered identity and roles within couples – women felt under more pressure to be carers and men to be main wage-earners. The Peak couple which reversed roles (to the extent that the father had lost his job and the mother was the main breadwinner) felt uncomfortable with the situation, so much so that the father was studying full-time in order to reverse the situation back to 'normal' in the future. This discomfort was a phenomenon that we found in role reversal couples in other countries.

Gender is clearly relevant to the well-being of employed parents. In particular, the ability (or not) to work flexible hours disproportionately affected the well-being of mothers more than fathers at Peak, as in the other case study organizations. There remains a widespread assumption in Peak that work–family policies are policies for mothers. Some fathers were able to work flexibly, including a lone father, who like many mothers, worked below his capacity in order to have flexibility to fit in childcare. Part-time work, however, was an option only taken up by mothers, and one that was usually career limiting. In a context where gendered assumptions about ideal workers continued to prevail, despite the discourse of culture change, work-life policies such as the availability of part-time work can contribute to positive well-being in the short-term, helping parents to manage work–family boundaries at the individual and household level, but with less positive long-term consequences.

Parents as active and strategic in relation to work-life and well-being

Interpretist approaches to work-life integration and well-being conceive of people as active and strategic in managing work and family boundaries (Campbell Clarke 2000; Nippert-Eng 1996). Parents in our study developed proactive, personal strategies for managing boundaries between their work and family spheres. Strategies varied from complete segregation of work and family (for example not thinking about or engaging in work while at home and vice versa), to integration. The permeability of work–family boundaries tended to be more problematic for mothers than for fathers in our study and fathers were more likely to separate the world of paid work and family life, although a notable exception was a single father of three young children. Neither integration nor segregation work–family strategies were found to automatically lead to greater or lower levels of reported well-being in a simple way. More important for well-being appeared to be whether a parent has a choice and some control over temporal and spatial flexibility. Being able to successfully achieve the preferred strategy, be it largely segregation or integration of work and family, tended to be associated with more positive well-being. Often parents' support needs in this respect, in the workplace or the family, were fairly minimal. For example, autonomy to be able to leave work five minutes earlier in order to catch a train that runs every half-hour could make a big difference. However, work-life balance, well-being and the ability to achieve preferred strategies depended on experiences, supports and constraints at multiple levels of context.

The role of context on experiences of well-being

Family context and childcare

Among two-parent families, partner support plays a fundamental role in parents' well-being. Most of the fathers interviewed at Peak had considerable support from their partners to enable them to manage work and parenting. However, partner support available to mothers was more variable and mothers often expected less from their partners as discussed above. The one single father in the Peak case study had considerable support from his mother which along with his flexible job contributed to his enjoyment of working and parenting. Access to high affordable quality childcare is crucial to attitudes to, and experience of, employed parenthood, although this concerned Peak mothers rather than fathers. Intergenerational support for childcare alleviated the time and financial stress of many of the Peak parents. It can, however, be double-edged. For example, Charlotte was uneasy about her children being cared for by her mother-in-law and felt very guilty that she was not at home with her daughter. This affected her feelings about being at work:

> It was awful, of coming back (to work)...(I felt) I'm being a bad parent, I'm abandoning her and leaving her with someone else and I'm her mother and I should be doing it and that's what I went through, and I went through hell with it.

Other Peak mothers also talked about this constant feeling of guilt, which seems to reflect the ambiguous national context in which mothers are expected to work whilst simultaneously expected to be the primary carer for their young children in the context of limited public childcare provision.

Economic context producing well-being

Economic context matters, although the wider study illustrated that parents in less affluent contexts often found different ways of coping, tended to have lower expectations and did not necessarily have a poorer sense of well-being than more affluent parents. Nevertheless finance was a very real issue for the lower paid employers at Peak in the context of high house prices and childcare costs. This impacted on their well-being often because of long commutes from areas with lower house prices. Economic needs and values, however, interacted with other values. Some couples were willing to lose part of household salary during transition to parenthood, because they considered it more important for one parent (usually the mother) to work part-time and spend more time with the child. Other mothers and fathers were prepared to spend more time in paid work than they considered ideal from a family perspective, in order to provide more material benefits for their children. For some, this was what being a good parent was about. There was much evidence across all the case studies of an intensification of the expectations of parenting (Brannen and Moss 1999), which includes aspiration to provide not only more time and attention but also more material goods. To some extent, then, the parents' sense of well-being reflected their expectations of work and of their ability to attain their aspirations for themselves and their children – based on consumerism rather than citizenship (Sointu 2005). It is, however, worth noting that the finance sector participants were very different in their expectations and ambitions from the social services participants in the UK public sector case study (Brannen and Brockman 2005). They were relatively materialistic, and more likely to be working for instrumental rather than ideological reasons than the social services employees interviewed, and hence their well-being was more dependent on achieving material goals.

The role of national and organizational policy

Workplace policies and practices influence the permeability of boundaries and work–family strategies and can impact on well-being. These policies and practices are shaped by national and local regulations, but this study shows that they are also increasingly a matter of daily and informal negotiation with managers in local organizations. As discussed above, new UK regulation on, for example, parental leave and the right to request flexible working arrangements, together with the drive for culture change at Peak towards greater flexibility and trust, enhanced parents' sense of entitlement to support to some extent. However, the new ethos was inconsistently applied and while some parents were happy to be able to negotiate the flexibility that they needed, others were frustrated that their expectations were not met. Well-being for Peak parents varied across departments, highlighting the discretionary application of informal, trust-based policies. On the other hand, supportive colleagues and managers, responsive to the needs of parents (particularly when family emergencies arose) and social aspects of work, often mitigate against dissatisfaction with other aspects of the organization.

However, even when managers and their working practices did enhance parents' flexibility and autonomy over work and family boundaries, this tended to be undermined by other factors, particularly long hours and the intensification of work. Flexible working can increase the permeability of work–family boundaries, but in the context of intensified workloads can result in work intruding on family time and lead to overwork. Some parents used ICTs to blur the boundaries, for example by checking e-mail at home, or texting partners during the day, and this study demonstrates that technology can also be used by parents in proactive ways to support complex work–family strategies, combining elements of segregation and integration. Nevertheless, intensified workloads can make separation of work and family very difficult, especially when work cannot be accomplished during the working day, or when, for example, work-related training is organized during non-work time.

Despite these difficulties most parents derived some sense of well-being from their work at Peak. The very pleasant physical environment in which Peak is located contributed to positive well-being, as did social factors and opportunities for interesting and challenging work. However, opportunities for challenging work were denied to some employees with family commitments if they were demoted on moving to part-time work.

Conclusions and implications

We have argued that well-being is complex, multifaceted, fluctuating over time and influenced by the many layers of context in which individuals' lives are embedded. Context sensitive research designs are needed to avoid oversimplistic findings on well-being, its determinants and consequences.

There can be no simple answers to questions about how policy can enhance well-being for working parents. There are nevertheless a number of issues arising from this study that are relevant for policy-makers to consider. At the most basic level of being able to work and care, the availability of high quality, affordable childcare, paid parental leave and the right of parents to be supported when their children are ill, are crucial, though ineffective if they are not fully accepted by management and integrated into workplace practices. Gaps between policy (national and/or workplace) and practice were evident in Peak and indeed in all the case study organizations. Parents' experiences of well-being in organizations depends on fundamental requirements in terms of not just policies, but also culture and practice and especially the day-to-day support of line managers.

Beyond meeting basic needs, a focus on multiple layers of context as well as dimensions of time point to the need for a multilayered approach to policy. We have seen that changes in legislation alone are of limited value for enhancing well-being of new parents without shifts in organizational, family and community values and practices. Policies in flexible working need to be supported by questioning assumptions about ideal workers in organizations and assumptions about gender roles and identities in families and wider society, if they are to have maximum impact on well-being. Policy-making to address well-being would therefore need to be integrated and collaborative at many levels

There are also significant questions to be considered about whose well-being is to be addressed, at what point of time, in what context. A life course approach would focus on the potential long-term as well as short-term impact of polices and practices on well-being in given contexts. For example, there is a dilemma that policies that meet parents' currently articulated needs – for example part-time work for mothers – can enhance mothers' well-being in the short term but also reproduce gender inequalities and potentially undermine well-being in the long term, unless change occurs in workplace values and practices and the gendered construction of organizational commitment in terms of full-time work.

Finally, it must be remembered that social reproduction is necessary for the long-term social sustainability of societies. If working and parenting become too difficult in the context of intensified work-loads in contemporary organizations this often becomes associated with declining birth rates (Fagnini et al. 2004; Lewis and Smithson

2006). Overall this project indicates that rapidly changing conditions in European workplaces in the global market require the ongoing evaluation of the impact – both long-term and short-term – of a range of policies and practices on the well-being of parents and their employing organizations, taking into account the roles of the most relevant actors: state, employers, trade unions and workers.

Notes

1. See www.workliferesearch.org/transitions We acknoweldge the collaboration of the other members of the UK Transitions team, Janet Smithson, Julia Brannen and John Haworth as well as our transnational partners: Ann Nilsen, Nevenka Cernigoj Sadar, Siyka Kovacheva, Maris das Dores Guerreiro, Anneka den Doornes-Huiskes, Margareta Back-Wicklund and Jeanne Fagnani.
2. The eight countries involved in the study were Bulgaria, France, Norway, Portugal, Slovenia, Sweden, the Netherlands and the UK (see Fagnani et al. 2004).

References

6, Perry (2002) *Sense and Solidarities: a Neo-Durkheimian Instutional Theory of Well-Being and its Implications for Public Policy*. ESRC seminar series, 'Well-Being: Situational and Individual Determinants', 2001–2 (www.wellbeing-esrc.com), Research and Policy for Well-Being.

Brannen, J. and Brockman, M. (2005) *UK Social Services Interview Study* (www.workliferesearch.org/transitions).

Brannen, J. and Moss, P. (1999) 'The Polarisation and Intensification of Parental Employment in Britain: Consequences for Parents, Children and the Community', *Community, Work and Family*, 1(3): 229–48.

Bunting, M. (2004) *Willing Slaves*. London: HarperCollins.

Campbell-Clarke, S. (2000) 'Work/Family Border Theory: a New Theory of Work/Family Balance', *Human Relations*, 53(6): 747–70.

DTI (2003) *Balancing Work and Family Life: Enhancing Choice and Support for Parents*. London: Department of Trade and Industry.

Fagnani, J., Houriet-Segard, G. and Bedouin, S. (2004) *Context Mapping for the EU Framework 5 Funded Study 'Gender, Parenthood and the Changing European Workplace'*. Manchester: Manchester Metropolitan University, Research Institute for Health and Social Change.

Gambles, R., Lewis, S. and Rapoport, R. (2006) *The Myth of Work–Life Balance: the Challenge of Our Time for Men, Women and Societies*. Chichester: Wiley.

Kossek, E. E. and Ozeki, C. (1999) 'Bridging the Work–Family Policy and Productivity Gap: a Literature Review', *Community, Work and Family*, 2(1): 7–32.

Lapido, D. and Wilkinson, F. (2002). 'More Pressure, Less Protection', in B. Burchell, D. Lapido and F. Wilkinson (eds), *Job Insecurity and Work Intensification*. London: Routledge.

Lewis, S. (1997) 'Family Friendly Policies: Organisational Change or Playing About at the Margins?', *Gender, Work and Organisations*, 4: 13–23.

Lewis, S. and Cooper, C. L. (1987) 'Stress in Two Earner Couples and Stage in the Life Cycle', *Journal of Occupational Psychology*, 60: 289–303.

Lewis, S. and Cooper, C. L. (1988) 'The Transition to Parenthood in Dual Earner Couples', *Psychological Medicine*, 18: 477–86.

Lewis, S. (2003) 'The Integration of Paid Work and the Rest of Life: Is Post-Industrial Work the New Leisure?', *Leisure Studies*, 22(4): 343–55.

Lewis, S. and Smithson, J. (2001) 'Sense of Entitlement to Support for the Reconciliation of Employment and Family Life', *Human Relations*, 55(11): 1455–81.

Lewis, S. and Smithson, J. (2006) *Final Report of the Transitions Project*. Manchester: Manchester Metropolitan University, Research Institute for Health and Social Change.

Nilsen, A. and Brannen, J. (2005) *Transitions Research Report No. 8: Negotiating Parenthood: Consolidated Interview Study Report*. Report for the EU Framework 5 funded study 'Gender, Parenthood and the Changing European Workplace'. ISBN 1-900139-32-4. Manchester: Manchester Metropolitan University, Research Institute for Health and Social Change.

Nippert-Eng, C. E. (1996) *Home and Work: Negotiating Boundaries Through Everyday Life*. Chicago: University of Chicago Press.

Noor, N. (2004) 'Work–Family Conflict, Work- and Family-Role Salience, and Women's Well-Being', *British Journal of Social Psychology*, 144(4): 389–406.

Osberg, L. and Sharpe, O. (2002) 'The Index of Economic Well-being', *Indicators: the Journal of Social Health*, 1(2): 24–62.

Rapoport, R., Bailyn, L., Fletcher, J. and Pruitt, B. (2002) *Beyond Work–Family Balance: Advancing Gender Equity and Work Performance*. Chichester: Wiley.

Reichle, B. (1996) 'From Is to Ought and the Kitchen Sink: On the Justice of Distributions in Close Relationships', in L. Montada and M. J. Lerner (eds), *Current Societal Concerns about Justice*. New York: Plenum.

Smithson, J., Lewis, S. and Purcell (eds) (2005) *Report on National Debates on the Reconciliation of Family and Employment. Transitions Research Report No. 9*. Manchester: Manchester Metropolitan University, Research Institute for Health and Social Change.

Sointu, E. (2005) 'The Rise of an Ideal: Tracing Changing Discourses on Well-Being', *Sociological Review*, 53(2): 255–74.

Swanson, V. (1999) 'Stress, Satisfaction and Role Conflict in Dual-Doctor Partnerships', *Community, Work and Family*, 2(1): 67–88.

Taylor, R. (2002) *Britain's World of Work-Myths and Realities*. ESRC Future of Work Programme Seminar Series. Economic and Social Research Council, Polaris House, Swindon. UK.

Thompson, J, and Bunderson, J. (2001) 'Work non-Work Conflict and the Phenomenology of Time', *Work and Occupations*, 28(1): 17–39.

13
Work, Leisure and Well-Being in Changing Social Conditions

John Haworth

Introduction

Profound transformations are occurring in the nature and organization of work with potentially far-reaching social and economic consequences. In many countries there is an intensification of workloads, and increasing job insecurity (Transitions 2006). Organizations are demanding greater efficiency and introducing new technologies and working practices in response to the pressures of competition in the private sector and efficiency drives in the public sector. In some organizations flexibility of working practices is being coupled with policies purporting to support the integration of work and non-work life, sometimes in response to new attitudes, values and aspirations of key workers; but also to enhance creativity, improve company loyalty, and reduce absenteeism and turnover (Lewis 2003b). Yet many employees are experiencing long working hours, intensified workloads, constantly changing work practices, and job insecurity (Burchall et al. 1999; Transitions 2006). Stress at work and home is viewed as a major problem (Worral and Cooper 2001; Schneider et al. 2004). But a gap exists in many Western societies between state policies on work-life balance and the implementation of polices in practice (Transitions 2006). Major social differentiation exists in relation to gender, class, occupation and other aspects of diversity (Taylor 2001, 2002), with resources in Western societies being increasingly unequally distributed, and significant variations arising in health, well-being and quality of life (Wilkinson 1996, 2000). In this context the meanings and concepts of work and leisure are being reappraised, and the relationships between work, leisure, social structure and well-being have emerged as challenging concerns for researchers, educators and policy-makers (Haworth and Veal 2004).

This chapter briefly discusses concepts and research in work and leisure as a context to summarize a model of well-being focusing on the characteristics of situations and persons. The pivotal role played by enjoyment in well-being is then examined. The chapter concludes with some recommendations for research and policy.

Work and leisure

Work has often been equated with labour. Yet work is important to human functioning. Kohn and Schooler (1983) indicate that where work has substantive complexity there is an improvement in mental flexibility and self-esteem. Csikszentmihalyi and LeFevre (1989), studying 'optimal experience' or 'flow' in a range of occupations, found that this came more from work than leisure. The historian of work, Applebaum (1992:ix), considers that 'Work is like the spine which structures the way people live, how they make contact with material and social reality, and how they achieve status and self-esteem. Work is basic to the human condition, to the creation of the human environment, and to the context of human relationships.' In modern society, paid work has been found to be important for well-being (Jahoda 1982; Warr 1987).

Leisure can be defined in a number of ways, for example as time left over from work or activities engaged in for intrinsic satisfaction. Today, the so-called 'residual' definition of leisure, that is time which is not occupied by paid work, unpaid work or personal chores and obligations, is widely accepted in research (Roberts 1999: 5). However, Roberts (1999: 3) notes that the residual definition of leisure proves difficult to apply to the unemployed and retired, as well as among women, regardless of their employment status. He also recognizes that technological, economic and social changes in society impact on leisure, making it 'necessary to ask repeatedly whether we need revise our notions about what leisure is' (1999: 5). This is particularly complex when considering work that is absorbing and identity affirming, where the boundaries between activities that can be considered work or leisure are blurred (Lewis 2003a). A distinction can also be made between serious leisure and other forms of leisure. For example, Stebbins (2004) discusses serious leisure, volunteerism and quality of life. His research shows that extended engagement in absorbing leisure activities which require effort can provide a range of rewards. But there are also costs involved, which entail a commitment to the pursuit. Stebbins argues that an optimal leisure lifestyle includes serious and 'unserious' leisure, the latter characterized as comprising immediately intrinsically rewarding, relatively short-lived pleasurable activity requiring little or no special training. Quality of leisure life is influenced by the people with whom leisure participants pursue their leisure (Csikszentmihalyi 1997). And leisure plays a part in establishing and maintaining social worlds (Unruh 1980), networks and friendships.

The amount of a person's total waking lifetime spent in non-work activities is now greater than the amount spent in paid work (Veal 1987: 16), so the importance of leisure for people's lives should not be under-estimated or obscured by the focus on paid work at certain points in the life course. A government report in the UK on *Life Satisfaction: the State of Knowledge and Implications for Government* (Donovan et al. 2002) cited strong links between work satisfaction and overall life satisfaction, and also between active leisure activities and overall satisfaction. The report noted the case for government intervention to boost life satisfaction, by encouraging a more leisured work-life balance. Recent research suggests that many people, especially in highly skilled jobs, prefer not to cease working altogether when they reach retirement age, but they do want to work less (Barnes et al. 2004). Leisure can provide an important part of life with implications for health and well-being.

Iso-Ahola and Mannell (2004), examine the reciprocal relationship between leisure and health in a contemporary context. They recognize that many people feel stressed because of financial difficulties and the dominance of work, and that in such situations leisure is used primarily for recuperation from work. The result is a passive leisure lifestyle and a reactive approach to personal health. They argue, on the basis of considerable research, that active leisure is important for health and well-being. Participation in both physical and non-physical leisure activities has been shown to reduce depression and anxiety, produce positive moods and enhance self-esteem and self-concept, facilitate social inter-action, increase general psychological well-being and life satisfaction, and improve cognitive functioning. Yet many people fail to discover active leisure. The authors argue that trying new things, and mastering challenges, is discouraged and undermined by the social system and environment.

However, the experiences of leisure and unpaid work in the house-hold are not gender neutral. Kay (2001) argues that within households, the capacity of male and female partners to individually exercise choice in leisure is highly contingent upon explicit or implicit negotiation between them. Many studies have shown that, even when both part-ners are working, women still make a significantly greater contribution to domestic tasks, and there are key differences between men's ability to preserve personal leisure time, and the much more limited capacity of women to do so; though recent research (see special issue of *Leisure Studies*, edited by Kay 2006) shows the importance that leisure can play in fatherhood. As individuals, men and women appear to give different priority to the work, family and leisure domains of their collective life, while simultaneously striving to achieve a mutually satisfying joint lifestyle. Kay (2001) argues that leisure is a significant domain of relative freedom and a primary site in which men and women can actively construct responses to social change. She considers that the recognition of this can contribute, at both a conceptual and empirical level, to a holistic understanding of contemporary lived experience; but that it raises the question about the extent to which we can realistically talk of families, collectively, being equipped to resolve the work-life dilemma.

Although experiences of work vary across different socio-political and cultural contexts, Haworth and Lewis (2005) drawing on two cross-national studies indicate that some general trends are nevertheless emerging across national boundaries. (Transitions[1] is a study looking at work, family and well being in young adults in eight European countries. *Looking Backwards to Go Forwards: the Integration of Paid Work and Personal Life*[2] is a recently completed study of the harmonization of paid work and personal life in seven countries in Europe, America, Africa and Asia.) The pervasiveness of the trend towards intensification of work, reducing time and energy for other activities, and the gendered impact of this trend are evident in both studies.

The Transitions study shows, for example, a drive for more efficiency and an intensification of work across all the countries as fewer people are expected to do more work. The study also reveals a widespread implementation gap between policies to support the reconciliation of work and family, whether at the state or workplace level, and actual practice; and persisting gender differences in work-life responsibilities and experiences in a range of social policy contexts. The Transitions case studies also show that both managers and work colleagues have a decisive role in creating the organizational climate and culture that contribute to the well-being of employed parents (see also Chapter 12 in this volume).

The study *Looking Backwards to Go Forwards* (see Lewis et al. 2003; Rapoport et al. 2006; Gambles et al. 2006) showed that the invasiveness of paid work into people's lives is moving from the 'developed' world to the 'developing' world. For example, people working in multinational companies in India tend to work long and intensive hours and report work-life balance as one of their major problems. The study found that many men and women in the countries studied report increased loneliness, and eroding support networks. The study also indicated that the barriers to satisfying and equitable harmonization of paid work and personal life are largely societal and global rather than residing within individuals.

Rapoport et al. (2006) argue that it is clear that current patterns of work create a lack of time and energy for the care of children, elders, and communities, as well as for pursuits that refresh the spirit and create the will and motivation for both employment and other activities. They consider that there is a need to see this as a central issue in the global economy and point to the need for fundamental change for people sustainability.

Work, leisure and well-being

Research into work and leisure has significantly informed the study of well-being. Jahoda (1982) has made a crucial case for the importance of the social institution of employment for well-being. She identified five categories of experience which employment automatically provides. These are: time structure, social contact, collective effort or purpose, social identity or status, and regular activity. Considerable research has shown the importance of these categories of experience for well-being (see Haworth 1997 for a summary). They have been incorporated in the nine environmental factors proposed by Warr (1987) as important for well-being.

Jahoda emphasizes that in modern society it is the social institution of employment which is the main provider of the five categories of experience. While recognizing that other institutions may enforce one or more of these categories of experience, Jahoda stresses that none of them combine them all with as compelling a reason as earning a living. Jahoda does recognize that the quality of experience of some jobs can be very poor and emphasizes the importance of improving and humanizing employment. Jahoda also emphasizes the important influence the institution of employment has on shaping thought and behaviour. She considers that since the industrial revolution employment has shaped the form of our daily lives, our experience of work and leisure, and our attitudes, values and beliefs. Jahoda (1986) agrees that human beings are striving, coping, planning, interpreting creatures, but adds that the tendency to shape one's life from the inside-out operates within the possibilities and constraints of social arrangements which we passively accept and which shape life from the outside-in. A great deal of life consists of passively following unexamined social rules, not of our making but largely imposed by the collective plans of our ancestors. Some of these rules meet basic human needs, even if we become aware of them only when they are broken by, for example, the enforced exclusion from an institution as in unemployment. Jahoda regards dependency on social institutions not as good or bad but as the *sine qua non* of human existence.

An influential model of the influence of characteristics of situations and persons on well-being has been proposed by Warr (1987, 1999). The model draws on that proposed by Jahoda (1982). It also encompasses features which Fryer and Payne (1984) highlight in their personal agency account of people coping well with unemployment. Warr (1987) identified nine 'situational' factors, or 'Principal Environmental Influences' important for well-being, measured on several dimensions. These factors are: opportunity for control, environmental clarity, opportunity for skill use, externally generated goals, variety, opportunity for interpersonal contact, valued social position, availability of money, and physical security. These features of the environment are considered to interact with characteristics of the person to facilitate or constrain psychological well-being or mental health. Warr produced a classification of 'enduring' personal characteristics which interact with situational factors on mental health. These person factors include baseline mental health, demographic factors such as age and gender, values and abilities. Baseline mental health includes several features often considered as elements of personality, such as neuroticism, self-confidence, hardiness and locus of control. It is recognized that well-being has many components (see Haworth 2004), and that what we view as important may be culturally determined. In his concept of mental health from a Western perspective, Warr (1987) advocates the measurement of affective well-being, competence, autonomy, aspiration and integrated functioning. However, it is the measure of affective well-being (Warr 1990) which has received the greatest empirical attention by Warr and colleagues. Warr (1987, 1990) devised a series of scales to measure affective well-being on three principal axes: the 'pleasure axis' (measuring displeasure to pleasure, by questions on enjoyment, satisfaction and happiness), the 'anxiety-contentment' axis, and the 'depression-enthusiasm' axis. The scales can be administered to measure affective well-being in work or in leisure.

Research conducted at Manchester University developing a questionnaire measure of the nine Principal Environmental Influences (PEIs) (summarized in Haworth 1997), shows strong associations between each of the nine PEIs and measures of mental health. Bryce and Haworth (2003) have also shown that the influence of control on well-being can operate by different pathways in males and females

An important development of the model, discussed in Haworth (1997, 2004), is the inclusion of the role of enjoyment. A study by Haworth et al. (1997) used questionnaires to measure the PEIs, the person factor: locus of control and well-being. The Experience Sampling Method was also used over a period of one week to measure positive subjective states, including enjoyment. The study indicated the important role enjoyment played in the link between person, situational factors and well-being. Rotter (1966, 1990) emphasizes that locus of control is a learned expectancy, rather than a fixed trait. Furnham and Steele (1993) also note that while locus of control beliefs may influence experience, the reverse may also be true. They suggest that positive successful life experiences probably increase internal locus of control beliefs through optimistic attributions. These may increase confidence, initiative and positive motivation, and thus lead to more successful experiences. Rotter (1982) indicates the possible importance of 'enhancement behaviours', which he viewed as specific cognitive activities that are used by those with an internal locus of control disposition to enhance and maintain good feelings. However, Uleman and Bargh (1989) also indicate the importance of subconscious processes in well-being, and Merleau-Ponty (1962) in his embodiment theory of consciousness indicates the importance of both non-reflective and reflective interactions in being (see Haworth 2000). Conceivably, positive subjective states could influence person factors, such as dispositions, coping styles etc. through both reflective and non-reflective interactions. In turn, person factors could influence well-being directly, or indirectly through access to situational factors important for well-being. The model can be investigated in both work and non-work situations, using the questionnaires given in Haworth (1997). Qualitative methods, including interviews, accounts, observation and ethnographic studies (Haworth 1996; Crossley 2000) can be used to investigate particular aspects in greater detail.

Extensive research shows that enjoyment in both leisure and work is important for well-being (e.g. Csikszentmihalyi and Csikszentmihalyi 1988; Clarke and Haworth 1994; Haworth and Evans 1995; Bryce and Haworth 2002). Delle Fave and Massimini (2003) note that creative activities in leisure, work, and social interaction can give rise to 'flow' or 'optimal' experiences. These experiences foster individual development and an increase in skills in the lifelong cultivation of specific interests and activities.

Enjoyment and flow

Seligman and Csikszentmihalyi (2000: 12) distinguish between pleasure and enjoyment. They note that

> Pleasure is the good feeling that comes from satisfying homeostatic needs such as hunger, sex, and bodily comfort. Enjoyment on the other hand, refers to the good feelings people experience when they break through the limits of homeostasis – when they do something that stretches them beyond what they were – in an athletic event, an artistic performance, a good deed, a stimulating conversation. Enjoyment, rather than pleasure, is what leads to personal growth and long term happiness.

Csikszentmihalyi has long considered enjoyment to play a pivotal role in well-being. In a pioneering study, Csikszentmihalyi (1975) set out to understand enjoyment in its own terms and to describe what makes an activity enjoyable. He found that when artists, athletes and creative professionals were asked to describe the best times experienced in their favourite activities they all mentioned a dynamic balance between opportunity and ability as crucial. Optimal experience, or 'flow' as some of the respondents described it, could be differentiated from states of boredom, in which there is less to do than one is capable of, and from anxiety, which occurs when things to do are more than one can cope with.

Csikszentmihalyi and Csikszentmihalyi (1988) report several in-depth accounts of flow and its importance for subjective well-being. They summarize the main dimensions of enjoyable flow as:

- Intense involvement
- Clarity of goals and feedback
- Deep concentration
- Transcendence of self
- Lack of self-consciousness
- Loss of a sense of time
- Intrinsically rewarding experience
- Balance between skill and challenge

Csikszentmihalyi (1991: 36) notes that in the flow state action follows upon action according to an internal logic that seems to need no conscious intervention by the actor. He expresses it as a unified flowing from one moment to the next in which one is in control of one's actions, and in which there is little distinction between self and environment, between stimulus and response, between past, present and future. It is considered that flow can be achieved in almost any activity, with the goals of activities serving as mere tokens that justify the activity by giving it direction and determining rules of action. Csikszentmihalyi emphasizes that flow activities need not be active in the physical sense, and that amongst the most frequently mentioned enjoyable activities are reading and being with other people. He also recognizes that the flow experience is not good in an absolute sense, and that whether the consequences of any particular instance of flow are good in the larger sense needs to be discussed in terms of more inclusive social criteria. Burglary, for example, can be a flow experience.

Flow has also been extensively investigated using the experience sampling method (ESM). Respondents answer questions about activity and subjective states on short scales in a diary several times a day in response to signals from a pre-programmed device such as a watch or radio pager. Several such studies are reported in Csikszentmihalyi and Csikszentmihalyi (1988). The defining characteristic of flow in these studies is a balance between skill and challenge. An important development of the three-channel model of flow (anxiety, flow, boredom) proposed by Csikszentmihalyi (1975) was made by Massimini and Carli (1988) by using the level of challenge as well as the skill challenge ratio (e.g. greater, equal and less) to give more differentiated models. A four-channel model showed that people were found to report the most positive subjective states when challenge and skills were in balance and when both were above the mean levels for the week of testing. Csikszentmihalyi and Csikszentmihalyi (1988: 260) note that when both challenges and skills are below what is customary for a person, it does not make sense to expect a person to be in flow, even if the two variables are perfectly balanced.

Studies by Clarke and Haworth (1994) and by Haworth and Evans (1995) showed that activities described as highly challenging with skill equal were highly enjoyable about only half of the time. Further, these studies showed that high enjoyment could be experienced when individuals engaged in activities which were described as only of a low challenge, such as watching TV. It is important to note, however, that high enjoyment was more often associated with high challenge met with equal skill (flow). Also, when high challenge met with equal skill is found to be enjoyable this seems to be beneficial for well-being. In the study of college students by Clarke and Haworth (1994) subjects who had flow experiences which were highly enjoyable were found to score significantly higher on several standard questionnaire measures of psychological well-being (Warr 1990; Warr et al. 1979; Goldberg 1978) than subjects who did not experience flow as highly enjoyable. The enjoyable flow group also experienced more happiness, relaxation and interest, on average, as measured by the ESM, than those who did not experience flow as highly enjoyable. Thus enjoyable flow seems to be important for psychological well-being, though this requires further exploration.

Enjoyable flow experiences come from a wide range of activities. In the study of young people by Haworth and Evans (1995) highly enjoyable flow experiences were most frequently associated with the job, followed by listening to music. Csikszentmihalyi and LeFevre (1989), in an ESM study, found, contrary to expectations, that the vast majority of flow experiences, measured as perceived balanced skill-challenge experiences above the person's average level, came when people were at work rather than in free time. A study by Haworth and Hill (1992) of young adult white-collar workers shows similar results.

A small study of working women by Allison and Duncan (1987, 1988) used a questionnaire they devised to measure enjoyable flow. The results showed work to be the primary source of flow for professional workers, whereas for blue-collar women it was leisure. The greatest source of flow in leisure was found to be in interpersonal relationships for both groups, particularly those with children. Using a similar questionnaire, a study of male and female office workers by Bryce and Haworth (2002) showed flow to be associated with well-being. Results also emphasized the importance of interpersonal relationships for flow in women. This is consistent with previous research indicating the importance of social interaction in leisure for women, arguably resulting from gender demands (Deem 1986; Green et al. 1990; Shaw 1994; Samuel 1996).

Work-life balance

Currently there is much concern with work-life balance. Primeau (1996), however, argues that it is not possible to say what is a healthy work-life balance. He suggests that occupational psychologists should examine the range of affective experiences that occur during engagement in one's customary round of occupations in daily life. He sites an important example being research into enjoyable, challenging ('flow') experiences in daily life. Greenhaus and Parasuraman (1999) indicate that while work and family can be in conflict, having negative effects on each other, they can also be integrated, having reciprocal positive effects. For example, positive attitudes and experiences in one domain may spill over to the other domain, permitting fuller and more enjoyable participation in that role. They note that 'Stressful, rigid work environments that demand extended commitments can interfere with family life, whereas flexible work environments that provide opportunities for self control can enrich family life' (1999: 409). They call for the adoption of a life stage perspective in research, and more research into dual earner families. Lewis (2003a) also notes that managing multiple work and non-work (especially family) roles can be very stressful, but can also create opportunities for multiple sources of satisfaction and well-being. Information technology is now increasingly allowing work to be done in almost any situation, creating pressures and opportunities.

Conclusions

The ways in which we conceptualize work, leisure and well-being are in flux, reflecting, in part, the changing societal, economic and community contexts in which work and leisure take place (Haworth and Lewis 2005). The conceptualization of well-being is shifting from a concern with stress and illness to include a focus on positive experiences.

Both work and leisure are important for well-being. Taylor (2002), in a report on the ESRC funded Future of Work programme, advocates that a determined effort is required to assess the purpose of paid work in all our lives, and the need to negotiate a genuine trade-off between the needs of job efficiency and leisure. Governments rightly place a very high priority on action to stimulate employment, for both economic and social reasons. Leisure facilites and opportunities are also provided by national and local government, and by educational institutions. Voluntary associations and groups also play an important role in leisure provision, occasionally funded by grants. But leisure opportunities are often cut back. While leisure is in many ways an individual phenomenon, the social and economic institution of leisure, arguably, needs to be more in balance with the social and economic institution of employment.

Taylor (2002) considers that class and occupational differences remain of fundamental importance to any understanding of the world of work. Class is also important in understanding the world of leisure (Critcher and Bramham 2004). It is thus important to monitor the distribution of resources available for work and leisure in different groups in society, whether these are analysed by class, gender, age, ethnicity or location. Equally important in societies characterized by diversity, is research into the experiences and motivations of individuals with varying work and leisure life styles.

Haworth (1997: ch. 7) argues that the diversity of individual experience and requirements is not merely a function of rational knowledge, but is built into the bodily fibre of experience and social networks of practice, reflecting both the social and temporal nature of human endeavour. Recognizing this means there is no one correct policy for work and leisure. In rapidly changing societies, time is needed for social practices to meet new requirements; and social practices need to be monitored and evaluated, using both quantitative and qualitative methods.

Notes

1. www.workliferesearch.org/transitions/. Professor Sue Lewis was project director. Dr John Haworth was a team member specializing in well-being.
2. The study *Looking Backwards to Go Forwards: the Integration of Paid Work and Personal Life* was funded by a grant from the Ford Foundation to Rhona Rapoport at the Institute for Family and Environment Research.

References

Allison, M. T. and Duncan, M. C. (1987) 'Women, Work and Leisure: the Days of our Lives', *Leisure Sciences*, 9: 143–62.

Allison, M. T. and Duncan, M. C. (1988) 'Women, Work and Flow', in M. Csikszentmihalyi and I. S. Csikszentmihalyi (eds), *Optimal Experience: Psychological Studies of Flow in Consciousness*. Cambridge: Cambridge University Press.

Applebaum, P. D. (1992) *The Concept of Work: Ancient, Medieval, and Modern*. Albany, NY: State University of New York Press.

Barnes, H., Parry, J. and Taylor, R. (2004) *Working After State Pensions Age: Qualitative Research*. London: Department of Work and Pensions.

Bryce, J. and Haworth, J. T. (2002) 'Wellbeing and Flow in a Sample of Male and Female Office Workers', *Leisure Studies*, 21: 249–63.

Bryce, J. and Haworth, J. T. (2003) 'Psychological Wellbeing in a Sample of Male and Female Office Workers', *Journal of Applied Social Psychology*, 33(3): 565–85.

Burchall, B., Day, D., Hudson, M., Lapido, D., Nolan, J., Reed, H., Wichert, I. and Wilkinson, E. (1999) *Job Insecurity and Work Intensification: Flexibility and the Changing Boundaries of Work*. York: Joseph Rowntree Foundation.

Clarke, S. G. and Haworth, J. T. (1994) '"Flow" Experience in the Daily Lives of Sixth Form College Students', *British Journal of Psychology*, 85: 511–23.

Critcher, C. and Bramham, P. (2004) 'The Devil Still Makes Work', in J. T. Haworth and A. J. Veal (eds), *Work and Leisure*. London: Routledge.

Crossley, M. (2000) *Introducing Narrative Psychology*. Buckingham: Open University Press.

Csikszentmihalyi, M. (1975) *Beyond Boredom and Anxiety*. San Francisco: Jossey-Bass.

Csikszentmihalyi, M. (1991) *Flow: the Psychology of Optimal Experience*. New York: Harper Perennial.

Csikszentmihalyi, M. (1997) *Finding Flow: the Psychology of Engagement with Everyday Life*. New York: Basic Books.

Csikszentmihalyi, M. and Csikszentmihalyi, I. S. (eds) (1988) *Optimal Experience: Psychological Studies of Flow in Consciousness*. Cambridge: Cambridge University Press.

Csikszentmihalyi, M. and LeFevre, J. (1989) 'Optimal Experience in Work and Leisure', *Journal of Personality and Social Psychology*, 56(5): 815–22.

Deem, R. (1986). *All Work and No Play: the Sociology of Women and Leisure*. Milton Keynes: Open University Press.

Delle Fave, A. and Massimini, F. (2003) 'Optimal Experience in Work and Leisure among Teachers and Physicians: Individual and Bio-cultural Implications', *Leisure Studies*, 22(4): 323–42.

Donovan, N., Halpern, D. and Sargeant, R. (2002) *Life Satisfaction: the State of Knowledge and Implications for Government*. London: Strategy Unit, Cabinet Office, Downing Street.

Fryer, D. and Payne, R. (1984) 'Proactive Behaviour in Unemployment Findings and Implications', *Leisure Studies*, 3: 273–95.

Furnham, A. and Steele, H. (1993) 'Measuring Locus of Control: a Critique of General, Children's, Health and Work Related Locus of Control Questionnaires', *British Journal of Psychology*, 84: 443–79.

Gambles, R., Lewis, S. and Rapoport, R.(2006) *The Myth of Work-Life Balance: the Challenge of Our Time for Men, Women and Society*. London: Wiley.

Goldberg, D. (1978) *The Detection of Psychiatric Illness by Questionnaire*. London: Oxford University Press.

Green, E., Hebron, S. and Woodward, D. (1990) *Women's Leisure, What Leisure?* Basingstoke: Macmillan.

Greenhaus, J. H. and Parasuraman, S. (1999) 'Research on Work, Family, and Gender: Current Status and Future Directions', in G.N. Powell (ed.), *Handbook of Gender and Work*. London: Sage.

Haworth, J. T. (1996) *Psychological Research: Innovative Methods and Strategies*. London: Routledge.

Haworth, J. T. (1997) *Work, Leisure and Well-Being*. London: Routledge.

Haworth, J. T. (2000) 'The Embodied Mind and Wellbeing', *Consciousness and Experiential Psychology*, 5: 14–19.

Haworth, J. T. (2004) 'Work, Leisure and Well-Being', in J. T. Haworth, and A. J. Veal (eds), *Work and Leisure*. London: Routledge.

Haworth, J. T. and Evans, S. (1995) 'Challenge, Skill and Positive Subjective States in the Daily Life of a Sample of YTS Students', *Journal of Occupational and Organisational Psychology*, 68: 109–121.

Haworth, J. T. and Hill, S. (1992) 'Work, Leisure and Psychological Well-Being in a Sample of Young Adults', *Journal of Community and Applied Social Psychology*, 2: 147–60.

Haworth, J. T., Jarman, M. and Lee, S. (1997). 'Positive Psychological States in the Daily Life of a Sample of Working Women', *Journal of Applied Social Psychology*, 27: 345–70.

Haworth, J. T. and Lewis, S. (2005) 'Work, Leisure and Well-Being', *British Journal of Guidance and Counselling*, 33(1): 67–79.

Haworth, J. T. and Veal, A. J. (eds) (2004) *Work and Leisure*. London: Routledge.

Iso-Ahola, S. E. and Mannell, R. C. (2004) 'Leisure and Health', in J. T. Haworth and A. J. Veal (eds), *Work and Leisure*. London: Routledge.

Jahoda, M. (1982) *Employment and Unemployment: a Social Psychological Analysis* Cambridge: Cambridge University Press.

Jahoda, M. (1986) 'In Defense of a Non-reductionist Social Psychology', *Social Behaviour*, 1: 25–9.

Kay, T. (2001) *Leisure, Gender and Family: Challenges for Work-Life Integration*. ESRC seminar series 'Wellbeing: Situational and Individual Determinants', 2001–2002 (www.wellbeing-esrc.com, Work, Employment, Leisure and Well-Being).

Kay, T. (2006) 'Where's Dad?, Fatherhood in Leisure Studies', *Leisure Studies*, 25(2): 133–52.

Kohn, M. and Schooler, M. (1983) *Work and Personality: an Enquiry into the Impact of Social Stratification*. Norwood, NJ: Ablex.

Lewis, S. (2003a) 'The Integration of Paid Work and the Rest of Life: Is Post Industrial Work the New Leisure?', *Leisure Studies*, 22(4): 343–55.

Lewis, S (2003b) 'Flexible Working Arrangements: Implementation, Outcomes and Management', in I. Roberson and C. Cooper (eds), *Annual Review of Industrial and Organisational Psychology*, Vol. 18. London: Wiley.

Lewis, S., Rapoport, R. and Gambles, R. (2003) 'Reflections on the Integration of Work and Personal Life', *Journal of Managerial Psychology*, 18: 824–41.

Massimini, F. and Carli, M. (1988) 'The Systematic Assessment of Flow in Daily Experience', in M. Csikszentmihalyi and I. S. Csikszentmihalyi (eds), *Optimal Experience: Psychological Studies of Flow in Consciousness*. Cambridge: Cambridge University Press.

Merleau-Ponty, M. (1962) *Phenomenology of Perception*. London: Routledge & Kegan Paul.

Primeau, C. A. (1996) 'Work and Leisure: Transcending the Dichotomy', *American Journal of Occupational Therapy*, 50: 569–77.

Rapoport, R., Lewis, S., Bailyn, L. and Gambles, R. (2006) 'Globalization and the Integration of Work with Personal Life', in S. Poelmans (ed.), *Work and Family: an International Research Perspective*. New Jersey: Erlbaum.

Roberts, K. (1999) *Leisure in Contemporary Society*. Wallingford, UK: CABI Publishing.

Rotter, J. B. (1966) 'Generalised Expectancies for Internal versus External Control of Reinforcement', *Psychological Monographs*, 80 (whole no.): 609.

Rotter, J. B. (1982) *The Development and Application of Social Learning Theory*. New York: Praeger.

Rotter, J. B. (1990) 'Internal versus External Locus of Control of Reinforcement: a Case History of a Variable', *American Psychologist*, 45(4): 489–93.

Samuel, N. (1996) *Women, Family and Leisure in Contemporary Society*. Wallingford, UK: CAB International.

Schneider, B., Ainbinder, A. M. and Csikszentmihalyi, M. (2004) 'Stress and Working Parents', in J. T. Haworth and A. J .Veal (eds), *Work and Leisure*. London: Routledge.

Seligman, M. E. P. and Csikszentmihalyi, M. (2000) 'Positive Psychology: an Introduction', *American Psychologist*, 55(1): 5–14.

Shaw, S. M. (1994). 'Gender, Leisure and Constraint: Towards a Framework for the Analysis of Women's Leisure', *Journal of Leisure Research*, 26: 8–22.

Stebbins, R. A. (2004) 'Serious Leisure, Volunteerism and Quality of Life', in J. T. Haworth and A. J .Veal (eds), *Work and Leisure*. London: Routledge.

Taylor, R. (2001) *The Future of Work-Life Balance*. ESRC Future of Work Programme Seminar Series. Swindon: Economic and Social Research Council, Polaris House.

Taylor, R. (2002) *Britain's World of Work-Myths and Realities*. ESRC Future of Work Programme Seminar Series. Swindon: Economic and Social Research Council, Polaris House.

Transitions (2006) *Final Report. Research Report No. 11*. Manchester, Manchester Metropolitan Universty: Research Institute for Health and Social Change.

Uleman, J. S. and Bargh, J. A. (eds) (1989) *Unintended Thought*. London: Guilford Press.

Unruh, D. R. (1980) 'The Nature of Social Worlds', *Pacific Sociological Review*, 23: 271–96.

Veal, A. J. (1987) *Leisure and the Future*. London: Allen & Unwin.

Warr, P. (1987) *Work, Unemployment and Mental Health*. Oxford: Clarendon Press.

Warr, P. (1990) 'The Measurement of Well-Being and Other Aspects of Mental Health', *Journal of Occupational Psychology*, 63: 193–210.

Warr, P. (1999) 'Well-Being and the Workplace', in D. Kahneman, E. Diener and N. Schwarz (eds), *Well-Being: the Foundations of Hedonic Psychology*. New York: Russell Sage Foundation.

Warr, P., Cook, J. and Wall, T. (1979) 'Scales for the Measurement of Some Work Attitudes and Aspects of Psychological Well-Being', *Journal of Occupational Psychology*, 52: 129–48.

Wilkinson, R. G. (1996) *Unhealthy Societies: the Afflictions of Inequality*. London: Routledge.

Wilkinson, R. G. (2000) *Mind the Gap: Hierarchies, Health and Human Evolution*. London: Weidenfeld & Nicolson.

Worrall, L. and Cooper, C. L. (2001) *Quality of Working Life: 2000 Survey of Managers' Changing Experiences*. London: Institute of Management.

14
Friendship, Trust and Mutuality

Ray Pahl

> A faithful friend is a strong defence, and he that hath found
> such an one hath found a treasure...A faithful friend is the
> medicine of life.
>
> Ecclesiasticus

Some years ago an American political scientist published a book entitled
Bowling Alone (Putnam 2000). It attracted considerable media attention
at the time – perhaps because the author was critical of aspects of American
society. It purported to show that Americans were becoming less
attached to society through their involvement in voluntary associations
and activities. A decline in the membership of bowling clubs became
an iconic illustration of this change: the picture on the cover of the
book showed a man literally bowling alone. However, this image was
misleading. Far from actually bowling alone, men were increasingly
playing with their friends and families. The activity could well involve
more and closer social relationships than would be the case in simply
playing as a member of a club team.

The decline in memberships of bowling teams was taken by Putnam
as an indication of a decline in civic engagement, which may or may
not be justifiable. However, it is certainly arguable that playing more
bowls with friends and family actually does more to increase personal
well-being.

However, before accepting too readily that our friendships provide us
with 'the medicine of life', we must first acknowledge that many sociologists
have been very sceptical about the social worth and significance
of modern friendships. In 1918 Georg Simmel believed that there had
been a shift in the quality of our social relationships associated with the
increased rationality and instrumentalism of modern life.

Modern man, possibly, has too much to hide to sustain a friendship in the ancient sense … The modern way of feeling tends more heavily toward differentiated friendship, which covers only one side of the personality, without playing into the other aspects of it. (Simmel in Wolff 1950: 326)

According to such a view, the putative medicine of life has become so diluted that it is no longer capable of enhancing our well-being – as may have been the case in some previous, unspecified, golden age.

Certainly Simmel's doubts are strongly endorsed by some contemporary sociologists such as Zygmunt Bauman, who, in his vigorous polemic on *Liquid Love*, claims that 'liquid modern individualized society has made long-term commitments thin on the ground, long-term engagement a rare expectation, and the obligation of mutual assistance "Come what may" a prospect that is neither realistic nor viewed as worthy of great effort' (Bauman 2003: 66). Of course, Bauman cannot deny that there still exists a world of solidarity which struggles to survive the assaults of market competitivism and individualization but, pessimistically, he argues that 'A world whose residents are neither competitors nor subjects of use and consumption' (2003: 70) has little hope of survival. He puts human solidarity and friendship in a 'grey area' which he describes as the kingdom of anarchy (2003: 71). So convinced is Bauman of the market offensive on what he terms the 'skills of sociality', that he believes that at best we shall come to value others as simply 'companions-in-the-essentially-solitary-activity of consumption' (2003: 75). Using the rhetorical stance of an Old Testament prophet, Bauman declares that 'Human solidarity is the first casualty of the triumphs of the consumer market' (2003: 76).

Professor Bauman writes with considerable verve and style and, if he is to be believed, then we have little hope that friendship, the medicine of life, will continue to be available to increase our well-being. However, fortunately, there are other stronger voices amongst political scientists, economists, specialists in social medicine, psychologists and sociologists who have presented solid empirical evidence to suggest that Simmel, Bauman and other pessimistic essayists may be mistaken (Cohen et al. 2000; Halpern 2005; Lane 1994, 2000; Layard 2005; Martin 1997; Pahl 2000; Spencer and Pahl 2006).

However, before drawing on this material, it is important to recognize that the solid evidence that links social support and friendship to individual well-being does not directly address the question of whether that social solidarity and support is either increasing or declining as a result of contemporary social trends. Demonstrating the contemporary significance of friendship, trust and mutuality may be taken as evidence that the glass is either half-full or half-empty. Social philosophers may argue whether social life is degenerating or improving and evidently the surrogate variables that are selected may substantially affect the outcome of the debate. Certainly, survey evidence can be adduced to indicate that social life is not what it used to be. In the case of trust, for example, in answer to the question 'would you say that most people can be trusted – or would you say that you can't be too careful in dealing with people?' 56 per cent of Britons in 1959 agreed that most people could be trusted. However, by 1998 the proportion had declined to 30 per cent (cited in Layard 2005: 81). Similar reductions in trust as measured by survey results have been reported for the United States.

However, let us be quite clear: such results are based on questions referring to 'most people'. The question is not about whether we now have less confidence in our best friends or our siblings. In much of the discussion about changing attitudes and trust the data used is actually about how we respond to strangers, not how we respond to 'our nearest and dearest'. Such a methodological caveat is not a mere quibble. There is no reason why an increasing distrust of 'most people' should not be paralleled by an increasing closeness and solidarity with that small circle of intimates who are most important to us.

Whilst it is not the purpose of this chapter to deal with social change and social relationships in broad terms, there is certainly evidence that friendships are becoming more important for certain social categories at certain stages of the life course. For example, it has been suggested that given the likelihood that around one in three marriages end in divorce, it is plausible that following such a disruption friends would increase in salience and importance. Evidence from the British Household Panel provides some confirmation of such a supposition. The proportion of those men who made contact with a 'close friend' (not a spouse or partner, but could be another relative), by writing, visiting or telephoning during the previous weeks increased from 68 per cent of those who were married to 79 per cent of those who were divorced (British Household Panel Study, Wave 4, 1994).

The importance of friends in helping individuals to cope with stressful life events has long been understood. For example, over a quarter of a century ago Professor George Brown and his colleagues at the University of London demonstrated the overwhelming importance of having a close, intimate and confiding relationship. They showed that women who had experienced life stress through a particular event or major difficulty were ten times more likely to be depressed without having such a confidante, than those who did have such a confidante (Brown et al. 1975).

In a more recent review of the literature on the importance of women's same-sex friends for their well-being and the importance of this for therapy, the authors reinforce the conclusion of the London study. The absence of friendship was linked to loneliness, depression and psychosomatic illness (Knickmeyer et al. 2002). The authors noted in particular a study that compared same-sex friendship with friendship within marriage for both men and women, which was based on measures of relationship quality and self-esteem.

> In comparing best friendships to friendships within marriage, women viewed their female friends and their spouses as equally encouraging and supportive, implying similar relational provisions. Women also reported feeling more secure and comfortable letting their guard down with best friends than with their spouses. (Knickmeyer et al. 2002: 49)

There has been much interest over the years by sociologists concerned with the problem of loneliness, since a concern with isolation is inevitably bound up with their traditional concern with social integration. The classic study *On Suicide* by Durkheim (1951) put the issue firmly in the mainstream sociological tradition. As Fischer and Phillips (1982: 21) remark, 'when a society has many isolated members, it is prone to crumble'. The authors report on a study carried out in 1977 based on a random sample of 1050 adults in northern California. They recognize that it is difficult in a large-scale social survey to determine precisely what 'alone' might mean, since the quantity of social contacts may say little about the quality of the social exchanges involved. They adopted the definition of social isolation as 'knowing relatively few people who are probable sources of rewarding exchanges' (1982: 22) and they asked questions about who had provided specific services or who had engaged in specific joint activities. The authors also included questions that measured respondents' well-being or happiness. From their analysis the authors conclude that 'isolated respondents – notably, those isolated from non kin – were less likely than others to express happiness' (1982: 36). However, in a significant footnote the authors acknowledge the perennial problem of causal direction, since psychological depression may cause an individual to withdraw from others and those who, for other reasons, lack social skills may not themselves be able to maintain adequate social support. This is an issue that has dominated the literature since the pioneering work by Fischer and his colleagues.

Nevertheless, Fischer and Phillips do demonstrate that isolation is socially patterned:

> Uneducated and poor people tend to be isolated from *non kin* (and confidants). Their relatively low risk of *kin* isolation does not make up for the deficit, since they remain relatively isolated in terms of total network; these are the high risk people. Stage in the life cycle reflects the other major pattern, albeit a complex one. For men, ageing increases the risk of all kinds of isolation, partly because of retirement, perhaps also because of decreased mobility and the death of friends. Marriage, however, protects them against kin isolation, and provides at least one confidant. Ageing has less effect on women but marriage has more: it tends to isolate women from non-kin. (1982: 37)

Later studies of isolation have reported very similar conclusions (Keith 1986). The significance of friendship for the emotional well-being of individuals is also well-established in the literature (Cohen et al. 2000; Lane 2000; Martin 1997). Gerontologists, in particular, have focused on the importance of friends for the morale and well-being of older people because friends were both confidants and companions (Larson 1978). This has encouraged programmes of practical social action to improve subjective happiness through forms of 'friend-like' interventions. This can range from relatively brief home visits to quasi-'friendly' relationships engineered by care workers.

A small qualitative study carried out in Buckinghamshire in 2001 provides some indications that a consciously provided 'befriending service' may also lead to the development of a reciprocal and balanced friendship. This is a difficult and delicate area, since the balance between the befriender's public and private roles is hard to maintain. If a true friendship does emerge, then it has to be sure to continue if the increase in well-being is to be maintained. The loss of a befriender could, in certain circumstances, be emotionally damaging (Andrews et al. 2003).

The literature on social support and well-being has developed considerably over the past twenty years, partly due to the availability of longitudinal panel studies such as the BHPS at Essex University. It is now robustly established that those with low support are far more likely to report common mental illness. Furthermore, low social support not only increases the probability of the onset of common mental illness but also decreases the probability of recovery (Pevalin and Goldberg 2003).

Research has also made it clear that it is the quality, not the quantity of friendship that makes for true happiness and well-being. In the words of Larson and his colleagues 'It is the spontaneous affection and joy of friends that makes them worth having' (Larson et al. 1986: 125). This is a theme that has echoed down the ages from the Book of Proverbs or Cicero to the philosophers, novelists and poets who have continued to celebrate friends and friendship (e.g. Konstan 1997; Pakaluk 1991; Ransome 1912; Vernon 2005).

Such universal agreement about the contribution of true friendship to our well-being and happiness is surely hard to refute. However, it may be claimed that spending time with our real or imaginary friends leads to a disengagement from a wider social or civic life and the responsibilities attached thereto. In a witty reference to Putnam's book, an article on 'Bowling With Our Imaginary Friends', Kanazawa suggested that a close involvement with TV soap operas focused on the friendly relations of small groups of peers could serve the same function as having real friends (Kanazawa 2002), but this argument was later strongly rebutted (Freese 2003). The debate continues.

The notion that enhanced personal well-being, through having close and supportive friendships, does not necessarily enhance societal well-being is an issue that has long been of concern. Alexis de Tocqueville writing in the 1830s recognized the problem from his observations of the American society of the time.

> Individualism is a mature and calm feeling, which disposes each member of the community to sever himself from the mass of his fellow-creatures; and to draw apart with his family and friends; so that after he has thus formed a little circle of his own, he willingly leaves society at large to itself. (de Tocqueville 1889, II: 90)

Such 'little circles' can indeed turn inwards but they can also serve as nuclei of intellectual ferment, as many accounts of revolutions in the nineteenth and twentieth centuries clearly demonstrate.

In an attempt to provide a sociological defence of the social importance of friendship in modern society, Allan Silver, in a very elegant essay, argues that it is a kind of inversion of wider values and ideals. In what Silver refers to as the Great Society, forms of association were built on explicit contract, rational exchange, formal division of labour and impersonal institutions. The ideal of friendship is based now on the mirror image of these. 'Especially in the urban core of western society, particularly in its more educated sectors, friendships are judged of high quality to the extent that they invert the ways of the larger society' (Silver 1989: 274).

Unlike contractual relations, friendships are based on open-ended commitments and generalized reciprocity. If the terms of exchange are monitored or finely defined, the quality of the friendship is thereby diminished. Silver argues:

> Friendships are grounded in the uniquely irreplaceable qualities of partners – their 'true' or 'real' selves, defined and valued independently of their place in public systems of power, utility and esteem. Friendships so conceived turn on intimacy, the confident revelation of the self to the other, the sharing of expressive and consummatory activities ... no body of law and administrative regulation brings sovereign authority to bear on friendships; while others may pass censure or render judgement, friends have the right and capacity to ignore them. (1989: 274–5)

As such, friendship provides a moral arena in which interpersonal trust can safely emerge. 'In transcending the unavoidable possibility of betrayal, personal trust achieves a moral elevation, lacking in contractual or other engagements by third parties' (1989: 275). Silver's main thesis is that this is a distinctively modern ideal of friendship, which inverts the wider institutionalized structures of society and is based on the intrinsic, not extrinsic, qualities of the other.

Here we have the central paradox in the sociological theory of friendship. On the one hand there are those, such as Simmel and Bauman, who argue that the institutions and values of market society and consumerism destroy the conditions in which the true ideal can flourish. Yet, on the other hand, Silver argues that it is only under the conditions of modern society that the distinctive ideal can possibly emerge. I recognize that I have done considerably less than justice to the arguments deployed on either side of the debate. This is a problem that requires a long and extended discussion. Perhaps one way to resolve the problem would be to suggest that Bauman is making assertions about how he observes or imagines individuals actually behaving in their personal relationships, whereas Silver is limiting himself to an ideal.

One way to make this distinction clear would be to consider the case of a monk, nun or friar. Such a person might have a true understanding of the highest ideal of friendship. They may be kindly, understanding, sympathetic and fully endowed with all the qualities inherent in a truly friendly disposition. They may be free of the constraints of competitive consumerism and instrumentalism in personal relationships. They may be said to be good people in the deepest sense, putting the highest value on trust and mutuality. However, and this is very often the case, they may have no true individual friends or soul mates. They may share their most intimate thoughts in prayers or with their confessor but they have no close individual friends (Carmichael 2004).

It is evident that discussion about friendship as an ideal or as a disposition may reveal very little about how people actually behave in their private lives. One might as well expect all philosophers to live lives of the greatest moral purity. The biography of Bertrand Russell is but one example to suggest that such an expectation is unlikely to be fulfilled.

The distinctions I have been making are not simply matters of theoretical interest: they have intense practical importance. There may be general approval of the idea that friendship is the medicine of life. We may recognize the importance of trust and the positive value of mutuality. We may be convinced that, indeed, market solutions to the deficit of companionship in modern society have failed. We may even consider that, in Cicero's words, 'friendship is the one good thing' and can do more for our well-being than any of the more conventional sources of happiness. However, if we limit ourselves to ideals and dispositions we are getting little understanding of the actual empirical reality of the friendly relationships most people have in their everyday lives.

In the remaining part of this chapter I draw on the research undertaken by Liz Spencer and myself over the past decade. Our project was concerned with 'Rethinking Friendship' and we were determined to avoid having preconceptions about the meanings of the varying terms people used to describe their range of actual, existing personal relationships. There are plenty of clichés in contemporary discussions referring to 'the decline of the extended family', 'the emergence of families of choice', 'the transformation of intimacy', 'liquid love' and so on. We devised a purposive sample, geographically based in Greater Manchester, the south-east and the West Midlands. The research design was rigorously qualitative and at its heart was the exploration and analysis of the people whom respondents considered 'were important to them now'. This small collection of people was explored in detail on a diagram representing an individual's 'personal community'.

Full details of our methods, analytical framework and findings appear elsewhere (Spencer and Pahl 2006). However, perhaps the most significant finding was the diverse nature of friendship that we were able to document for Britain today. Some of the friendly relationships were so close that they could be described as being quasi-family. Other friendships, by contrast, were casual, shallow and short-lived. It is probably these latter kind of relationships that have caught the attention of the pessimistic commentators who have, perhaps, been over-ready to generalize on partial information. Certain kinds of friends – associates, neighbours or what we term 'fun friends' – may fade when people move, or follow different life-course trajectories. Yet it is also true that such fun friends can be immensely affectionate and last a lifetime. We also found that people varied in their range or repertoire of friendships. Some people had what we termed basic or narrow repertoires, where all their friends were fun friends or associates. For them more intimate, confiding relationships were confined to members of their families or partners – or, indeed, missing altogether from their personal community. Yet others, with broader types of repertoires, were able to include a range of different kinds of friendships from close confidants to more casual light-hearted friends.

Given this great diversity, we recognized that to argue that most informal personal relationships outside the family are more likely to be casual or fleeting did not conform to empirical reality. Even when we focused on those respondents who were the most reflexive or self-conscious about their social world and who might appear to be the prime candidates for 'liquid love', they were not involved in what critics have discussed as 'pick-up and put-down-again' relationships. Quite the contrary – they had a range of close and more distant family ties and broad friendship repertoires that included soul-mates, confidants, help mates, favour friends and also some purely sociable fun friends. Far from being dupes of the consumer-conscious market society, they were well aware of the circumstances whereby some friends could drift apart. Indeed, it seemed as though their personal communities almost needed some friendships to fade to a degree, so that other friendships could blossom and become more committed – and even more demanding. However, unlike the sociological Jeremiahs of contemporary opinion, such people did not consider their more light-hearted or short-lived friendships to be any the less valuable or worthwhile, a kind of vital counter-balance to other more serious or committed relationships. Such respondents referred to the contrast between their 'high maintenance' friends and their 'champagne bubble' friends.

In order to provide a more precise structure to our long and complex discussion of the different kinds of relationships that were revealed in

	High commitment	Low commitment
Given	Solid / foundational	Nominal
Given-as-chosen	Bonus	Neglected/abandoned
Chosen-as-given	Adopted	Heart sink
Chosen	Forged	Liquid

Figure 14.1: Commitment and choice in personal relationships

our study, we devised the diagram shown as Figure 14.1. We did not use the terms 'friend' or 'family', since we recognized and described a considerable suffusion between these too over-broad categories. Some friends were more family-like than were some actual given ties and some members of a family were merely nominal in terms of their personal commitment.

Among *solid, foundational* ties we expect to find immediate family, for example, parents, children and siblings, who enjoy a close bond. *Nominal* ties are likely to refer to more distant relatives who, for whatever reason, are on the periphery of each other's social world, such as cousins or step-relations whose existence we scarcely register. With *bonus* relationships, given ties become *as chosen*; here we find cases where the special quality of certain given relationships is recognized and, for example, a favourite sibling is seen as more than a brother or sister and assigned the honorary status of friend. By contrast, with *neglected* or *abandoned* ties the element of choice serves to weaken rather than strengthen the relationship (which is still given): here we find relatives who have fallen out because of irreconcilable differences in values or social position, or parents who have lost touch with their children after a messy divorce.

Adopted ties are highly committed chosen-as-given relationships, such as very close friendships which have taken on an almost family-like status: for example, a friend may also be considered a sister or brother. Also in this category are fictive kin: the unrelated 'uncles' and 'aunts' who may be part of a child's given social world. *Forged* relationships, on the other hand, are strong chosen ties and this is where we would expect to find close, established, lifelong friendships. Finally, *liquid* ties are likely to be light-hearted, casual friends and acquaintances, or, alternatively, casual sexual partners.

In our analysis of personal communities we did find that some people had examples of all eight kinds of relationships on their map. Others included distinctive combinations of high and low commitment, given and chosen ties. We found no evidence that personal relationships today are uniformly casual. Indeed, crucially, we did not find a single example in our study of a personal community made up entirely of nominal, neglected or liquid ties.

However, it is true that certain social categories were not captured in our sample. We did not interview any footballers' wives, minor actresses or people who have been in Big Brother's house. Conceivably such people could fit the stereotypical notion of liquid lovers with all their relationships in the low-commitment column. However, this is doubtful. Even those with the most transitory and fleeting of friends have close and fulfilling relationships with a parent, child or sibling. If someone says that their mother or their brother is their closest friend with whom they can share their deepest thoughts and emotions, this is often conveniently overlooked when categorizing their set of relationships as a whole.

In the light of these remarks on the diversity of ties we documented in our study, I return now to the central theme of this chapter, namely how far can the social support given by actual – not ideal – friends and friendships provide us with the medicine of life essential for our well-being? This is an issue we specifically addressed in our book (Spencer and Pahl 2006: 199–202).

We chose as our empirical measure of well-being the General Health Questionnaire (GHQ) which all our participants completed. This is a well-tried, robust and standardized method of measuring mental well-being. Across all our participants, scores of this measure varied widely but when we related the scores to our typology of personal communities, some interesting patterns emerged. The most vulnerable personal communities were those we described as 'partner-based' and 'professional based'.

In those personal communities we termed 'friend-based' and 'family-based' there were no clusters of people whose GHQ scores indicated poor mental health, although there were inevitably certain isolated cases with higher scores indicating poorer well-being. These individual cases could be understood in terms of particular or unusual circumstances and did not undermine our overall conclusions.

We were thus able to conclude that some types of personal communities are more likely than others to provide the necessary 'medicine of life' or social support, which is such a crucial part of most people's well-being. People with friend-like, friend-enveloped and family-like personal communities have a range of people – friends, family members, neighbours – to whom they can turn for a whole range of emotional and material support. It is this *diversity of ties* that a number of studies had previously identified as being associated with better physical and mental health (Cohen et al. 2000; Uchino et al. 1996). By contrast, those with partner-based and professional-based personal communities lack such diverse sources. Evidently, those 'with all their eggs in one basket' are more likely to be vulnerable if their partner leaves them, for whatever reason, or if the services on which they depend are withdrawn. This last point is particularly relevant in connection with the befriending scheme mentioned above.

We found cases where people had fragile personal communities because they had failed to give the time and energy to nurture friendships. One such example would be those women who had left the area where their friends and family lived in order to follow their husband's employment. By putting all their energies into being a wife and mother of small children they became vulnerable and registered a higher GHQ score. A similar situation could arise for men who might move to a 'better' environment, for the sake of their children's education perhaps, only to find that the length of time spent commuting to work helped to cut them off, so that they had no time left to keep up with old friends or to make new ones.

It is important to recognize that there is no inevitable determinism linking specific circumstances – such as divorce or relocation – to fragile social support. Those embedded in more diverse and robust 'little circles' or personal communities are much better placed to withstand the vicissitudes of a rapidly changing and turbulent world.

Rethinking Friendship: Hidden Solidarities Today is a long and complex study and my references to our work have, of necessity, been highly compressed. However, our main themes of the *diversity* of different forms of friendship, the *suffusion* of family and non-family forms of relationship and the distinctive *personal communities* that we have described stand out clearly. And the implications are equally clear. Despite what the gloomy polemicists might claim, there are deep and enduring friendships of great complexity alive and flourishing in Britain today. Liz Spencer and I were much heartened by what we found. However, it is significant that these solidarities still remain largely hidden, largely because those commenting on social trends in our society are looking with the wrong lens in the wrong places. This is a theme we develop in our book.

If, then, friendship is such a self-evidently social good maybe some practical policy outcomes could be devised? Should we be arguing for a Prime Minister's Task Force on the Medicine of Life? Simply to state the question provides the answer. The strength of friendship is that it is private, an inversion of the institutional arrangements of the Great

Society, subversive even. Certainly, the authorities could provide more formal spaces in which the informal could flourish. If we are to give friendship priority over commodities then 'governments would have to alter firms' cost and profit calculations so that they would themselves seek to foster companionship (if not workmen's solidarity!) and reciprocal affection in family life' (Lane 1994: 545).

All this may seem idealistic and unrealistic. However, if the greater well-being of people in society depends on the quality and diversity of friendship as much as anything, then surely, governments concerned with promoting well-being should at least consider how society could become more 'friend conscious'. One way to help towards this would be to make the study of friends and friendship part of the National Curriculum. Young people are more likely to be interested in the topic, since it is directly related to their everyday social life. The topic can be approached from a variety of perspectives – that of philosophy being one of the richest. But the historical, sociological, anthropological, psychological and literary approaches are deep and complex. If young people were to understand more about the rich diversity of friendship, this would carry with it explicit and implicit guidance on how we should treat each other morally. Friendship flourishes amongst the young and the old, the rich and the poor and in all creeds, cultures and faiths. It is truly universal. Perhaps educationists have underestimated the true depth and diversity of the topic. Certainly it has been trivialized in much journalistic commentary. However, a topic that was central to the philosophy and politics of Aristotle and is now also central to the practical concerns of marketing and media executives deserves a wider understanding of its importance and contemporary significance.[1]

Not only is friendship essential for our individual and collective well-being, its disciplined study and exploration can help us as a society to be more conscious of the processes of which we form a part.

Notes

1. Those interested in the pratical, commercial aspects of friendship may get more information from www.thefriendshipproject.com

References

Andrews, G. J., Galvin, N., Begley, S. and Brodie, D. (2003) 'Assisting Friendships, Combating Loneliness: Users' Views on a "Befriending" Scheme', *Ageing and Society*, 23: 349–62.

Bauman, Z. (2003) *Liquid Love*. Cambridge: Polity Press.

Brown, G. W., Bhrolchain, M. N. and Harris, T. (1975) 'Social Class and Psychiatric Disturbance Among Women in an Urban Population', *Sociology*, 9: 225–54.

Carmichael, L. (2004) *Friendship: Interpreting Christian Love.* London and New York: T. and T. Clark International.

Cohen, S., Underwood, L. G. and Gottleib, B. H. (eds) (2000) *Social Support: Measurement and Intervention.* Oxford: Oxford University Press.

Durkheim, E. (1951) *Suicide,* trans. J. A. Spaulding and G. Simpson. Glencoe: Free Press.

Fischer, C. S. and Phillips, S. L. (1982) 'Who is Alone? Social Characteristics of People with Small Networks', in L. A. Poplau and D. Perlman (eds), *Loneliness: a Source Book of Current Theory, Research and Therapy.* New York: Wiley-Interscience.

Freese, J. (2003) 'Imaginary Imaginary Friends? Television Viewing and Satisfaction with Friendships', *Evolution and Human Behaviour,* 24: 65–9.

Halpern, D. (2005) *Social Capital.* Cambridge: Polity Press.

Kanazawa, S. (2002) 'Bowling With Our Imaginary Friends', *Evolution and Human Behaviour,* 23: 167–71.

Keith, P. M. (1986) 'Isolation of the Unmarried in Later Life', *Family Relations,* 35: 389–95.

Knickmeyer, N., Sexton, K. and Nishimura, N. (2002) 'The Impact of Same-Sex Friendships on the Well-Being of Women: a Review of the Literature', *Women and Therapy,* 25(1): 37–59.

Konstan, D. (1997) *Friendship in the Classical World.* Cambridge: Cambridge University Press.

Lane, R. E. (1994) 'The Road Not Taken: Friendship, Consumerism and Happiness', *Critical Review,* 8(4): 521–54.

Lane, R. E. (2000) *The Loss of Happiness in Market Democracies.* New Haven and London: Yale University Press.

Larson, R. (1978) 'Thirty Years of Research on the Subjective Well-Being of Older Americans', *Journal of Gerontology,* 33: 109–25.

Larson, R., Mannell, R. and Zuzanek, J. (1986) 'Daily Well-Being of Older Adults with Friends and Family', *Psychology and Ageing,* 1(2): 117–26.

Layard, R. (2005) *Happiness.* London: Allen Lane.

Martin, P. (1997) *The Sickening Mind.* London: HarperCollins.

McMahon, D. M. (2006) *Happiness: a History.* New York: Atlantic Monthly Press.

Pahl, R. (2000) *On Friendship.* Cambridge: Polity Press.

Pakaluk, M. (ed.) (1991) *Other Selves: Philosophers on Friendship.* Indianapolis/ Cambridge: Hackett Publishing Company, Inc.

Pevalin, D. J. and Goldberg, D. P. (2003) 'Social Precursors to Onset and Recovery from Episodes of Common Mental Illness', *Psychological Medicine,* 33: 299–306.

Putnam, R. D. (2000) *Bowling Alone.* New York and London: Simon & Schuster.

Ransome, A. (ed.) (1912) *The Book of Friendship: Essays, Maxims and Prose Passages.* London and Edinburgh: T. C. and E. C. Jack.

Silver, A. (1989) 'Friendship and Trust as Moral Ideals: an Historical Approach', *European Journal of Sociology,* 30: 274–97.

Spencer, L. and Pahl, R. (2006) *Rethinking Friendship: Hidden Solidarities Today.* Princeton and Oxford: Princeton University Press.

Tocqueville, A. de (1889) *Democracy in America.* 2 volumes. London: Longman, Green and Co.

Vernon, M. (2005) *The Philosophy of Friendship.* Basingstoke and New York: Palgrave Macmillan.

Uchino, B. N., Cacioppo, J. T. and Kiecolt-Glaser, J. K. (1996) 'The Relationship Between Social Support and Psychological Processes: a Review with Emphasis on Underlying Mechanisms and Implications for Health', *Psychological Bulletin*, 119: 488–531.

Wolff, K. H. (ed.) (1950) *The Sociology of Georg Simmel*. Glencoe: Free Press.

Index